New Perspectives in Infectious Diseases

Editor

ROBERT H. MEALEY

VETERINARY CLINICS OF NORTH AMERICA: EQUINE PRACTICE

www.vetequine.theclinics.com

Consulting Editor
A. SIMON TURNER

December 2014 • Volume 30 • Number 3

ELSEVIER

1600 John F. Kennedy Boulevard • Suite 1800 • Philadelphia, Pennsylvania, 19103-2899

http://www.vetequine.theclinics.com

VETERINARY CLINICS OF NORTH AMERICA: EQUINE PRACTICE Volume 30, Number 3
December 2014 ISSN 0749-0739, ISBN-13: 978-0-323-32686-5

Editor: Patrick Manley
Developmental Editor: Donald Mumford

Veterinary Clinics of North America: Equine Practice (ISSN 0749-0739) is published in April, August, and December by Elsevier Inc., 360 Park Avenue South, New York, NY 10010-1710. Business and Editorial Offices: 1600 John F. Kennedy Blvd., Suite 1800, Philadelphia, PA 19103-2899. Subscription prices are $270.00 per year (domestic individuals), $431.00 per year (domestic institutions), $130.00 per year (domestic students/residents), $315.00 per year (Canadian individuals), $543.00 per year (Canadian institutions), $365.00 per year (international individuals), $543.00 per year (international institutions), and $180.00 per year (international and Canadian students/residents). To receive student/resident rate, orders must be accompanied by name of affiliated institution, date of term, and the signature of program/residency coordinator on institution letterhead. Orders will be billed at individual rate until proof of status is received. Foreign air speed delivery is included in all *Clinics* subscription prices. All prices are subject to change without notice. **POSTMASTER:** Send address changes to *Veterinary Clinics of North America: Equine Practice*, 3251 Riverport Lane, Maryland Heights, MO 63043. Customer Service (orders, claims, online, change of address): Elsevier Health Sciences Division, Subscription Customer Service, 3251 Riverport Lane, Maryland Heights, MO 63043. Tel: 1-800-654-2452 (U.S. and Canada); 314-447-8871 (outside U.S. and Canada). Fax: 314-447-8029. E-mail: journalscustomerservice-usa@elsevier.com (for print support); E-mail: journalsonlinesupport-usa@elsevier.com (for online support).

Reprints. For copies of 100 or more of articles in this publication, please contact the Commercial Reprints Department, Elsevier Inc., 360 Park Avenue South, New York, NY 10010-1710. Tel.: 212-633-3874; Fax: 212-633-3820; E-mail: reprints@elsevier.com.

Veterinary Clinics of North America: Equine Practice is covered in *MEDLINE/PubMed (Index Medicus), Excerpta Medica, Current Contents/Agriculture, Biology and Environmental Sciences, and ISI.*

Contributors

CONSULTING EDITOR

A. SIMON TURNER, BVSc, MS, DVSc
Department of Clinical Sciences, College of Veterinary Medicine and Biomedical Sciences, Colorado State University, Fort Collins, Colorado

EDITOR

ROBERT H. MEALEY, DVM, PhD
Diplomate of the American College of Veterinary Internal Medicine (Large Animal); Professor, Department of Veterinary Microbiology and Pathology, College of Veterinary Medicine, Washington State University, Pullman, Washington

AUTHORS

UDENI B.R. BALASURIYA, BVSc, MS, PhD
Department of Veterinary Science, Maxwell H. Gluck Equine Research Center, College of Agriculture, Food and Environment, University of Kentucky, Lexington, Kentucky

BRANDY A. BURGESS, DVM, MSc, PhD
Diplomate of the American College of Veterinary Internal Medicine (Large Animal); Diplomate of the American College of Veterinary Preventive Medicine; Department of Population Health Sciences, Virginia-Maryland Regional College of Veterinary Medicine, Virginia-Tech, Blacksburg, Virginia

NOAH D. COHEN, VMD, MPH, PhD
Diplomate of the American College of Veterinary Internal Medicine; Professor, Department of Large Animal Clinical Sciences, College of Veterinary Medicine and Biomedical Sciences, Texas A&M University, College Station, Texas

R. FRANK COOK, PhD
Associate Professor, Department of Veterinary Science, Gluck Equine Research Center, University of Kentucky, Lexington, Kentucky

DAVID W. HOROHOV, MS, PhD
Jes E. and Clementine M. Schlaikjer Endowed Chair & Professor, Department of Veterinary Science, Maxwell H. Gluck Equine Research Center, University of Kentucky, Lexington, Kentucky

DANIEL K. HOWE, PhD
Department of Veterinary Science, Professor, M.H. Gluck Equine Research Center, University of Kentucky, Lexington, Kentucky

GISELA SOBOLL HUSSEY, DVM, PhD
Department of Pathobiology and Diagnostic Investigation, College of Veterinary Medicine, Michigan State University, East Lansing, Michigan

CHARLES J. ISSEL, DVM, PhD
Wright-Markey Chair of Equine Infectious Diseases, Department of Veterinary Science, Gluck Equine Research Center, University of Kentucky, Lexington, Kentucky

DONALD P. KNOWLES, DVM, PhD
Diplomate of the American College of Veterinary Practitioners; Professor, Department of Veterinary Microbiology and Pathology; Research Leader, USDA ARS ADRU, Washington State University, Pullman, Washington

GABRIELE A. LANDOLT, Dr med vet, MS, PhD
Diplomate of the American College of Veterinary Internal Medicine; Associate Professor, Department of Clinical Sciences, College of Veterinary Medicine and Biomedical Sciences, Colorado State University, Fort Collins, Colorado

MAUREEN T. LONG, DVM, PhD
Diplomate of the American College of Veterinary Internal Medicine (Large Animal); Fern Audette Associate Professorship in Equine Studies, Department of Infectious Diseases and Pathology, College of Veterinary Medicine, University of Florida, Gainesville, Florida

ROBERT J. MACKAY, BVSc, PhD
Professor of Large Animal Medicine, Department of Large Animal Clinical Sciences, College of Veterinary Medicine, University of Florida, Gainesville, Florida

ROBERT H. MEALEY, DVM, PhD
Diplomate of the American College of Veterinary Internal Medicine (Large Animal); Professor, Department of Veterinary Microbiology and Pathology, College of Veterinary Medicine, Washington State University, Pullman, Washington

DEBORAH MIDDLETON, BVSc, MVSc, PhD
Senior Veterinary Pathologist, Australian Animal Health Laboratory, CSIRO, Geelong, Victoria, Australia

PAUL S. MORLEY, DVM, PhD
Diplomate of the American College of Veterinary Internal Medicine (Large Animal); Department of Clinical Sciences, James L. Voss Veterinary Teaching Hospital, Colorado State University, Fort Collins, Colorado

ALLEN E. PAGE, DVM, PhD
Post-Doctoral Fellow, Department of Veterinary Science, University of Kentucky, Lexington, Kentucky

ANGELA M. PELZEL-McCLUSKEY, DVM
Equine Epidemiologist, Surveillance, Preparedness, and Response Services, USDA APHIS Veterinary Services, Fort Collins, Colorado

NICOLA PUSTERLA, DVM, PhD
Department of Medicine and Epidemiology, School of Veterinary Medicine, University of California, Davis, California

STEPHEN M. REED, DVM
Adjunct Professor, Department of Veterinary Science, M.H. Gluck Equine Research Center, University of Kentucky; Rood and Riddle Equine Hospital, Lexington, Kentucky

NATHAN M. SLOVIS, CHT, CHT-V
Diplomate of the American College of Veterinary Internal Medicine; Director, McGee Medicine Center, Hagyard Equine Medical Institute, Lexington, Kentucky

ANDREW P. STRINGER, BVSc, PhD, MRCVS
Director of Veterinary Programmes, Society for the Protection of Animals Abroad
(SPANA), London, United Kingdom

ANDREW S. WALLER, BSc, PhD
Head of Bacteriology, Centre for Preventive Medicine, Animal Health Trust, Lanwades
Park, Kentford, Newmarket, Suffolk, United Kingdom

L. NICKI WISE, DVM, MS
Diplomate of the American College of Veterinary Internal Medicine (Large Animal);
Associate Professor, Department of Large Animal Medicine and Surgery, St. George's
University, USDA ARS ADRU, Grenada, West Indies

Contents

Equine myeloencephalopathy (EHM), an uncommon manifestation of equine herpesvirus 1 (EHV-1) infection, can cause devastating losses on individual farms, boarding stables, veterinary hospitals, and show and racing venues. An improved understanding of EHM has emerged from experimental studies and from data collected during field outbreaks at riding schools, racetracks, horse shows, and veterinary hospitals throughout North America and Europe. These outbreaks have highlighted the contagious nature of EHV-1 and have prompted a reevaluation of diagnostic procedures, treatment modalities, preventative measures, and biosecurity protocols for this disease. This article focuses on recent data related to the cause, epidemiology, pathogenesis, immunity, diagnosis, treatment, and prevention of EHV-1 infection with emphasis on EHM.

For decades the horse has been viewed as an isolated or "dead end" host for influenza A viruses, with equine influenza virus being considered as relatively stable genetically. Although equine influenza viruses are genetically more stable than those of human lineage, they are by no means in evolutionary stasis. Moreover, recent transmission of equine-lineage influenza viruses to dogs also challenges the horse's status as a dead-end host. This article reviews recent developments in the epidemiology and evolution of equine influenza virus. In addition, the clinical presentation of equine influenza infection, diagnostic techniques, and vaccine recommendations are briefly summarized.

Mosquito-borne diseases affect horses worldwide. Mosquito-borne diseases generally cause encephalomyelitis in the horse and can be difficult to diagnose antemortem. In addition to general disease, and diagnostic and treatment aspects, this review article summarizes the latest information on these diseases, covering approximately the past 5 years, with a focus on new equine disease encroachments, diagnostic and vaccination aspects, and possible therapeutics on the horizon.

Equine arteritis virus (EAV), the causative agent of equine viral arteritis (EVA), is a respiratory and reproductive disease that occurs throughout the world. EAV infection is highly species-specific and exclusively limited to members of the family *Equidae*, which includes horses, donkeys, mules, and zebras. EVA is an economically important disease and outbreaks could cause significant losses to the equine industry. The primary objective of this article is to summarize current understanding of EVA, specifically the disease, pathogenesis, epidemiology, host immune response, vaccination and treatment strategies, prevention and control measures, and future directions.

In the absence of an effective vaccine, the success of the test and removal approach for the control of equine infectious anemia (EIA) cannot be overstated, at least in those areas where testing has been traditionally routine. This article addresses 4 main aspects: what has been learned about EIA virus, host control of its replication, and inapparent carriers; international status regarding the control of EIA; diagnostic and laboratory investigation; and reducing the spread of blood-borne infections by veterinarians. An attempt is made to put these issues into practical contemporary perspectives for the equine practitioner.

Hendra virus infection of horses occurred sporadically between 1994 and 2010 as a result of spill-over from the viral reservoir in Australian mainland flying-foxes, and occasional onward transmission to people also followed from exposure to affected horses. An unprecedented number of outbreaks were recorded in 2011 leading to heightened community concern. Release of an inactivated subunit vaccine for horses against Hendra virus represents the first commercially available product that is focused on mitigating the impact of a Biosafety Level 4 pathogen. Through preventing the development of acute Hendra virus disease in horses, vaccine use is also expected to reduce the risk of transmission of infection to people.

Strangles, characterized by abscessation of the lymph nodes of the head and neck, is the most frequently diagnosed infectious disease of horses worldwide. The persistence of the causative agent, *Streptococcus equi*, in a proportion of convalescent horses plays a critical role in the recurrence and spread of disease. Recent research has led to the development of effective diagnostic tests that assist the eradication of *S equi* from local horse populations. This article describes how these advances have been made and provides advice to assist the resolution and prevention of

have reliably induced antibody responses in challenged horses but have not consistently produced acute neurologic disease. Diagnosis and options for treatment of EPM have improved over the past decade.

Equine piroplasmosis, caused by the parasites *Theileria equi* and *Babesia caballi*, is a globally important disease, affecting a large percentage of the world's horses. This article serves as a review of these divergent parasites. Discussed are the clinical presentation of disease, diagnosis, and treatment. Special attention is given to the current disease status specifically in North America.

Most working equids reside in low-income countries where they have an essential role in the livelihoods of their owners. Numerous infectious diseases negatively impact the health and productivity of these animals. There are considerable technical, social-behavioral, and institutional impediments globally to reducing the burden of infectious diseases on working equids. One the greatest remaining challenges is the lack of funding for research, resulting from the low priority assigned to working equids by funding bodies. Changing the attitudes of decision makers will require data-driven advocacy, and global networks of collaborators have a vital role in building this more robust evidence base.

VETERINARY CLINICS OF
NORTH AMERICA: EQUINE PRACTICE

THE CLINICS ARE NOW AVAILABLE ONLINE!
Access your subscription at:
www.theclinics.com

VETERINARY CLINICS OF NORTH AMERICA: EQUINE PRACTICE

Foreword

A Farewell and Thanks

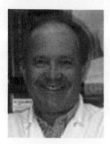

A. Simon Turner, BVSc, MS, DVSc
Consulting Editor

It is with quite some sadness that I step down as Consulting Editor for Elsevier's *Veterinary Clinics of North America: Equine Practice* (*VCNA*). I have been in this position for 26 years and I have seen it gain a lot of popularity with busy practicing veterinarians. The other *VCNA* series from Elsevier are also gaining in popularity for the same reasons as the Equine Practice issues.

I have thoroughly enjoyed thinking up what topics would be attractive to veterinarians that have devoted a lot of their lives caring for horses. Many veterinarians who have had a very busy day dealing with ailing pets and their demanding owners may be simply too exhausted to sift through a pile of veterinary journals that have accumulated in their office. With the *VCNA* they can pick the subject they are interested in simply by reading the titles on the spines. They can then turn to the table of contents and go straight to the article on *exactly* what they need to focus in on. This saves them from thumbing through piles of journals and their necessary advertisements looking for that specific topic. Time is money for these people and they cannot waste it.

What also attracts the busy equine veterinarian is that the material presented is so fresh compared with a textbook that has taken several years to get on their shelves. A large comprehensive textbook may take several years to complete and as many as 20 authors may be involved. Such textbooks are perfect to teach new veterinary students what's what in that subject. But for the busy veterinarian who wants the latest information, and has to make a quick decision so the animal gets the correct diagnosis and treatment, these textbooks may not be the best way to go. This, I think, is one of the key advantages of the *VCNA*. The material is as current as it could be. The cost to readers compared with a big, fat, heavy textbook is much lower too.

I chose the guest editors by reading who had recently chaired a local, national, or international symposium on a particular subject. They were chosen to do that because they knew the key issues and the experts in a particular subject.

Finally, I am very grateful for John Vassallo at Elsevier for working with me on these issues. He certainly taught me what publishing and printing issues I could not ignore.

Vet Clin Equine 30 (2014) xiii–xiv
http://dx.doi.org/10.1016/j.cveq.2014.10.002   **vetequine.theclinics.com**
0749-0739/14/$ – see front matter © 2014 Elsevier Inc. All rights reserved.

I wish Dr Tom Divers at Cornell University good luck as my replacement as consulting editor of the *VCNA*. I hope that he has as much fun and personal satisfaction in that position as I had.

A. Simon Turner, BVSc, MS, DVSc
Department of Clinical Sciences
College of Veterinary Medicine and Biomedical Sciences
Colorado State University
300 West Drake Road
Fort Collins, CO 80523-1678, USA

E-mail address:
Anthony.Turner@colostate.edu

Preface

New Perspectives in Infectious Diseases

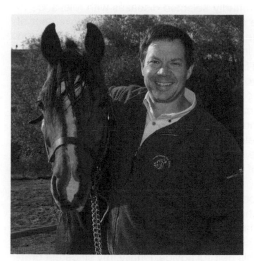

Robert H. Mealey, DVM, PhD
Editor

The last issues of *Veterinary Clinics of North America: Equine Practice* that focused on infectious diseases were the December 2000 issue edited by Dr Peter Timoney titled, "Emerging Infectious Diseases," and the August 1993 issue edited by Dr Josie Traub-Dargatz titled, "Update on Infectious Diseases." Since these issues were published, there have been significant improvements made in the ability to diagnose, treat, and prevent infectious diseases in the horse. Despite the advances of the last two decades however, many of the same diseases remain important threats to equine health today and will continue to pose significant challenges in the future. As specific examples, improved diagnostics and therapeutic protocols for equine protozoal myeloencephalitis and *Rhodococcus equi* pneumonia have had a tremendous impact, but these diseases continue to be significant causes of morbidity and death, effective vaccines have not yet been produced, and, in the case of *R equi*, antimicrobial resistance is now an emerging problem. Likewise, improved vaccines are needed to protect against equine herpesvirus myeloencephalopathy, strangles, and equine arteritis virus and to overcome the antigenic drift of equine influenza virus. Even though effective vaccines are available against the encephalitis viruses and West Nile virus, some strains are expanding in distribution and epizootics continue to occur. Salmonella outbreaks continue to shut down hospitals. Not much was known about equine proliferative enteropathy at the time the last infectious disease issue was published, but it has become an increasingly important problem in North America and worldwide.

The articles in this issue deal with the topics highlighted above and more. Unfortunately, it was not possible to include all infectious diseases, and there are many important diseases we were not able to cover, including some emerging diseases for which the story continues to unfold (enteric coronavirus and flaviviruses associated with hepatitis are examples). Although we have primarily selected diseases with relevance to North America, we live in a highly mobile society and the international movement of horses is commonplace. Thus, knowledge of infectious diseases that are considered exotic or otherwise affect domestic and international movement is prudent. The re-emergence of piroplasmosis in the United States is a good example. Equine infectious anemia is another. Hendra virus is noteworthy because it is a serious emerging zoonotic pathogen for which an effective vaccine has recently been developed. Finally, putting things in perspective, North American horses represent only 9% of the approximate 112 million equids in the world, and the majority of these are working equids residing in some of the world's least developed regions. These working horses, donkeys, and mules do not benefit from the level of care available in more developed countries, and they suffer from a variety of infectious diseases for which we have provided an overview.

The contributors to this issue and I hope you find these articles a useful reference. I would like to sincerely thank each of the authors for their hard work in providing comprehensive and cutting-edge information. All are experts and leaders in their respective fields and working with them has been a very rewarding and educational experience. I also thank Dr Paul Lunn for his helpful advice. Finally, my sincerest gratitude goes to Dr Simon Turner for the opportunity to put this issue together.

Robert H. Mealey, DVM, PhD
Department of Veterinary Microbiology and Pathology
College of Veterinary Medicine
Washington State University
Pullman, WA 99164-7040, USA

E-mail address:
rhm@vetmed.wsu.edu

Equine Herpesvirus 1 Myeloencephalopathy

Nicola Pusterla, DVM, PhD[a],*, Gisela Soboll Hussey, DVM, PhD[b]

KEYWORDS

- Equine herpesvirus 1 • Equine herpesvirus myeloencephalopathy • Etiology
- Epidemiology • Pathogenesis • Clinical signs • Diagnosis • Treatment

KEY POINTS

- EHV-1 is ubiquitous in horses worldwide and greater than 80% of horses are estimated to be latently infected with the virus. Because of this the elimination of the virus from the population is unlikely, and efforts need to focus on prevention and treatment of clinical diseases associated with EHV-1.
- Clinical disease manifestations of EHV-1 include respiratory disease, late-term abortion, neonatal foal death, chorioretinopathy, and EHM.
- Sudden onset of signs including ataxia, paresis, and urinary incontinence; involvement of multiple horses on the premises; and a recent history of fever, abortion, or viral respiratory disease in the affected horse or herdmates are typical features of EHM outbreaks, although there is considerable variation between outbreaks with respect to epidemiologic and clinical findings.
- The mechanism underlying CNS endothelial infection is unknown, as are the risk factors that determine its occurrence. Although viral factors are certain to be important, host and environmental factors also play a critical role.
- An antemortem diagnosis of EHM is supported by ruling out other neurologic conditions; demonstrating xanthochromia and an elevated cerebrospinal fluid protein concentration; and identifying or isolating EHV-1 from the respiratory tract, buffy coat, or CSF.
- The equine ocular fundus is physiologically and anatomically similar to that of the CNS, but the eye's unique anatomic features permits observation of the chorioretinal vasculature in vivo and may allow for using the eye as a surrogate to study aspects of EHM pathogenesis.
- The treatment of EHM is challenging and directed toward supportive nursing and nutritional care and reducing CNS inflammation.
- Immunity following infection or vaccination offers limited protection in particular in regards to EHM. This lack of induction of protective immunity to EHV-1 is likely caused by immunomodulatory properties of the virus. Early recognition of suspected cases and the close monitoring of high-risk horses represent the most reliable measures at preventing outbreaks of EHM.

[a] Department of Medicine and Epidemiology, School of Veterinary Medicine, University of California, One Shields Avenue, Davis, CA 95616, USA; [b] Department of Pathobiology and Diagnostic Investigation, College of Veterinary Medicine, Michigan State University, 736 Wilson Road, East Lansing, MI 48824, USA
* Corresponding author.
E-mail address: npusterla@ucdavis.edu

Vet Clin Equine 30 (2014) 489–506
http://dx.doi.org/10.1016/j.cveq.2014.08.006
vetequine.theclinics.com

INTRODUCTION

Equine herpesvirus 1 (EHV-1) myeloencephalopathy (EHM), although a relatively uncommon manifestation of EHV-1 infection, can cause devastating losses on individual farms, boarding stables, veterinary hospitals, and show and racing venues. Although outbreaks of EHM have been recognized for centuries in domestic horse populations, many aspects of this disease remain poorly characterized. In recent years, an improved understanding of EHM has emerged from experimental studies and from data collected during field outbreaks at riding schools, racetracks, horse shows, and veterinary hospitals throughout North America and Europe. These outbreaks have highlighted the contagious nature of EHV-1 and have prompted a reevaluation of diagnostic procedures, treatment modalities, preventative measures, and biosecurity protocols for this disease. This article focuses on the recent data related to the cause, epidemiology, pathogenesis, immunity, diagnosis, treatment, and prevention of EHV-1 infection with emphasis on EHM.

ETIOLOGY

EHV-1 is an important, ubiquitous equine viral pathogen that exerts its major impact by inducing abortion storms or sporadic abortions in pregnant mares, early neonatal death in foals, respiratory disease in young horses, and myeloencephalopathy.[1] Although EHM is a sporadic and relatively uncommon manifestation of EHV-1 infection, it can cause devastating losses and severely impact the equine industry, as exemplified by recent outbreaks at riding schools, racetracks, horse shows, and veterinary hospitals throughout North America and Europe.[2–4]

EHV-1 and EHV-4 are α-herpesviruses and are distinguishable from EHV-2, EHV-3, and EHV-5 by biologic properties and virus neutralization tests, and from each other by restriction endonuclease fingerprinting of DNA, DNA sequences, and several immunologic tests based on monoclonal antibodies to each virus.[1,5,6] EHV-1 and EHV-4 are closely related but genetically and antigenically different and associated with distinct disease profiles.

EHV-1 is a DNA virus that possesses linear double-stranded genomes composed of a unique long region, joined to a unique short region that is flanked by an identical pair of inverted repeat regions, the terminal repeat and the internal repeat regions.[7] The EHV-1 genome is 150 kilobases in size and encodes for 76 open reading frames or genes. Expression of these genes within infected cells is tightly ordered into a highly controlled cascade.[8] One complete replication cycle takes approximately 20 hours during which well-ordered sequential events occur, including attachment to the host cell membrane, membrane fusion and penetration, translocation of viral DNA to the nucleus, viral DNA replication and protein synthesis, assembly of the capsid, envelopment, and lysis of the cell with release of progeny virions.

Virulence markers distinguishing EHV-1 strains that induce EHM and/or abortion have recently been determined. The most important discovery may be the association with a single nucleotide polymorphism at position 2254 in the DNA polymerase gene (ORF 30) and the occurrence of EHM.[9] Analysis of more than 100 EHV-1 outbreaks with various clinical presentations demonstrated that variability of a single amino acid residue at position 752 of the DNA polymerase was found to be strongly associated with the occurrence of EHM, with EHV-1 strains associated with neurologic outbreaks involving a D_{752} genotype, whereas most nonneurologic outbreaks involved a N_{752} genotype.[9,10] The observation that EHV-1 viruses of the D_{752} genotype have a greater potential to induce EHM was recently supported by an experimental study using recombinant viruses with differing polymerase sequences.[11] The N_{752} mutant virus caused no neurologic signs and was associated with reduced levels of viremia, whereas viral shedding was similar between both virus mutants. From an epidemiologic standpoint it seems that most EHV-1 viruses circulating in the field are of the N_{752} genotype.[12,13] Although EHV-1 D_{752} genotype viruses are more commonly associated with EHM, viruses with a N_{752} genotype are certainly not apathogenic; they have been responsible for approximately 81% to 98% of abortion outbreaks in the United States, United Kingdom, and other countries, and between 15% and 26% of neurologic outbreaks (**Fig. 1**).

EPIDEMIOLOGY

According to Allen and colleagues[14] the main epidemiologically relevant features of EHV-1 include high incidence of respiratory infection early in life; establishment of latency in a high percentage of infected horses; and frequent reactivation of latent virus with subsequent shedding, resulting in transmission to naive hosts. Currently, it is estimated that 80% of all horses are latently infected; however, prevalence may vary depending on geographic region and age.[15] Furthermore, testing technology and tissues sampled for detection of latency affect sensitivity of testing and actual numbers of latently infected horses may be even higher.[12,13]

Primary infection of the respiratory tract typically occurs around the time of weaning, but has been reported in the first weeks of life irrespective of vaccination status.[14,16,17] Infection occurs by way of respiratory secretions, contact with aborted fetuses or placentas, and fomites. Presence of EHV-1 has also been reported in testis and semen of infected stallions but a venereal transmission has not been reported.[18]

Following primary infection, a cell-associated viremia is established and several weeks later a transition from viremic-infected cells to latently infected cells occurs. In contrast to other α-herpesviruses, latency for EHV-1 is established in the lymphoreticular system and the trigeminal ganglion, and reactivation occurs from these sites, often in the absence of any clinical signs.[15] Nasal viral shedding can be detected at 1 day postinfection and occurs by the respiratory secretions for 1 to 3 weeks postinfection, although the duration of shedding depends on pre-existing immunity and viral properties.[14] Similarly, duration of shedding following recrudescence varies.[19]

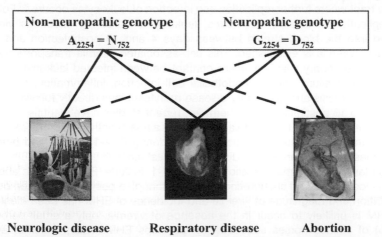

Fig. 1. Association of EHV-1 genotypes of the DNA polymerase with various disease presentations. The dashed lines represent EHV-1 genotypes with greater potential for the development of specific disease forms.

Because prolonged shedding has been detected particularly in cases of EHM outbreaks, current recommendations by the American Association of Equine Practitioners are to wait 28 days before lifting quarantine measures. This period starts from the resolution of all clinical signs on affected premises and is based on the fact that viral shedding typically ceases by 21 days postinfection and EHV-1 is an enveloped virus, which does not survive in a cell-free environment. Treatment with disinfectants, detergents, heat, or lipid solvents is effective. Experimentally, there is some evidence for viral survival for up to 1 month under selected conditions; however, viral survival for more than 21 days after depopulation of infected horses is very unlikely.[20]

Although primary respiratory infection is common in horses younger than 2 years of age, it is of much lesser significance in older horses, particularly in the presence of pre-existing immunity.[14] However, nasal shedding and transmission of EHV-1 can occur despite the absence of clinical signs of respiratory disease. Conversely, the risk for abortions in the third trimester of pregnancy and outbreaks of neurologic disease is of greater significance in middle-aged or older horses. In recent years, there has been an increase in outbreaks of EHM in North America (http://www.fas.org/promed). Because of this, in January 2007 the Center for Emerging Issues released an emerging disease notice report regarding the neurologic form of EHV-1. Despite this knowledge and strong efforts to control this disease, EHM outbreaks continue to be a problem and in May of 2011 the largest outbreak ever was reported.[21] The reason for this increase in the prevalence of EHM is not clear, and there are several identified viral, host, and environmental components that factor into the incidence of EHM (**Table 1**).

PATHOGENESIS

The pathogenesis of EHV-1 is illustrated in **Fig. 2**. Primary infection with EHV-1 occurs by the respiratory tract.[14] Following infection, replication in the respiratory airway epithelium causes erosion of the respiratory mucosa and shedding of virus by the nasal secretions into the environment. Within 12 to 24 hours the virus spreads quickly by the basement membrane to the cells of the lamina propria and the underlying tissues. By 24 to 48 hours the virus can be detected in the local lymph nodes of the respiratory tract where further replication and infection of leukocytes occurs.[20] Following viral replication in local lymph nodes, leukocytes harboring infectious virus are released into the blood stream between days 4 and 10 postinfection and a cell-associated viremia is established. This cell-associated viremia transports the virus to sites of secondary infection where contact between infected leukocytes and the vascular endothelium leads to endothelial cell infection, inflammation, thrombosis, and tissue necrosis and secondary disease manifestations directly following viremia on days 9 to 13 postinfection. Furthermore, recent studies have identified increased presence of D dimers during viremia, supporting a role of activation of the coagulation cascade and deposition/degradation of fibrin during EHV-1 viremia and potentially early stages of secondary EHV-1 disease manifestations.[22]

Secondary disease manifestations for EHV-1 include EHM, EHV-1 abortions, neonatal foal death, and chorioretinopathies. Although a positive correlation between the duration and magnitude of viremia and incidence of EHM has been identified,[23] and EHM is unlikely to occur in the absence of viremia, only a small percentage (~10%) of viremic horses subsequently develops EHM. Thus, a combination of host and viral factors likely determines whether EHM occurs (see **Table 1**).

The incidence of late-term abortions caused by EHV-1 is higher (~50%) than incidence of EHM. This may be related to the hormonal milieu and altered immune system

Table 1
Risk factors for disease associated with EHV-1

Respiratory Disease	Abortion	EHM
Age <2 y		Age >3 y, further increase in risk in mares older than 20 y of age (66%)
	Infection with N725	Infection with D752 genotype
		Season: late autumn, spring, winter
		Breed and gender
		Geographic region
Past exposure	Past exposure	Past exposure
		Secondary fever several days following primary exposure
		Magnitude and duration of viremia
Stress associated with weaning, transport, introduction of new horses, secondary infection, immune suppression	Stress associated with weaning, transport, introduction of new horses, secondary infection, immune suppression	Stress associated with weaning, transport, introduction of new horses, secondary infection, immune suppression
	Pregnancy in the last trimester	Pregnancy or foal at foot
		Keep in stable
Presence of EHV-1 and/or a shedding horse together with susceptible horses	Presence of EHV-1 and/or a shedding horse together with susceptible horses	Presence of EHV-1 and/or a shedding horse together with susceptible horses
		Greater number of biosecurity risks and classes competed in at an event
		Vaccination against EHV-1 in the 5 wk before the event

in the last trimester of pregnancy. The pathogenesis of EHM and EHV-1 abortion at the vascular endothelium is, however, considered to be similar. Infection of endothelial cells of the endometrium follows viremia and leads to vasculitis, thrombosis, microcotyledonary infarction, perivascular cuffing, and transplacental spread of virus at the sites of vascular lesions.[24]

The vasculature of the eye is another site of secondary infection for EHV-1. Most ocular infections are subclinical and rarely lead to loss of function or even immediate symptoms. Although EHV-1 chorioretinopathies are much less significant economically and clinically, they may offer a unique opportunity to examine EHV-1 infection of the vascular endothelium and provide a surrogate model to study EHM pathogenesis.[25] The equine ocular fundus is physiologically and anatomically similar to that of the central nervous system (CNS) with similar tight junctions analogous to the blood-brain barrier, but importantly, the eye's unique anatomic features permit observation of the chorioretinal vasculature in vivo. Furthermore, prevalence of ocular lesions can be greater than 50% following experimental and natural infection.[25] The reason that EHV-1 chorioretinopathies are observed in a much larger percentage of horses than EHM is likely because one can observe subclinical infection in the eye, which is not

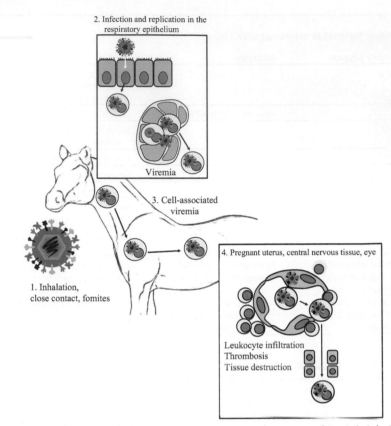

Fig. 2. EHV-1 pathogenesis following primary exposure. (*Courtesy of* Dr Gabriele Landolt, Fort Collins, CO).

possible in the spinal cord. Of note is that although postmortem acute inflammation and viral antigen can be detected in the choroidal vasculature at the onset of EHM, ocular lesions are not visible in vivo until the acute disease processes have led to focal disruption of the retinal pigmented epithelium, allowing light to reflect off the tapetum and resulting in the appearance of focal or multifocal shotgun lesions (**Fig. 3**).

CLINICAL SIGNS

Clinical manifestations of EHV-1 infection include primary respiratory disease, late-term abortions, neonatal foal death, EHM, and chorioretinopathy (**Fig. 4**). Differences in pathogenic potential of viral strains may influence clinical outcome, as can several additional host and environmental factors (see **Table 1**).

Respiratory Disease

Infection of the respiratory tract with EHV-1 can be mild or asymptomatic in older or previously exposed horses.[14] In contrast, the respiratory disease observed in young immunologically naive horses is often severe; lasts for 2 to 3 weeks; and is characterized by a biphasic fever, depression, anorexia, coughing, and nasal and ocular discharge that is initially serous and then becomes mucopurulent. Horses commonly develop a significant lymphadenopathy of the respiratory tract lymph nodes that is

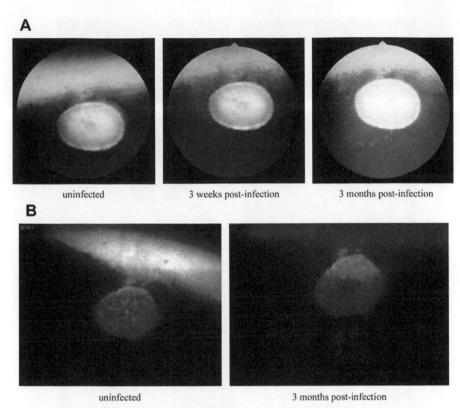

uninfected   3 weeks post-infection   3 months post-infection

uninfected   3 months post-infection

Fig. 3. Development of ocular lesions following experimental infection with EHV-1. (*A*) Fundus photography. (*B*) Fluorescent angiography.

accompanied by lymphopenia and neutropenia and lasts for several days. Lower respiratory tract disease associated with secondary bacterial infection, tachypnea, anorexia, and depression can be observed in young foals.

Abortion

EHV-1 is also a cause of late-term abortions and premature delivery of foals that die soon after birth. Mares infected with EHV-1 can appear healthy and abort 2 weeks to several months after infection or reactivation of the virus.[14] Abortion usually occurs in the last trimester of pregnancy without warning and the placenta is expelled together with the fetus, which has died from asphyxia or dies shortly after birth. Sporadic abortions in individual mares are most common, but EHV-1 outbreaks with high attack rates have been reported and depend on herd management, immune status, and viral factors. Long-term effects of EHV-1 abortion are not common and most mares deliver a healthy foal in the following breeding season. Occasionally, apparently healthy foals are delivered that become ill within 2 days of delivery and show respiratory distress, fever, failure to nurse, weakness, diarrhea, and leukopenia and do not respond well to treatment. These foals were likely infected perinatally or during birth.

Equine Herpesvirus Myeloencephalopathy

EHM is a devastating manifestation of EHV-1 infection that affects the CNS. Outbreaks are characterized by a large number of horses affected with mild to moderate

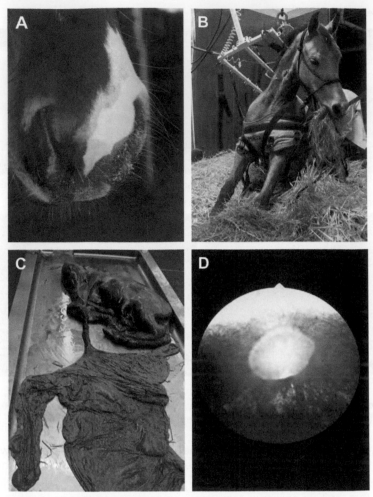

Fig. 4. Clinical signs associated with EHV-1. (*A*) Respiratory disease. (*B*) Neurologic disease. (*C*) Abortion. (*D*) Chorioretinopathy.

respiratory disease and a fever, with 10% to 40% of infected horses developing EHM. Clinical signs of EHM appear following the onset of viremia, often following a secondary fever spike and in the absence of respiratory disease. Onset of EHM typically occurs between 6 and 10 days, often suddenly, and reaches peak severity within 2 to 3 days. Experimentally, EHM occurs during or at the end of the cell-associated viremia.[26] Clinical signs range from mild, temporary ataxia to paralysis that can lead to recumbency and urinary incontinence, often resulting in euthanasia. Commonly, the caudal spinal cord is affected more severely, resulting in weakness of hind limbs, bladder dysfunction, and sensory deficits in the perineal area. Severe cases of EHM can show paresis, paralysis, or even tetraplegia. Less frequently horses with EHM can develop cortical, brainstem, or vestibular disease characterized by depression, recumbency, head tilt, ataxia, and cranial nerve deficits. One of the central questions remaining is whether the initial infection of CNS endothelial cells (which may be common) is sufficient for neuropathogenicity, or whether a "second hit" imparted by proinflammatory, procoagulant, or other host factors drives EHM pathogenesis.

Equine Herpesvirus 1 Chorioretinopathy

It has been known for more than 25 years that EHV-1 infection can lead to chorioretinopathy causing permanent shotgun lesions of the retina in a substantial proportion of infected horses. However, the connection between ocular lesions and EHV-1 infection is often not made. Recently, it has been shown that up to 80% of yearling horses can exhibit classical shotgun lesions following experimental infection with EHV-1.[25] Ocular lesions primarily affect the choroidal vasculature and appear between 4 weeks and 3 months after primary infection (see **Fig. 3**). Lesions can be focal, multifocal, or in rare occasions diffuse, which affects the entire eye. Clinically, only diffuse lesions have a significant impact and cause loss of vision.

DIAGNOSIS

An antemortem diagnosis of EHM is supported by (1) ruling out other neurologic conditions; (2) demonstrating xanthochromia and an elevated cerebrospinal fluid (CSF) protein concentration; (3) identifying or isolating EHV-1 from the respiratory tract, buffy coat, or CSF; and (4) demonstrating a four-fold increase in antibodies using serum neutralizing (SN), complement fixation, or enzyme-linked immunosorbent assay tests performed on acute and convalescent serum from affected or in-contact horses 7 to 21 days apart.

Cell Blood Count

Hematologic abnormalities in horses with EHM are inconsistent and may include mild anemia and lymphopenia in the early stages, followed a few days later by mild hyperfibrinogenemia.[27] Azotemia and hyperbilirubinemia may occur secondary to dehydration and anorexia, respectively.

Cerebrospinal Fluid Analysis

CSF fluid analysis typically reveals xanthochromia, an increased protein concentration (100–500 mg/dL), and an increased albumin quotient (ratio of CSF to serum albumin concentration), which reflects vasculitis with protein leakage into the CSF. The nucleated cell count in the CSF is usually normal (0–5 cells/µL) but is occasionally increased.[27] Location of CSF collection may also influence the cytologic results. It is important that the CSF collection matches the neuroanatomic disease location.

Virus Isolation and Detection

Virus isolation is considered the gold standard test for making a laboratory diagnosis of EHV-1 infection and should be attempted, especially during outbreaks of EHM, concurrent with use of rapid diagnostic tests, such as quantitative polymerase chain reaction (qPCR), to achieve retrospective biologic and molecular characterization of the viral isolate. The likelihood of isolating EHV-1 during outbreaks of neurologic disease is increased by monitoring in-contact horses and collecting nasal or nasopharyngeal swab and buffy coat samples from these animals during the prodromal febrile phase before neurologic signs develop.

Polymerase Chain Reaction Testing

PCR has become the diagnostic test of choice because of its high sensitivity and specificity and PCR detection of EHV-1 is routinely performed on secretions from nasal or nasopharyngeal swabs or from uncoagulated blood samples. Because of the risk of carry-over contamination, conventional molecular platforms have been replaced by qPCR. Advantages of qPCR include quick analytical turn-around time, high sensitivity and specificity, and cost-effectiveness. Furthermore, qPCR represents a major improvement in the detection of infectious pathogens by allowing character-ization of disease stage, assessment of risk of exposure to other animals, and moni-toring of response to therapy.[28] However, research and diagnostic laboratories should use quantitative methods with the least evidence of variability between samples and extraction protocols. Protocols normalizing results against a preselected volume (ie, eluted DNA or volume of nasal secretions) are more prone to interlaboratory variations than protocols standardizing viral load to the entire swab, a house-keeping gene, or an arbitrarily chosen amount of extracted DNA.[29] It is important that diagnostic labora-tories use an internal quality control system to increase the reliability of results and minimize the risk of reporting false-negative results. qPCR has recently been used to document differences in viral loads between disease stages in adult horses and be-tween clinically and subclinically infected horses.[30] This study found high viral loads in the nasal secretions of horses with EHM confirming their importance as a potential source of infection for other horses and highlighted the need for imposition of strict biosecurity when horses were identified with suspected or confirmed EHM (**Fig. 5**). Follow-up assessment of viral loads in blood and nasal or nasopharyngeal secretions can guide modifications to control measures, including the lifting of quarantine for in-dividual horses that test negative on subsequent sampling.

A recently identified variable region in the EHV-1 genome correlates with neurologic disease.[9] This sequence variation occurs in the DNA polymerase gene (ORF 30) involved in initial viral replication within cells. PCR assays based on ORF 30 have recently been developed and used to differentiate between EHV-1 isolates from neurologically and nonneurologically affected horses. However, the genotyping of field isolates needs to be interpreted carefully because between approximately 14% and 24% of EHV-1 isolates from horses with EHM do not have this neuropathogenic marker.[9,10] Strain characterization may be important given that the potential of EHM development is greater in horses infected with a neuropathogenic genotype (D_{752}).

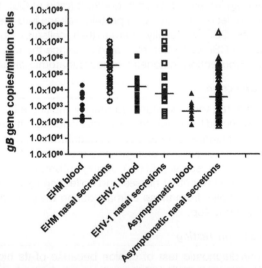

Fig. 5. Viral loads expressed as gB gene copies/million cells in blood (solid shapes) and nasal secretions (open shapes) of 27 horses with EHM (circles); 28 horses with EHV-1 infection but no neurologic signs (squares); and 52 asymptomatic, infected horses (triangles). Horizontal bars represent medians.

Furthermore, detection of a neurotropic EHV-1 strain may influence therapy, especially in the use of antiviral drugs, such as valacyclovir, used to decrease viremia and prevent the development of neurologic sequelae.

Serologic Analysis

Serology that demonstrates a four-fold or greater increase in serum antibody titer between acute and convalescent samples collected 7 to 21 days apart provides presumptive evidence of infection.[31] However, many horses with EHM do not exhibit a four-fold rise in SN titer. This may occur when titers rise rapidly and peak by the time neurologic signs appear. Although serology is limited in confirming EHM in an individual horse, testing of paired serum samples from in-contact animals is recommended given that a significant proportion of these horses seroconvert, providing indirect evidence of EHV-1 infection. Interpretation of serology is complicated because SN and complement fixation tests used at most diagnostic laboratories do not distinguish between antibodies to EHV-1 and -4.

Histopathologic Examination

Histopathologic examination of the brain and spinal cord is essential in confirming EHV-1 infection in a horse with suspected EHM. Vasculitis and thrombosis of small blood vessels in the spinal cord or brain are consistent histopathologic changes and virus antigen detection in the CNS is achieved using immunohistochemistry, in situ hybridization, and PCR.

THERAPEUTIC STRATEGIES

The treatment of EHM is challenging and the outcome is directly related to the severity of the neurologic deficits in the affected horse. Because no specific treatment is available, the management of affected animals is directed toward supportive nursing and nutritional care and in reducing CNS inflammation.

Nonrecumbent horses should be encouraged to stand and should be protected from self-inflicted trauma by the provision of good footing, such as a grass paddock; by placement of food and water in accessible locations at a convenient height above ground level; and by other measures including the use of padded hoods and the removal of obstacles. Patients that become recumbent should be maintained in a sternal position on a thick cushion of dry absorbent bedding and should be rolled at least every 2 to 4 hours to reduce the risk of developing myonecrosis, decubital ulcers, and aspiration pneumonia. Whenever possible, horses should be lifted to, and supported in the standing position using an appropriately fitted sling. Slings are most beneficial for moderately affected horses that are too weak to rise but are able to maintain a standing position with minimal assistance.

Affected horses usually maintain a good appetite, even when recumbent, although hand feeding may be necessary to encourage some animals to eat. Maintenance of hydration is important, and provision of a laxative diet or the administration of laxatives, such as bran mashes, mineral oil, or psyllium, may be necessary to reduce intestinal impaction.

If affected horses are unable to stand and urinate or if bladder function is significantly impaired, manual evacuation of the bladder by application of pressure per rectum may be necessary. If these measures are unsuccessful, judicious urinary catheterization is indicated and should be performed aseptically with the collection tubing attached to a sterile closed bag to minimize the risk of urinary tract infection. Urine scalding can become a major problem, particularly in mares dribbling urine. Prevention of such scalding involves the regular washing of the perineum, tail, and hind legs with water; the application of water-repellent ointments; and the braiding or wrapping of the tail to simplify cleaning. Administration of enemas or manual emptying of the rectum may also be necessary to promote defecation and improve patient comfort.

The medical treatment of horses with EHM focuses mainly on decreasing the inflammation associated with the induced vasculitis and preventing thromboembolic sequelae. Most drugs used for the treatment of EHM are listed in **Table 2**. One must keep in mind that the effectiveness of any of these drugs is unproved for the treatment of EHM and their justification is theoretic. Corticosteroids could aid in the control or prevention of the cellular response adjacent to infection of CNS endothelial cells, thereby potentially reducing vasculitis, thrombosis, and the resultant neural injury.[32] A short course of treatment with corticosteroids, such as prednisolone acetate or dexamethasone for 2 to 3 days, is frequently recommended for severely affected animals. Among nonsteroidal anti-inflammatory drugs, flunixin meglumine is commonly used for the treatment of CNS vasculitis. Recent in vitro work shows that flunixin meglumine, firocoxib, and dexamethasone suppress cellular interactions between infected lymphocytes and endothelial cells.[33] Several drugs have been used anecdotally for the prevention of thromboembolic events associated with vasculitis, including dimethyl sulfoxide, acetylsalicylic acid, unfractionated or low-molecular-weight heparin, and pentoxifylline. Because of the high risk of development of cystitis, especially in horses requiring bladder catheterization, it is advisable to administer broad-spectrum antimicrobials.

Antiviral drugs are of theoretic value for the treatment of EHV-1 and have demonstrated in vitro efficacy against EHV-1.[34] There are, however, limited data describing

Table 2
Drugs commonly used in the treatment of equine herpesvirus 1 myeloencephalopathy

Drug	Dosages[a]	Regiment, Route, and Duration of Treatment[a]
Anti-inflammatories		
Flunixin meglumine	1.1 mg/kg	Twice daily, PO or IV, for 5–10 d
Dexamethasone	0.05–0.25 mg/kg	Daily, IM or IV, for 3 d
Prednisolone acetate	1–2 mg/kg	Daily, PO, for 3 d
Free-radical scavengers		
Dimethyl sulfoxide	0.5–1 g/kg	Daily, IV or PO, for 3 d
Antimicrobials		
Trimethoprim-sulfamethoxazole	30 mg/kg	Twice daily, PO, for 5–7 d
Sodium ceftiofur	2.2 mg/kg	Once to twice daily, IM or IV, for 5–7 d
Antithrombotic/rheologic drugs		
Pentoxifylline	7.5–10 mg/kg	Twice daily, PO for 5–10 d
Acetylsalicylic acid	15–20 mg/kg	Every other day, PO, for 5–10 d
Unfractionated heparin	40–100 IU/kg	Four times daily SC, for 3–5 d
Low-molecular-weight heparin	50 IU/kg	Once daily, SC, for 3–5 d
Antiherpetic drugs		
Acyclovir	10–20 mg/kg	Three to five times daily, PO, for 7 d
Valacyclovir	30–40 mg/kg	Twice to three times daily, PO, for 7 d

Abbreviations: IM, intramuscular; IV, intravenous; PO, per os; SC, subcutaneous.
[a] Dosage, regiment, route, and duration of treatment represent a compilation of published data.

the in vivo efficacy of acyclovir against EHV-1 infection and controlled clinical studies have yet to be carried out. Pharmacokinetic studies in adult horses with single oral administrations of 10 and 20 mg/kg of acyclovir indicated poor bioavailability of the drug (2.8%) and great variability in serum acyclovir time profiles.[35] Recent data indicate that another nucleoside analog, valacyclovir, may have promise in the treatment of EHV-1–affected horses and in the prophylaxis and containment of EHV-1 outbreaks.[34,36] The bioavailability of the prodrug valacyclovir is in the order of 35% to 40% and has been administered per os at 30 to 40 mg/kg two to three times daily. Currently, the effects of timing of valacyclovir administration relative to the onset of natural EHV-1 infection or EHM development on treatment outcome are unknown.

Affected horses that remain standing have a good prognosis, and improvement is generally apparent within a few days. Several weeks to more than a year may be required before horses with severe neurologic deficits completely recover. Some horses may be left with permanent residual neurologic deficits, including urinary incontinence and ataxia.

IMMUNITY AND IMMUNE EVASION
Immunity to Equine Herpesvirus 1

In the past decade, much progress has been made toward an understanding of the adaptive immunity to EHV-1. For example, it is known that following infection there is only a short period of immunity that protects against reinfection with EHV-1. Although virus-neutralizing antibodies play a role in reduction of nasal viral shedding, cytotoxic T lymphocytes (CTLs) are most critical for protection from clinical disease, viremia, and viral shedding.[37] More recently, innate immunity to EHV-1 infection has been investigated based on the premise that early immunity is not only critically important for immediate protection but likely shapes subsequent adaptive immune responses.[38] Despite these efforts, immunity following infection or vaccination is insufficient and offers limited protection, especially against EHM. This lack of induction of protective immunity to EHV-1 is likely caused by immunomodulatory properties of the virus.[39]

Immune Evasion by Equine Herpesvirus 1

Immune evasion strategies used by EHV-1 include interference and modulation of natural killer cell lysis, alteration of cytokines regulating B- and T-cell responses, alteration of the chemokine network resulting in loss of efficient antigen presentation and chemoattraction of immune cells, inhibition of antibody-dependent cytotoxicity, induction of T-regulatory cells, and alteration of CTL responses.[40] All of these mechanisms can contribute to and explain the short-lived immunity following infection and it is critical to understand the effects of viral immune evasion strategies on the immune response to infection, because they are likely to be key targets for successful preventative or therapeutic approaches. Research in recent years has identified several EHV-1 candidate immunomodulatory genes including the UL49.5 and ORF1 gene that interfere with major histocompatibility complex-I antigen presentation and induction of CTL responses.[41] Another viral modulatory gene identified is glycoprotein G. This gene has been found to function as a viral chemokine-binding protein that selectively inhibits interleukin-8 and CCL-3 mediated chemotaxis of phagocytes (neutrophils and macrophages).[42] Other viral modulatory genes are likely present and may be identified in the future.

Given what has been learned about EHV-1 immunity and immune evasion, future vaccination approaches to prevent EHV-1 infection and protect horses from EHM will likely have to go beyond current inactivated vaccines that are unlikely to induce strong CTL responses or modified life vaccines that contain active immune modulatory viral genes.

CONTROL STRATEGIES

Currently available vaccines do not reliably block infection, the development of viremia, or the establishment of latency and EHM has been observed in horses regularly vaccinated against EHV-1.[2,4] Furthermore, vaccination has been cited as a potential risk factor for the development of EHM, although the supporting evidence is far from conclusive.[15] The significant reduction in viral shedding observed in vaccinated horses provides reasonable justification for booster vaccination of nonexposed horses at risk for infection to reduce viral shedding in the event of exposure to EHV-1. By enhancing herd immunity, it is hoped that the level of infectious virus circulating in the at-risk population and, in turn, that the risk of individual horses in the population developing disease, will be reduced. This approach also relies on the assumption that the immune system of most mature horses has been primed by prior exposure to EHV-1 antigens through field infection or vaccination and can therefore be boosted within 7 to 10 days of administration of a single dose of vaccine. Although the validity of this approach has not been critically evaluated for the prevention of EHM, its implementation seems rational when faced with one or more horses with confirmed clinical EHV-1 infection of any form. Whereas booster vaccination of horses that are likely to have been exposed is not recommended, it is rational to booster vaccinate nonexposed horses, and those that must enter the premises, if they have not already been vaccinated against EHV-1 during the previous 90 days. Horse owners must develop an understanding of the concept of boosting herd immunity to help protect individual horses rather than having an as yet unattainable expectation that the attending veterinarian can reliably protect an individual horse from developing potentially fatal EHM by administering one of the currently available vaccines.

Although there is no reliable method of preventing EHM, implementation of routine management practices aimed at reducing the likelihood of introducing and disseminating EHV-1 infection is justified. To prevent EHM within veterinary clinics and hospitals, all horses presenting with significant fevers and nonspecific symptoms that may or may not include neurologic signs should be strictly isolated until a diagnosis is secured. Such an approach can prevent the later quarantine of an entire hospital should EHV-1 infection be diagnosed subsequently. The blood and nasal secretions of suspect horses should be tested by qPCR for EHV-1 and other infectious agents until these tests and accompanying clinical signs confirm or rule out active EHV-1 infection. Once EHV-1 infection is confirmed, strict isolation procedures and secondary quarantine of the clinic and the source stable of the particular horse should be used. At stables and farms, all newly arrived horses should be isolated for at least 3 weeks. Foot-baths, boot covers, and coveralls should be provided and adequately maintained for sanitary purposes. Separate equipment, tack, bedding, and feedstuffs should be used in the care of these animals. Grooms and other personnel should be instructed to work with these animals last in the course of their daily routine. Exercise periods should be confined to a time when other horses are not present in the training areas and riders should wear protective clothing and clean and thoroughly disinfect their boots, tack, and hands after contact with such animals. Horses returning from shows or extended traveling events should be isolated according to their particular circumstances. Minimum isolation precautions include the prevention of fomite transmission through nose-to-nose contact or the indirect transmission of infective nasal secretions by mechanical transmission through stable employees or horse owners. All horse vans and trailers should be thoroughly cleaned and disinfected after use. Prevention of EHM following horse shows, races, or other athletic events is problematic. Although the requirement of an "active vaccination status" before admittance and during extended stays at such events may lessen the probability of outbreaks of the respiratory form of EHV-1 infection, no vaccine currently offers protection against the development of EHM. Consequently, the effectiveness of any such strategy in this context is questionable. The examination of at-risk horses for clinical signs of disease, including twice-daily assessment of rectal temperature, remains the most effective tool in determining possible sources of virus introduction.

Following the identification of a horse with clinical signs consistent EHM, such as fever, nasal discharge, and the acute onset of neurologic deficits, measures must be instituted immediately to confirm the diagnosis and control disease spread. It is known that the nasal secretions of horses with EHM contain extremely large amounts of replicating virus and these secretions particularly contribute to the spread of disease to other susceptible individuals. As a consequence, horses suspected of having EHM must be removed from the stable environment as quickly as possible and placed in strict isolation. Failure to remove these animals facilitates the continued viral contamination of the environment and contributes to the spread of disease. Clinically affected horses should remain in strict quarantine until such time as they are proved either not to have EHV-1 infection or have fully recovered and are asymptomatic for 21 days. Horses known to have had direct contact with a suspected EHM case should be maintained in their existing barns and segregated from other horses during exercise periods until a diagnosis is made. Once confirmed, appropriate quarantine restricting the movement of all potentially exposed horses is necessary to prevent the spread of disease to other locations. Aerosol transmission is considered less important than direct contact or spread of secretions on fomites between horses by handlers. These procedures may begin with the focal quarantine of individuals in the immediate area of exposure, such as a single barn or other unit of housing within a facility. Horses in the immediate focal contact area of the clinically affected (index) individual should be monitored twice daily for fever and if found to be febrile should be tested for EHV-1 infection by qPCR. If after focal quarantine measures additional clinically ill or EHV-1–positive horses are identified at other locations within the facility, additional quarantine of exposed horses should be instituted and the area under quarantine may be expanded to include other affected barns or the entire stable area. An optimum strategy is the imposition of a series of focal quarantine procedures in an expanding series of concentric rings of disease control. Individual animals that have tested positive for EHV-1 infection within the designated quarantine area, whether symptomatic or not, should be periodically retested until disease is confirmed or eliminated based on lack of clinical signs and a negative PCR test result. Quarantine should be maintained until absence of further clinical cases and positive tests from exposed horses suggest no new cases are occurring. At this point areas of the facility under focal quarantine may have their restrictions rescinded in a reverse concentric ring approach.

The effectiveness of medical intervention to reduce the likelihood of EHM development in horses with early signs (fever) is unproved and the justification is theoretic. The goal of such medical strategy is aimed at decreasing viremia with the use of antiviral drugs, at preventing interactions between infected peripheral blood mononuclear cells and endothelial cells of the CNS by using nonsteroidal anti-inflammatory drugs, and at minimizing sequelae resulting from infected endothelial cells by using antithrombotic or rheologic drugs. The random treatment of exposed but asymptomatic horses with any of the previously listed drugs should be discouraged.

SUMMARY

Although EHM is an uncommon manifestation of EHV-1 infection, it can cause devastating losses during outbreaks. Antemortem diagnosis of EHM relies mainly on PCR detection of EHV-1 in nasal secretions and blood. Management of horses affected by EHM is aimed at supportive nursing and nutritional care, at reducing CNS inflammation, and at preventing thromboembolic sequelae. Horses exhibiting sudden and severe neurologic signs consistent with a diagnosis of EHM pose a definite risk to the surrounding horse population. Consequently, early intervention to prevent the spread of infection is required. Disease control measures, such as isolation of affected horses, segregation and monitoring of exposed horses, and quarantine measures, should be established to prevent the spread of the virus. Although there are several vaccines available against the respiratory and abortigenic forms of EHV-1 infection, currently no vaccines are protective against the neurologic strain of the virus.

REFERENCES

1. Ostlund EN. The equine herpesviruses. Vet Clin North Am Equine Pract 1993; 9(2):283–94.
2. Henninger RW, Reed SM, Saville WJ, et al. Outbreak of neurologic disease caused by equine herpesvirus-1 at a university equestrian center. J Vet Intern Med 2007;21(1):157–65.
3. Burgess BA, Tokateloff N, Manning S, et al. Nasal shedding of equine herpesvirus-1 from horses in an outbreak of equine herpes myeloencephalopathy in Western Canada. J Vet Intern Med 2012;26(2):384–92.
4. Traub-Dargatz JL, Pelzel-McCluskey AM, Creekmore LH, et al. Case-control study of a multistate equine herpesvirus myeloencephalopathy outbreak. J Vet Intern Med 2013;27(2):339–46.
5. Allen GP, Bryans JT. Molecular epizootiology, pathogenesis, and prophylaxis of equine herpesvirus-1 infections. Prog Vet Microbiol Immunol 1986;2:78–144.
6. Crabb BS, Studdert MJ. Expression of small regions of equine herpesvirus 1 glycoprotein C in Escherichia coli. Vet Microbiol 1995;46(1–3):181–91.
7. Telford EA, Watson MS, McBride K, et al. The DNA sequence of equine herpesvirus-1. Virology 1992;189(1):304–16.
8. Gray WL, Baumann RP, Robertson AT, et al. Regulation of equine herpesvirus type 1 gene expression: characterization of immediate early, early, and late transcription. Virology 1987;158(1):79–87.
9. Nugent J, Birch-Machin I, Smith KC, et al. Analysis of equid herpesvirus 1 strain variation reveals a point mutation of the DNA polymerase strongly associated with neuropathogenic versus nonneuropathogenic disease outbreaks. J Virol 2006; 80(8):4047–60.
10. Perkins GA, Goodman LB, Tsujimura K, et al. Investigation of the prevalence of neurologic equine herpes virus type 1 (EHV-1) in a 23-year retrospective analysis (1984-2007). Vet Microbiol 2009;139(3–4):375–8.
11. Goodman LB, Loregian A, Perkins GA, et al. A point mutation in a herpesvirus polymerase determines neuropathogenicity. PLoS Pathog 2007;3(11):e160.
12. Allen GP, Bolin DC, Bryant U, et al. Prevalence of latent, neuropathogenic equine herpesvirus-1 in the Thoroughbred broodmare population of central Kentucky. Equine Vet J 2008;40(2):105–10.
13. Pusterla N, Mapes S, Wilson WD. Prevalence of equine herpesvirus type 1 in trigeminal ganglia and submandibular lymph nodes of equids examined postmortem. Vet Rec 2010;167(10):376–8.

14. Allen GP. Equid herpesvirus 1 and equid herpesvirus 4 infections. In: Coetzer JA, Tustin RC, editors. Infectious diseases of livestock. Newmarket (ON): Oxford University Press; 2004. p. 829–59.
15. Dunowska M. A review of equid herpesvirus 1 for the veterinary practitioner. Part B: pathogenesis and epidemiology. N Z Vet J 2014;62(4):179–88.
16. Gilkerson JR, Whalley JM, Drummer HE, et al. Epidemiological studies of equine herpesvirus 1 (EHV-1) in Thoroughbred foals: a review of studies conducted in the Hunter Valley of New South Wales between 1995 and 1997. Vet Microbiol 1999;68(1–2):15–25.
17. Gilkerson JR, Whalley JM, Drummer HE, et al. Epidemiology of EHV-1 and EHV-4 in the mare and foal populations on a Hunter Valley stud farm: are mares the source of EHV-1 for unweaned foals. Vet Microbiol 1999;68(1–2):27–34.
18. Walter J, Balzer HJ, Seeh C, et al. Venereal shedding of equid herpesvirus-1 (EHV-1) in naturally infected stallions. J Vet Intern Med 2012;26(6):1500–4.
19. Pusterla N, Hussey SB, Mapes S, et al. Molecular investigation of the viral kinetics of equine herpesvirus-1 in blood and nasal secretions of horses after corticosteroid-induced recrudescence of latent infection. J Vet Intern Med 2010;24(5):1153–7.
20. Lunn DP, Davis-Poynter N, Flaminio MJ, et al. Equine herpesvirus-1 consensus statement. J Vet Intern Med 2009;23(3):450–61.
21. Equine Herpesvirus (EHV-1) Situation Report 2011. Accessed June 2, 2011. Available at: http://www.aphis.usda.gov/vs/nahss/equine/ehv/ehv_2011_sitrep_060211.pdf.
22. Goehring LS, Soboll Hussey G, Gomez Diez M, et al. Plasma D-dimer concentrations during experimental EHV-1 infection of horses. J Vet Intern Med 2013;27(6):1535–42.
23. Allen GP. Risk factors for development of neurologic disease after experimental exposure to equine herpesvirus-1 in horses. Am J Vet Res 2008;69(12):1595–600.
24. Gardiner DW, Lunn DP, Goehring LS, et al. Strain impact on equine herpesvirus type 1 (Ehv-1) abortion models: viral loads in fetal and placental tissues and foals. Vaccine 2012;30(46):6564–72.
25. Hussey GS, Goehring LS, Lunn DP, et al. Experimental infection with equine herpesvirus type 1 (EHV-1) induces chorioretinal lesions. Vet Res 2013;44:118.
26. Lunn DP, Mayhew I. Neurological examination of the horse. Equine Vet Educ 1989;1:94–101.
27. Wilson WD. Equine herpesvirus 1 myeloencephalopathy. Vet Clin North Am Equine Pract 1997;13(1):53–72.
28. Pusterla N, Wilson WD, Mapes S, et al. Characterization of viral loads, strain and state of equine herpesvirus-1 using real-time PCR in horses following natural exposure at a racetrack in California. Vet J 2009;179(2):230–9.
29. Pusterla N, Hussey SB, Mapes S, et al. Comparison of four methods to quantify equid herpesvirus 1 load by real-time polymerase chain reaction in nasal secretions of experimentally and naturally infected horses. J Vet Diagn Invest 2009; 21(6):836–40.
30. Pusterla N, Mapes S, Wilson WD. Use of viral loads in blood and nasopharyngeal secretions for the diagnosis of EHV-1 infection in field cases. Vet Rec 2008; 162(22):728–9.
31. McCartan CG, Russell MM, Wood JL, et al. Clinical, serological and virological characteristics of an outbreak of paresis and neonatal foal disease due to equine herpesvirus-1 on a stud farm. Vet Rec 1995;136(1):7–12.
32. Wilson WD, Pusterla N. Equine herpesvirus-1 myeloencephalopathy. In: Reed SM, Bayly WM, Sellon DC, editors. Equine Internal Medicine. St. Louis: Saunders Elsevier; 2010. p. 615–22.

33. Goehring LS, Brandes KM, Wittenburg L, et al. Anti-inflammatory drugs decrease the rate of endothelial cell infection with EHV-1 in vitro. In: Proceedings of 2012 Veterinary Symposium. New Orleans (LA): American College of Veterinary Internal Medicine; 2012.

34. Garré B, van der Meulen K, Nugent J, et al. *In vitro* susceptibility of six isolates of equine herpesvirus 1 to acyclovir, ganciclovir, cidofovir, adefovir, PMEDAP and foscarnet. Vet Microbiol 2007;122(1–2):43–51.

35. Bentz BG, Maxwell LK, Erkert RS, et al. Pharmacokinetics of acyclovir after single intravenous and oral administration to adult horses. J Vet Intern Med 2006;20(3): 589–94.

36. Maxwell LK, Bentz BG, Bourne DW, et al. Pharmacokinetics of valacyclovir in the adult horse. J Vet Pharmacol Ther 2008;31(4):312–20.

37. Kydd JH, Wattrang E, Hannant D. Pre-infection frequencies of equine herpesvirus-1 specific, cytotoxic T lymphocytes correlate with protection against abortion following experimental infection of pregnant mares. Vet Immunol Immunopathol 2003;96(3–4):207–17.

38. Soboll Hussey G, Hussey SB, Wagner B, et al. Evaluation of immune responses following infection of ponies with an EHV-1 ORF1/2 deletion mutant. Vet Res 2011; 42:23.

39. Ambagala AP, Gopinath RS, Srikumaran S. Peptide transport activity of the transporter associated with antigen processing (TAP) is inhibited by an early protein of equine herpesvirus-1. J Gen Virol 2004;85(2):349–53.

40. van der Meulen KM, Favorell HW, Pensaert MB, et al. Immune escape of equine herpesvirus 1 and other herpesviruses of veterinary importance. Vet Immunol Immunopathol 2006;111(1–2):31–40.

41. Soboll Hussey G, Ashton LV, Quintana AM, et al. Equine herpesvirus type 1 pUL56 modulates innate responses of airway epithelial cells. Virology 2014; 464–465:76–86. http://dx.doi.org/10.1016/j.virol.2014.05.023.

42. Van de Walle GR, May ML, Sukhumavasi W, et al. Herpesvirus chemokine-binding glycoprotein G (gG) efficiently inhibits neutrophil chemotaxis in vitro and in vivo. J Immunol 2007;179(6):4161–9.

Equine Influenza Virus

Gabriele A. Landolt, Dr med vet, MS, PhD

KEYWORDS

- Influenza A virus • Virus evolution • Epidemiology • Diagnosis • Control

KEY POINTS

- Despite extensive use of vaccines, equine influenza virus continues to be one of the most important equine viral respiratory pathogens.
- Control of equine influenza virus is hampered by continued genetic evolution of the virus (antigenic drift).
- Antigenic drift negatively affects the degree of immunoprotection evoked by inactivated vaccines.
- Isolation and genetic characterization of currently circulating equine influenza viruses remains a priority, and is essential for vaccine strain selection.

INTRODUCTION

Influenza is a well-known and ancient disease. In fact, a disease resembling influenza was described by Hippocrates in 412 BC. Yet hardly a month goes by without a new headline about influenza in the media. Although millions of dollars have been spent on research, influenza virus continues to challenge our understanding of its ecology and our ability to control its spread. Two key reasons why influenza virus has remained one of the most important causes of viral respiratory disease are its potential for establishing genetic and antigenic diversity and its ability to occasionally transmit between different host species.[1]

For decades the horse has been viewed as an isolated or "dead-end" host for influenza A viruses, with equine influenza virus being considered as relatively stable genetically. Although equine influenza viruses are genetically more stable than their human-lineage counterparts, they are by no means in evolutionary stasis. Moreover, recent transmission of equine-lineage influenza viruses to dogs also challenges the horse's status as a dead-end host. This article reviews recent developments in the epidemiology and evolution of equine influenza virus. In addition, the clinical presentation of equine influenza infection, diagnostic techniques, and vaccine recommendations are briefly summarized.

Funding Sources: Merck Animal Health.
Conflict of Interest: None.
Department of Clinical Sciences, College of Veterinary Medicine and Biomedical Sciences, Colorado State University, 300 West Drake Road, Fort Collins, CO 80523, USA
E-mail address: Landoltg@colostate.edu

ETIOLOGY

Equine influenza virus is a member of the influenza A viruses, which belong to the Orthomyxoviridae family. The Orthomyxoviridae family comprises 5 genera (**Fig. 1**), all containing enveloped viruses with segmented, single-stranded, negative-sense RNA genomes. In contrast to the rather narrow host ranges of influenza B and C viruses, influenza A viruses can infect a wide variety of species (see **Fig. 1**).

Influenza A viruses possess a host-cell–derived lipid envelope, which contains 3 envelope glycoproteins: the hemagglutinin (HA), neuraminidase (NA), and M2 ion channel protein (**Fig. 2**). Both the HA and NA are major surface antigens of the virus, and antibodies to these proteins are associated with resistance to infection.

- Based on antigenic properties of the HA and the NA, influenza A viruses are divided into subtypes.
- Cross-protection between subtypes (heterotypic immunity) is weak.
- Eighteen HA subtypes (H1–H18) and 11 NA subtypes (N1–N11) have been found.
- Equine influenza has been caused by viruses of H7N7 (A/equine/1) and H3N8 (A/equine/2) subtypes.

In addition to the envelope glycoproteins, the influenza A virus genome encodes for an additional 5 structural (M1 matrix protein, nucleoprotein [NP], and polymerase complex [PA, PB1, PB2]) and 3 "nonstructural" proteins (NS1, NS2 [also referred to as the NEP "nuclear export protein"], and PB1-F2) (see **Fig. 2**).

During infection antibodies are also produced to the internal proteins, but these antibodies are not protective. Similarly, the cytotoxic T-cell (CTL) response, primarily

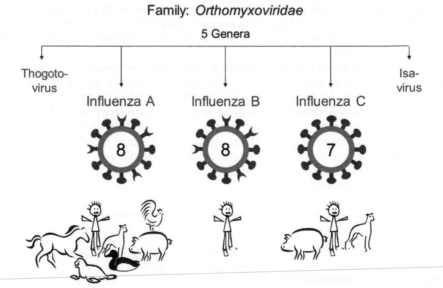

Family: *Orthomyxoviridae*

5 Genera

Thogoto-virus   Influenza A   Influenza B   Influenza C   Isa-virus

Fig. 1. The 5 Orthomyxoviridae genera. In contrast to the wide host range of influenza A viruses, influenza B and C viruses have a more narrow host range. Whereas influenza A and B contain 8 separate segments of single-stranded RNA, influenza C viruses possess only 7.

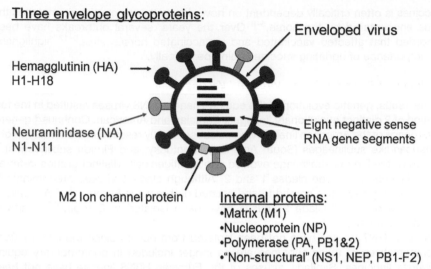

Three envelope glycoproteins:

Enveloped virus

Hemagglutinin (HA)
H1-H18

Neuraminidase (NA)
N1-N11

Eight negative sense
RNA gene segments

M2 Ion channel protein

Internal proteins:
•Matrix (M1)
•Nucleoprotein (NP)
•Polymerase (PA, PB1&2)
•"Non-structural" (NS1, NEP, PB1-F2)

Fig. 2. The influenza A virus virion. The 3 envelope glycoproteins hemagglutinin (HA), neur-aminidase (NA), and the M2 ion channel protein are embedded in a host-cell–derived lipid envelope. In addition, the influenza A virus genome encodes for 5 structural (M1, NP, PA, PB1, PB2) and 3 nonstructural (NS1, NEP, PB1-F2) proteins.

directed against M, NP, and PB2, does not prevent infection but seems to play a role in recovery and virus clearance.[2] In contrast to the humoral response that provides only limited heterotypic immunity, the CTL response is cross-reactive between influenza A virus subtypes.[3,4]

GENETIC DIVERSITY OF INFLUENZA A VIRUS

Both the RNA-based genome and its segmented configuration confer influenza A viruses with the capacity for vast genetic diversity. As viral RNA polymerases lack proofreading functions, RNA viruses generally demonstrate high mutation rates, with resultant potential for rapid evolution. This genetic diversity allows adaptation to a new environment (eg, a new host species) or immune escape.

Mechanisms of generating antigenic diversity by influenza A viruses:

- Antigenic drift: Selection, driven by the host immune system, of viruses with mutations affecting the antigenic sites in the HA (and NA) protein

- Antigenic shift: Exchange of gene segments (genetic reassortment) between 2 influenza viruses during replication resulting in the switch of the progeny virus' HA (or NA) subtype

Although there is no evidence to date that equine viruses have participated in genetic reassortment events, it is clear that they undergo some degree of antigenic drift. Despite the rate of genetic diversion of equine influenza viruses being small compared with human influenza viruses,[1] the sustained genetic and antigenic evolution has an impact in terms of immunization. It has long been recognized that the antigenic distance between 2 influenza virus strains affects the extent of cross-protection provided by antibodies raised to 1 strain. Therefore, the level of protection provided by vaccines is often critically dependent on how closely the vaccine strain matches the virus encountered by the horse.[5–8] Over the years, several outbreaks have been recorded that affected vaccinated and unvaccinated horses alike,[9–12] highlighting the importance of updating vaccine strains periodically.

Evolution of Equine Influenza Virus and Vaccine Composition

In the 1980s, genetic evolution of the equine-lineage H3N8 viruses resulted in the formation of 2 distinct evolutionary lineages, Eurasian and American. Continued genetic divergence of the American lineage viruses subsequently resulted in the formation of 3 American-like sublineages (South American, Kentucky, and Florida sublineages).[13] Recently, the Florida sublineage evolved into 2 antigenically distinct groups, referred to as Florida sublineage clades 1 and 2. Although clade 1 viruses predominate in America, they have also spread to and caused outbreaks in Europe,[14–16] Australia,[17] Africa,[18] and Asia.[19] Clade 2 viruses have been isolated in Europe,[20,21] parts of Africa,[22] and Asia.[23–25]

As the H7N7 viruses have not been isolated from horses since the late 1970s,[26] representatives of these subtypes are no longer included in contemporary equine influenza vaccines. Similarly, viruses of the Eurasian H3N8 lineage have not been isolated since 2005.[11] Thus, the OIE Expert Panel for equine influenza advised that there was no longer a need to include these viruses in equine influenza vaccines. By contrast, with the divergence of the Florida sublineage viruses into 2 antigenically distinct clades, the panel recommended that killed vaccines should include strains representative of both Florida clade 1 and clade 2. As the sustained genetic evolution of the equine H3N8 viruses will likely continue to result in suboptimal vaccine protection in the future, inclusion of viral antigens representative of contemporary circulating viruses has to remain a priority.

Cross-Species Transmission of Equine Influenza

It has long been recognized that influenza A viruses exhibit partial restriction of their host range, meaning that viruses from one host species occasionally can transmit to infect another host.[1] It is generally accepted that the HA protein has an important role in determining the species specificity of influenza A viruses.[27] Serving as the viral receptor-binding protein, the HA mediates the fusion of the virus envelope with the host-cell membrane, with the subsequent release of the virus into the cytoplasm.[28]

Binding of the HA protein to sialic acid (SA) receptor on the host cell is determined by the SA species (N-acetylneuraminic acid [Neu5Ac] or N-glycolneuraminic acid [Neu5Gc]) and its linkage to galactose residues (α2,6 linkage or α2,3 linkage).[27]

- Human influenza viruses prefer binding to SAα2,6-gal in NeuAc form, matched by SAα2,6-gal expression on the human upper respiratory tract epithelium.

- Avian, equine, and canine viruses prefer binding to SAα2,3-gal (NeuGc and NeuAc [avian]; NeuGc [equine]), mirrored by a predominance of SAα2,3-gal expression on the epithelial cells of horse trachea and duck intestine.

As already stated, the horse has been viewed as an isolated host for influenza A viruses, meaning that exchange of viruses or their gene segments between horses and other species is limited.[1] However, the transmission H3N8 equine influenza viruses to dogs in the United States,[29] the United Kingdom,[30,31] and Australia[32] clearly challenges this notion. In addition to these naturally occurring cross-species transmission events, equine influenza virus has also been found to spread from an experimentally infected horse to a dog that was housed in the same stall,[33] and experimental inoculation of dogs with equine influenza virus resulted in nasal virus shedding and subsequent seroconversion.[34] In this regard it is interesting that recent studies showed that dogs predominantly express SAα2,3-linked residues throughout the respiratory tract,[30,34] which is matched by the preferential binding of both canine and equine influenza viruses to this type of receptor.[34,35] On first glance, these findings provide an attractive explanation for the apparent susceptibility of dogs to infection with equine H3N8 viruses. Despite this fact, there are subtle differences in binding specificity among these viruses. Although equine and canine isolates prefer binding to SAα2,3-gal, Yamanaka and colleagues[36] found that whereas equine influenza viruses display a clear binding preference for the Neu5Gc receptor moiety, canine H3N8 isolates did not appear to have a preference for either the Neu5Gc or the Neu5Ac sialic acid analogue.[36]

In light of these similarities in receptor-binding preference, one could expect influenza viruses to spread also in the reverse direction, meaning from dog to horse. Intriguingly recent studies found that 2 distinct isolates of H3N8 canine influenza viruses were unable to infect, replicate, and spread among influenza-naïve equids.[36,37] Moreover, inoculation of horses with these canine isolates did not result in clinical disease in either study. These results suggest that factors other than receptor-binding preference likely contribute to species specificity of canine and equine H3N8 influenza viruses.

EPIDEMIOLOGY

Although horses of all ages are susceptible to infection, disease incidence is lower in young foals[38–41] and is thought to be due to the presence of maternally derived antibodies. Influenza-specific serum antibody concentration is often used as a correlate for protection against infection and disease, and animals with high concentrations of homologous antibody are almost always protected against experimental challenge.[42–46]

Following experimental inoculation:

- Horses begin to shed virus in nasal secretions within 24 to 48 hours
- Nasal virus shedding typically lasts between 6 and 7 days
- Partially immune animals might shed less virus for shorter durations
- Morbidity is often high with low mortality

Outbreaks of disease occur most often when susceptible animals are congregated and housed in close contact with each other (eg, horse shows, racetracks, sale barns).[47] Anecdotal evidence suggests that disease can spread rapidly through a group of immunologically naïve animals (ie, in a matter of hours to days). In partially immune animals the spread of disease is often considerably slower, and outbreaks may last as long as 3 to 4 weeks.[48] In contrast to the seasonal pattern of human influenza epidemics, equine influenza may occur at any time of the year.

Spread of virus among susceptible animals may occur through 3 modes: direct contact with infected animals or fomites, droplet transmission (droplets >10 μm and capable of being projected over moderate distances by coughing and sneezing), and aerosol transmission (droplet nuclei <5 μm, capable of wide dissemination and of reaching the lower respiratory tract).[49] Although aerosol transmission unquestionably has the greatest impact in regard to influenza virus infection control, the importance of bioaerosol transmission in the spread of influenza virus has not been well characterized. Depending on the prevailing environmental conditions (humidity, temperature, exposure to sun light, and so forth), the virus can remain infectious for days on contaminated surfaces.[50] Meteorologic factors associated with an increased risk of spread of equine influenza virus between premises during a recent outbreak were relative humidity of less than 60% and wind speeds of greater than 30 km/h from the direction of a barn with infected horses.[51]

RECENT EQUINE INFLUENZA OUTBREAKS

Since 2000 several widespread equine influenza outbreaks have occurred, which highlight the continued threat equine influenza viruses poses to the health of horses worldwide. In 2003 an outbreak affecting generally well-vaccinated horses occurred in the United Kingdom, with infection being confirmed in at least 12 locations and at least 21 training yards in Newmarket.[9,52] In contrast to previously published observations suggesting that younger horses are likely to develop more severe disease,[8,46] this outbreak was characterized by an apparent increased risk of infection and more severe clinical disease in older horses.[9] This seeming discrepancy in epidemiology appeared to be linked to the length of time since last vaccination. As the level of protection elicited by vaccination likely peaked within the first 3 months of vaccine administration and subsequently declined, more recently vaccinated horses (in this case the younger horses) were better protected. Based on these data, the investigators concluded that vaccination during an outbreak, even using traditional inactivated vaccines, could have merit to reduce the risk of infection.[9] In addition, this study highlighted the importance of the timing of first vaccine administration in determining later serologic responses. As suggested by previous studies,[7,53–55] the investigators found that administration of an equine influenza vaccine early in life, most likely in the face of existing maternally derived antibodies, increased the risk of influenza infection later in life.[9]

Between 2003 and 2009, sizable equine influenza outbreaks were also reported in South Africa,[56] India,[57] Japan,[19] and, for the first time, in Australia.[17] The outbreak in Australia was caused by a virus introduced by importation of a subclinically infected vaccinated horse from Japan.[17,19,58] Subsequent breakdown in quarantine protocols allowed the virus to enter the native horse population.[58] This incident highlights an important point in terms of equine influenza infection control. Although vaccination reduces or even eliminates clinical signs of disease, it may not prevent infection and subsequent virus shedding.[59] This aspect is likely of particular relevance with increasing antigenic distance between vaccine strain and infecting virus.[6] Despite the fact that nasal virus-shedding titers are often lower in vaccinated animals, the infected vaccinated horse may still shed infectious virus, and thus pose a risk of introducing influenza virus into a population.[11,60,61]

The equine influenza outbreak in Australia resulted in approximately 70,000 infected horses in New South Wales and in southeastern Queensland.[58] Promptly initiated control measures, consisting of stringent horse movement control, quarantine of affected and suspect premises, targeted vaccination, and on-farm biosecurity measures (personal hygiene, equipment hygiene, and access control measures), were successful at containing the outbreak to these 2 states.[62] More importantly, these control measures resulted in the eradication of the virus from the Australian horse population, and Australia regained its equine influenza-free status in December 2008.[63,64]

Given that this outbreak had a substantial impact on the equine industry, there are several conclusions concerning biosecurity practices that can be drawn. For example, the most important risk factor for virus introduction was proximity to the nearest infected premises.[62] The use of footbaths before introduction of infection onto the premises, which may have been a reflection of the overall on-site biosecurity standards, was associated with a 4-fold reduction of risk of infection.[62] Furthermore, farm owners who believed that these measures were effective were more likely to demonstrate a high level of compliance with general recommended biosecurity measures.[65] This finding supports data from other studies on human behavior, which suggest that having more confidence in the efficacy of the preventive behavior is associated with a greater likelihood of taking action.[66,67] Finally, it appeared that horse owners who received infection control information from a veterinarian (rather than the media, governmental sources, other horse owners, and so forth) were more likely to perceive equine influenza biosecurity measures as effective.[65]

PATHOGENESIS AND CLINICAL DISEASE

After influenza virus attaches to the respiratory epithelial cell, it enters the cell by receptor-mediated endocytosis. After virus replication and the release of progeny virus from the host cell, the virus spreads rapidly throughout the respiratory tract. As virus replication leads to cell death, mostly through apoptosis,[68–70] the ciliated respiratory epithelium in the trachea and bronchial tree is lost (**Fig. 3**).[71] Reduced mucociliary clearance,[72–74] in addition to the disruption of the superficial layers of the respiratory epithelium, predisposes the affected animal to the development of secondary bacterial complications such as bacterial bronchopneumonia.[71,75] In uncomplicated cases, complete resolution of the epithelial damage takes a minimum of 3 weeks.[74,76]

Clinical signs of equine influenza virus infection consist of fever, anorexia, lethargy, nasal discharge, and cough. Pyrexia is often the first symptom present, with body temperatures peaking somewhere between 48 and 96 hours after infection. In some cases, a second peak of pyrexia may occur approximately 7 days after infection. Nasal discharge is typically serous early on, but may become mucopurulent later. Concurrently a dry, hacking cough develops. In general, uncomplicated cases of influenza resolve within 1 to 2 weeks, although the cough may persist for several weeks after

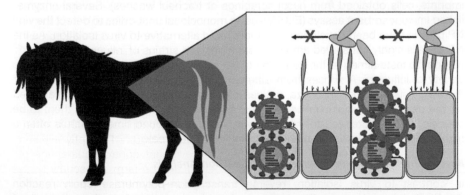

Fig. 3. Pathogenesis of influenza virus. The virus spreads throughout the respiratory tract, damaging the respiratory epithelial cells largely through virus-induced apoptosis. Impairment of mucociliary clearance predisposes the affected animal to the development of secondary bacterial infections.

infection. The disease is rarely fatal, but deaths have been reported during some epidemics, particularly in donkeys and, rarely, in neonatal foals.[39,77,78]

Complications of equine influenza can be severe and include secondary bacterial pneumonia, myositis, myocarditis, and limb edema.[73,74,79] During the 2003 outbreak in the United Kingdom, 2 influenza-infected horses developed neurologic disease.[80] Necropsy results of one horse revealed the presence of nonsuppurative encephalitis. Influenza-associated encephalopathy is an uncommon complication in humans and is more common in children.[81,82] The pathogenesis of influenza-associated encephalopathy is unclear. As the virus is rarely detected in the central nervous system, direct neuroinvasion of influenza is not thought to be the cause of the encephalopathy.[82]

DIAGNOSIS

The basic approaches for the laboratory diagnosis of equine influenza infection are the isolation of the etiologic agent, demonstration of the virus, virus genome, or viral products in clinical specimens, and the detection of virus-specific antibodies. The *Manual of Diagnostic Tests and Vaccines for Terrestrial Animals*, published by the World Organization for Animal Health (OIE; http://www.oie.int) provides an in-depth review of the currently available diagnostic testing strategies.

Virus Isolation

Despite equine influenza virus isolation from clinical specimens being difficult and typically time consuming, it is crucial for epidemiologic investigation and vaccine strain selection. The best results for virus isolation are often achieved by culturing nasal or nasopharyngeal swab samples collected in the first 24 to 48 hours after onset of clinical disease. As the duration of nasal virus shedding is often brief in partially immune animals, it may prove useful to sample immunologically less protected individuals in a group (eg, younger horses, poorly vaccinated or unvaccinated animals) to increase the likelihood of isolating virus.

Antigen Detection

Assays aimed at detecting viral antigen have a faster turnaround time than virus isolation. Immunofluorescence (fluorescent antibody [FA] test) can be used to detect viral antigen in a broad range of clinical samples (eg, frozen sections of tissues, tissue imprints, cells obtained from nasal scrapings or tracheal washes). Several enzyme-linked immunosorbent assays (ELISAs) using monoclonal antibodies to detect the viral NP protein have been developed as a more rapid alternative to virus isolation. As the NP gene is highly conserved among all subtypes and strains of influenza A viruses,[83] diagnostic tests aimed at the detection of NP are often capable of identifying a wide variety of influenza A viruses from different host species. Originally developed for the diagnosis of human influenza, antigen-capture ELISAs have since been validated for the detection of equine influenza virus, and many studies have found them to be specific.[61,84–87] Moreover, they have a very rapid turnaround time, which is often a highly desirable feature during an equine influenza outbreak.

Reverse Transcription–Polymerase Chain Reaction Analysis

In contrast to virus isolation, reverse transcription–polymerase chain reaction (RT-PCR) does not require the presence of viable virus; therefore, the sensitivity of RT-PCR methods is often substantially higher than that for virus isolation. However, because of the assay's high sensitivity, this technique is also susceptible to the production of false-positive results. Any influenza virus nucleic acid contaminant, for example, the administration of an inactivated whole-virus vaccine at the time of sample collection,[88] may produce a false-positive result. Real-time RT-PCR assays use a target-specific fluorescent probe and provide results more rapidly than conventional RT-PCR methods. In addition, real-time PCR can also be used for quantification of virus in clinical samples.[89–91]

Antibody Detection

Serologic tests have remained a key tool in equine influenza diagnosis and surveillance. However, to demonstrate active influenza infection, paired samples collected 10 to 21 days apart (acute and convalescent titer) must be tested. Seroconversion, as defined by at least a 4-fold increase in antibody titers between the acute and convalescent sample, must be present to confirm active infection.

Most serologic tests do not provide information as to whether existing antibodies were produced in response to infection or vaccination. To address this shortcoming, an ELISA to detect antibodies directed against the influenza NS1 protein was recently developed.[92] As antibodies to the nonstructural NS1 protein are only produced in response to influenza virus replication,[93] and the protein is highly conserved among influenza A viruses,[94] NS1 has been found to serve as a diagnostic marker to differentiate infected from vaccinated animals (DIVA). In fact, the assay was found to perform well in a recent study, and was able to differentiate experimentally infected horses from horses vaccinated with an inactivated equine influenza virus.[92]

A different DIVA approach was taken in the 2007 equine influenza outbreak in Australia.[95,96] As the canarypox-vectored vaccine (Recombitek Influenza, Merial) only contains the influenza virus hemagglutinin gene, it raises only HA-specific antibodies in the vaccinated animal (**Fig. 4**). Using an influenza virus NP-based blocking

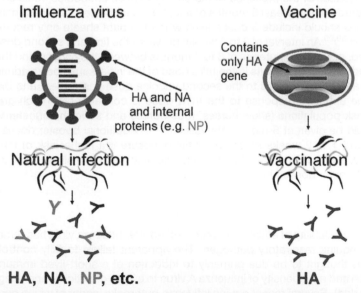

Fig. 4. The approach to differentiate infected from vaccinated animals (DIVA), used during the 2007 equine influenza outbreak in Australia. As the canarypox-vectored vaccine only contains the influenza virus HA gene, only HA-specific antibodies are detected in the vaccinated animal. By contrast, natural infection results in production of antibodies against HA, NA, and the internal proteins. Using an NP-based serologic assay provides DIVA capability.

ELISA for the serologic testing, this strategy was successful at distinguishing vaccinated from infected horses.[97,98]

CONTROL

Control of equine influenza primarily relies on adequate husbandry procedures and vaccination. Prevention of equine influenza virus introduction into a group of horses can likely be accomplished by following the biosecurity guidelines (eg, isolation of horses for 4 weeks before introduction into the horse population) published by the OIE (published in the Terrestrial Animal Health Code, Volume II, 2013; http://www. oie.int/). However, as these criteria may be difficult to achieve for most barns, 2 weeks of strict isolation and adequate vaccination may serve as an adequate compromise. Unfortunately even these measures are often not taken, and vaccination is the primary modality used for infection control.

A wide variety of equine influenza vaccine formulations are currently available for use, and include inactivated whole virus, modified live virus, and recombinant vectored vaccines (reviewed in Refs.[99,100]). However, despite the fact that the vaccines are generally very efficacious, outbreaks of equine influenza continue to occur. As discussed previously, one of the reasons for this is that the virus undergoes antigenic drift. In addition, vaccination seldom induces the same immunity as natural infection, and vaccine-induced antibodies may not persist very long,[100] which is particularly true for vaccines based on inactivated whole virus. By contrast, vaccines using modified live virus and recombinant vectored virus technologies (eg, poxvirus-based vaccines) stimulate both humoral and cellular immune responses, and mimic immunity elicited by natural infection more closely.[100]

Recommendations for equine vaccination are available from a variety of sources.[59,99] Because of the presence of maternally derived antibodies, foals should not be vaccinated before at least 6 months of age.[55] For inactivated vaccines, initial vaccination series should include 3 doses even when the data sheets only recommend 2 initial doses.[59,99] An interval of 3 to 4 weeks between the first and second dose is recommended, but a longer interval of 3 to 4 months between the second and third dose is preferred. This hiatus results in the third dose of the initial series being administered when the antibody response to the second vaccine dose has waned, and the amplitude of the antibody response to the third dose is consequently much greater.[101] For high-risk populations (show horses, race horses and so forth), booster vaccinations should be given at 6-month intervals.[59,99,102] Additional booster doses may be administered 1 to 2 weeks before potential exposure if a higher risk of infection is anticipated. The modified live intranasal vaccine only requires a single initial dose, followed by booster doses at 6-month intervals.

SUMMARY

Despite the availability of efficacious vaccines, equine influenza virus has remained an important equine respiratory pathogen. The apparent failure to fully control equine influenza is thought to be due primarily to induction of a short-lived immunity after vaccination and a propensity of influenza A virus to evolve genetically and antigenically (antigenic drift). Several recent equine influenza outbreaks, some of which occurred in vaccinated horses, clearly highlight the need for continued equine influenza virus surveillance and the periodic updating of vaccines (particularly the inactivated products) with relevant contemporary equine influenza virus strains. Moreover, analyses of the 2009 equine influenza outbreak in Australia indicate that on-site biosecurity measures (such as footbaths), put in place before introduction of the disease onto the premises, were clearly effective in reducing the risk of infection.

REFERENCES

1. Webster RG, Bean WJ, Gorman OT, et al. Evolution and ecology of influenza A viruses. Microbiol Rev 1992;56:152–79.
2. McMichael AJ, Michie CA, Gotch FM, et al. Recognition of influenza A virus nucleoprotein by human cytotoxic T lymphocytes. J Gen Virol 1986;67:719–26.
3. Hemann EA, Kang SM, Legge KL. Protective CD8 T cell-mediated immunity against influenza A virus infection following influenza virus-like particle vaccination. J Immunol 2013;191:2486–94.
4. McKinstry KK, Dutton RW, Swain SL, et al. Memory CD4 T cell-mediated immunity against influenza A virus: more than a little helpful. Arch Immunol Ther Exp 2013;61:341–53.
5. Daly JM, Yates PJ, Newton JR, et al. Evidence supporting the inclusion of strains from each of the two co-circulating lineages of H3N8 equine influenza virus in vaccines. Vaccine 2004;22:4101–9.
6. Daly JM, Yates RJ, Browse G, et al. Comparison of hamster and pony challenge models for evaluation of effect of antigenic drift on cross protection afforded by equine influenza vaccines. Equine Vet J 2003;35:458–62.
7. Newton JR, Lakhani KH, Wood JL, et al. Risk factors for equine influenza serum antibody titres in young thoroughbred racehorses given an inactivated vaccine. Prev Vet Med 2000;46:129–41.
8. Newton JR, Verheyen K, Wood JL, et al. Equine influenza in the United Kingdom in 1998. Vet Rec 1999;145:449–52.
9. Barquero N, Daly JM, Newton JR. Risk factors for influenza infection in vaccinated racehorses: lessons from an outbreak in Newmarket, UK in 2003. Vaccine 2007;25:7520–9.
10. Burrows R, Goodridge D, Denyer M, et al. Equine influenza infections in Great Britain, 1979. Vet Rec 1982;110:494–7.
11. Elton D, Cullinane A. Equine influenza: antigenic drift and implications for vaccines. Equine Vet J 2013;45:768–9.
12. Mumford JA, Wood J, Chambers T. Consultation of OIE and WHO experts on progress in surveillance of equine influenza and application to vaccine strain selection. In Report of a meeting held at the Animal Health Trust. Newmarket (United Kingdom), September 18-19, 1995.
13. Lai AC, Chambers TM, Holland RE Jr, et al. Diverged evolution of recent equine-2 influenza (H3N8) viruses in the Western Hemisphere. Arch Virol 2001;146:1063–74.
14. Bryant NA, Rash AS, Russell CA, et al. Antigenic and genetic variations in European and North American equine influenza virus strains (H3N8) isolated from 2006 to 2007. Vet Microbiol 2009;138:41–52.
15. Bryant NA, Rash AS, Woodward AL, et al. Isolation and characterization of equine influenza viruses (H3N8) from Europe and North America from 2008 to 2009. Vet Microbiol 2011;147:19–27.
16. Gildea S, Quinlivan M, Arkins S, et al. The molecular epidemiology of equine influenza in Ireland from 2007-2010 and its international significance. Equine Vet J 2012;44:387–92.
17. Watson J, Halpin K, Selleck P, et al. Isolation and characterization of an H3N8 equine influenza virus in Australia, 2007. Aust Vet J 2011;89:35–7.

18. King EL, MacDonald D. Report to the Board of Inquiry appointed by the Board of the National Horseracing Authority to conduct enquiry into the causes of the equine influenza with started in the Western cape in early December 2003 and spread to the Eastern Cape and Gauteng. Aust Vet J 2004;23:139–42.
19. Yamanaka T, Niwa H, Tsujimura K, et al. Epidemic of equine influenza among vaccinated racehorses in Japan in 2007. J Vet Med Sci 2008;70:623–5.
20. Legrand LJ, Pitel PH, Marcillaud-Pitel CJ, et al. Surveillance of equine influenza viruses through the RESPE network in France from November 2005 to October 2010. Equine Vet J 2013;45:776–83.
21. Woodward AL, Rash AS, Blinman D, et al. Development of a surveillance scheme for equine influenza in the UK and characterisation of viruses isolated in Europe, Dubai and the USA from 2010-2012. Vet Microbiol 2014;169: 113–27.
22. Laabassi F, Lecouturier F, Amelot G, et al. Epidemiology and genetic characterization of H3N8 equine influenza virus responsible for clinical disease in Algeria in 2011. Transbound Emerg Dis 2014. [Epub ahead of print].
23. Bera BC, Virmani N, Shanmugasundaram K, et al. Genetic analysis of the neuraminidase (NA) gene of equine influenza virus (H3N8) from epizootic of 2008-2009 in India. Indian J Virol 2013;24:256–64.
24. Yondon M, Heil GL, Burks JP, et al. Isolation and characterization of H3N8 equine influenza A virus associated with the 2011 epizootic in Mongolia. Influenza Other Respir Viruses 2013;7:659–65.
25. Zhu C, Li Q, Guo W, et al. Complete genomic sequences of an H3N8 equine influenza virus strain isolated in China. Genome Announc 2013;1.
26. Webster RG. Are equine 1 influenza viruses still present in horses? Equine Vet J 1993;25:537–8.
27. Ito T, Kawaoka Y. Host-range barrier of influenza A viruses. Vet Microbiol 2000; 74:7 1–5.
28. Skehel JJ, Wiley DC. Receptor binding and membrane fusion in virus entry: the influenza hemagglutinin. Annu Rev Biochem 2000;69:531–69.
29. Crawford PC, Dubovi EJ, Castleman WL, et al. Transmission of equine influenza virus to dogs. Science 2005;310:482–5.
30. Daly JM, Blunden AS, MacRae S, et al. Transmission of equine influenza virus to English foxhounds. Emerg Infect Dis 2008;14:461–4.
31. Newton JR, Cooke A, Elton D, et al. Canine influenza virus: cross-species transmission from horses. Vet Rec 2007;161:142–3.
32. Kirkland PD, Finlaison DS, Crispe E, et al. Influenza virus transmission from horses to dogs, Australia. Emerg Infect Dis 2010;16:699–702.
33. Yamanaka T, Nemoto M, Tsujimura K, et al. Interspecies transmission of equine influenza virus (H3N8) to dogs by close contact with experimentally infected horses. Vet Microbiol 2009;139:351–5.
34. Pecoraro HL, Bennett S, Garretson K, et al. Comparison of the infectivity and transmission of contemporary canine and equine H3N8 influenza viruses in dogs. Vet Med Int 2013;2013:874521. http://dx.doi.org/10.1155/2013/874521.
35. Suzuki Y, Ito T, Suzuki T, et al. Sialic acid species as a determinant of the host range of influenza A viruses. J Virol 2000;74:11825–31.
36. Yamanaka T, Tsujimura K, Kondo T, et al. Infectivity and pathogenicity of canine H3N8 influenza A virus in horses. Influenza Other Respir Viruses 2010;4:345–51.
37. Quintana AM, Hussey SB, Burr EC, et al. Evaluation of infectivity of a canine lineage H3N8 influenza A virus in ponies and in primary equine respiratory epithelial cells. Am J Vet Res 2011;72:1071–8.

38. Nyaga PN, Wiggins AD, Priester WA. Epidemiology of equine influenza, risk by age, breed and sex. Comp Immunol Microbiol Infect Dis 1980;3:67–73.
39. Peek SF, Landolt G, Karasin AI, et al. Acute respiratory distress syndrome and fatal interstitial pneumonia associated with equine influenza in a neonatal foal. J Vet Intern Med 2004;18:132–4.
40. Smith BP. Influenza in foals. J Am Vet Med Assoc 1979;174:289–90.
41. Happold J, Rubira R. Equine influenza: patterns of disease and seroprevalence in Thoroughbred studs and implications for vaccination. Aust Vet J 2011; 89(Suppl 1):135–7.
42. Heldens JG, Pouwels HG, van Loon AA. Efficacy and duration of immunity of a combined equine influenza and equine herpesvirus vaccine against challenge with an American-like equine influenza virus (A/equi-2/Kentucky/95). Vet J 2004;167:150–7.
43. Mumford JA, Jessett D, Dunleavy U, et al. Antigenicity and immunogenicity of experimental equine influenza ISCOM vaccines. Vaccine 1994;12:857–63.
44. Mumford JA, Wood JM, Folkers C, et al. Protection against experimental infection with influenza virus A/equine/Miami/63 (H3N8) provided by inactivated whole virus vaccines containing homologous virus. Epidemiol Infect 1988;100: 501–10.
45. Mumford JA, Wood JM, Scott AM, et al. Studies with inactivated equine influenza vaccine. 2. Protection against experimental infection with influenza virus A/equine/Newmarket/79 (H3N8). J Hyg (Lond) 1983;90:385–95.
46. Newton JR, Townsend HG, Wood JL, et al. Immunity to equine influenza: relationship of vaccine-induced antibody in young Thoroughbred racehorses to protection against field infection with influenza A/equine-2 viruses (H3N8). Equine Vet J 2000;32:65–74.
47. Morley PS, Townsend HG, Bogdan JR, et al. Risk factors for disease associated with influenza virus infections during three epidemics in horses. J Am Vet Med Assoc 2000;216:545–50.
48. Morley PS, Townsend HG, Bogdan JR, et al. Descriptive epidemiologic study of disease associated with influenza virus infections during three epidemics in horses. J Am Vet Med Assoc 2000;216:535–44.
49. Bridges CB, Kuehnert MJ, Hall CB. Transmission of influenza: implications for control in health care settings. Clin Infect Dis 2003;37:1094–101.
50. Boone SA, Gerba CP. The occurrence of influenza A virus on household and day care center fomites. J Infect 2005;51:103–9.
51. Firestone SM, Cogger N, Ward MP, et al. The influence of meteorology on the spread of influenza: survival analysis of an equine influenza (A/H3N8) outbreak. PLoS One 2011;7:e35284.
52. Newton JR, Daly JM, Spencer L, et al. Description of the outbreak of equine influenza (H3N8) in the United Kingdom in 2003, during which recently vaccinated horses in Newmarket developed respiratory disease. Vet Rec 2006;158:185–92.
53. van Maanen C, Bruin G, de Boer-Luijtze E, et al. Interference of maternal antibodies with the immune response of foals after vaccination against equine influenza. Vet Q 1992;14:13–7.
54. Van Oirschot JT, Bruin G, de Boer-Luytze E, et al. Maternal antibodies against equine influenza virus in foals and their interference with vaccination. Zentralbl Veterinarmed B 1991;38:391–6.
55. Wilson WD, Mihalyi JE, Hussey S, et al. Passive transfer of maternal immunoglobulin isotype antibodies against tetanus and influenza and their effect on the response of foals to vaccination. Equine Vet J 2001;33:644–50.

56. Guthrie AJ. Equine influenza in South Africa, 2003 outbreak. In 9th International Congress of World Equine Veterinary Association. International Veterinary Information Service. Marrakech, Morrocco, January 22-26, 2006.

57. Virmani N, Bera BC, Gulati BR, et al. Descriptive epidemiology of equine influenza in India (2008-2009): temporal and spatial trends. Vet Ital 2010;46:449–58.

58. Callinan I. Equine influenza: The August 2007 outbreak in Australia. Report of the Equine Influenza Inquiry. 2008. Available at: http://pandora.nla.gov.au/pan/47126/20100421-1408/www.aph.gov.au/library/intguide/law/eiiexhibits/REP.0001.001.0001.pdf.

59. Lunn DP, Townsend HG. Equine vaccination. Vet Clin North Am Equine Pract 2000;16:199–226.

60. Daly JM, Newton JR, Mumford JA. Current perspectives on control of equine influenza. Vet Res 2004;35:411–23.

61. van Maanen C, Cullinane A. Equine influenza virus infections: an update. Vet Q 2002;24:79–94.

62. Firestone SM, Schemann KA, Toribio JA, et al. A case-control study of risk factors for equine influenza spread onto horse premises during the 2007 epidemic in Australia. Prev Vet Med 2011;100:53–63.

63. Garner MG, Scanlan WA, Cowled BD, et al. Regaining Australia's equine influenza-free status: a national perspective. Aust Vet J 2011;89:169–73.

64. Scott-Orr H. Proof of freedom from equine influenza infection in Australia in 2007-08. Aust Vet J 2011;89:163–4.

65. Schemann K, Firestone SM, Taylor MR, et al. Horse owners'/managers' perceptions about effectiveness of biosecurity measures based on their experiences during the 2007 equine influenza outbreak in Australia. Prev Vet Med 2012;106:97–107.

66. Bish A, Michie S. Demographic and attitudinal determinants of protective behaviours during a pandemic: a review. Br J Health Psychol 2010;15:797–824.

67. Schemann K, Taylor MR, Toribio JA, et al. Horse owners' biosecurity practices following the first equine influenza outbreak in Australia. Prev Vet Med 2011;102:304–14.

68. Lin C, Holland RE Jr, Donofrio JC, et al. Caspase activation in equine influenza virus induced apoptotic cell death. Vet Microbiol 2002;84:357–65.

69. Lin C, Zimmer SG, Lu Z, et al. The involvement of a stress-activated pathway in equine influenza virus-mediated apoptosis. Virology 2001;287:202–13.

70. Schultz-Cherry S, Dybdahl-Sissoko N, Neumann G, et al. Influenza virus ns1 protein induces apoptosis in cultured cells. J Virol 2001;75:7875–81.

71. Wilson WD. Equine influenza. Vet Clin North Am Equine Pract 1993;9:257–82.

72. Coggins L. Viral respiratory disease. Vet Clin North Am Large Anim Pract 1979;1:59–72.

73. Gerber H. Clinical features, sequelae and epidemiology of equine influenza. In: Bryans JT, Gerber H, editors. Equine infectious disease. 2nd edition. New York: Karger; 1969. p. 63–80.

74. Willoughby R, Ecker G, McKee S, et al. The effects of equine rhinovirus, influenza virus and herpesvirus infection on tracheal clearance rate in horses. Can J Vet Res 1992;56:115–21.

75. Wright PF, Webster RG. Orthomyxoviruses. In: Knipe D, Howley PM, editors. Field's virology. Philadelphia: Lippincott-Raven; 2007. p. 1647–90.

76. Hall WJ, Douglas RG Jr, Hyde RW, et al. Pulmonary mechanics after uncomplicated influenza A infection. Am Rev Respir Dis 1976;113:141–8.

77. Alexander DJ, Brown IH. Recent zoonoses caused by influenza A viruses. Rev Sci Tech 2000;19:197–225.

78. Gilkerson JR. Equine influenza in Australia: a clinical overview. Aust Vet J 2011; 89(Suppl 1):11–3.
79. Powell DG. Viral respiratory disease of the horse. Vet Clin North Am Equine Pract 1991;7:27–52.
80. Daly JM, Whitwell KE, Miller J, et al. Investigation of equine influenza cases exhibiting neurological disease: coincidence or association? J Comp Pathol 2006;134:231–5.
81. Newland JG, Laurich VM, Rosenquist AW, et al. Neurologic complications in children hospitalized with influenza: characteristics, incidence, and risk factors. J Pediatr 2007;150:306–10.
82. Steininger C, Popow-Kraupp T, Laferl H, et al. Acute encephalopathy associated with influenza A virus infection. Clin Infect Dis 2003;36:567–74.
83. Lamb R, Krug R. Orthomyxoviruses: the viruses and their replication. In: Knipe D, Howley PM, editors. Field's virology. Philadelphia: Lippincott-Raven Publishers; p. 1691–740.
84. Adam EN, Morley PS, Chmielewski KE, et al. Detection of cold-adapted vaccine-strain influenza virus using two commercial assays. Equine Vet J 2002; 34:400–4.
85. Chambers TM, Shortridge KF, Li PH, et al. Rapid diagnosis of equine influenza by the Directigen FLU-A enzyme immunoassay. Vet Rec 1994;135:275–9.
86. Livesay GJ, O'Neill T, Hannant D, et al. The outbreak of equine influenza (H3N8) in the United Kingdom in 1989: diagnostic use of an antigen capture ELISA. Vet Rec 1993;133:515–9.
87. Morley PS, Bogdan JR, Townsend HG, et al. Evaluation of Directigen Flu A assay for detection of influenza antigen in nasal secretions of horses. Equine Vet J 1995;27:131–4.
88. Diallo IS, Read AJ, Kirkland PD. Potential of vaccination to confound interpretation of real-time PCR results for equine influenza. Vet Rec 2011;169:252.
89. Foord AJ, Selleck P, Colling A, et al. Real-time RT-PCR for detection of equine influenza and its evaluation using samples from horses infected with A/equine/ Sydney/2007 (H3N8). Aust Vet J 2009;89(Suppl 1):37–8.
90. Soboll G, Hussey SB, Minke JM, et al. Onset and duration of immunity to equine influenza virus resulting from canarypox-vectored (ALVAC) vaccination. Vet Immunol Immunopathol 2010;135:100–7.
91. Pusterla N, Madigan JE, Leutenegger CM. Real-time polymerase chain reaction: a novel molecular diagnostic tool for equine infectious diseases. J Vet Intern Med 2006;20:3–12.
92. Ozaki H, Sugiura T, Sugita S, et al. Detection of antibodies to the nonstructural protein (NS1) of influenza A virus allows distinction between vaccinated and infected horses. Vet Microbiol 2001;82:111–9.
93. Birch-Machin I, Rowan A, Pick J, et al. Expression of the nonstructural protein NS1 of equine influenza A virus: detection of anti-NS1 antibody in post infection equine sera. J Virol Methods 1997;65:255–63.
94. Nakajima K, Nobusawa E, Nakajima S. Evolution of the NS genes of the influenza A viruses. II. Characteristics of the amino acid changes in the NS1 proteins of the influenza A viruses. Virus Genes 1990;4:15–26.
95. Kirkland PD, Delbridge G. Use of a blocking ELISA for antibodies to equine influenza virus as a test to distinguish between naturally infected and vaccinated horses: proof of concept studies. Aust Vet J 2011;89:45–6.
96. Perkins NR, Webster RG, Wright T, et al. Vaccination program in the response to the 2007 equine influenza outbreak in Australia. Aust Vet J 2011;89:126–34.

97. Kirkland PD. Role of the diagnostic laboratories during the 2007 equine influenza outbreak in Australia. Aust Vet J 2011;89(Suppl 1):29–32.
98. Sergeant ES, Cowled BD, Bingham P. Diagnostic specificity of an equine influenza blocking ELISA estimated from New South Wales field data from the Australian epidemic in 2007. Aust Vet J 2011;89(Suppl 1):43–5.
99. Myers C, Wilson WD. Equine influenza virus. Clin Tech Equine Pract 2006;5: 187–96.
100. Paillot R, Hannant D, Kydd JH, et al. Vaccination against equine influenza: quid novi? Vaccine 2006;24:4047–61.
101. Townsend HG, Lunn DP, Bogdan J, et al. Comparative efficacy of commercial vaccines in naive horses: serologic responses and protection after influenza challenge. In 49th Annual AAEP Convention, American Association of Equine Practitioners. New Orleans, 2003. November 21-25, 2003.
102. Park AW, Wood JL, Newton JR, et al. Optimising vaccination strategies in equine influenza. Vaccine 2003;21:2862–70.

West Nile Virus and Equine Encephalitis Viruses
New Perspectives

Maureen T. Long, DVM, PhD

KEYWORDS

- Flavivirus • Alphavirus • Eastern equine encephalitis • West Nile virus • Arbovirus
- Horses

KEY POINTS

- Mosquito-borne disease viruses are the most common infection of the equine central nervous system (CNS) worldwide, with new epizootics occurring worldwide.
- New activity in alphaviruses demonstrates enhanced virulence of Eastern equine encephalitis virus (EEEV) strains in South America.
- Venezuelan equine encephalitis (VEE) continues to occur in horses, although there are prospects for newly engineered vaccines that are both safe and have enhanced protection.
- For flaviviruses, West Nile virus (WNV), lineage 2 (L2) strains, previously localized to Africa and of limited neurovirulence, are expanding.
- Work with vaccines and diagnostics demonstrates that there is cross-protection of current WNV L1 vaccine against WNV L2 encroaching strains.
- Continued development of treatment options is also ongoing with some viable compounds on the horizon.

EASTERN EQUINE ENCEPHALITIS
Etiology

The genus *Alphavirus* belongs to the family Togaviridae and includes several viruses that have been isolated from horses with neurologic disease. Of these alphaviruses, Eastern, Western, and Venezuelan equine encephalitis (EEE, WEE, and VEE) viruses are the most frequently isolated from epizootics of encephalitis in horses and humans in the Western Hemisphere; however, there are others throughout the world that either are known to cause disease in horses or have only been described as pathogenic to humans (**Table 1**).[1–3] The Togaviruses are single-stranded, enveloped, linear

Department of Infectious Diseases and Pathology, College of Veterinary Medicine, University of Florida, PO Box 11088, Gainesville, FL 32611-0880, USA
E-mail address: longm@ufl.edu

Vet Clin Equine 30 (2014) 523–542
http://dx.doi.org/10.1016/j.cveq.2014.08.009
0749-0739/14/$ – see front matter © 2014 Elsevier Inc. All rights reserved.

Table 1
Most common or known alphaviruses, flaviviruses, and bunyaviruses[a] that cause encephalomyelitis in horses

Virus Species	Geographic Location	Reservoir Species	Equine Syndrome
Alphavirus			
Eastern equine encephalitis virus	North/South/Central America, Caribbean	Birds, rodents, snakes?	Encephalomyelitis
Western equine encephalitis virus	North/South America	Birds, rodents, snakes	Encephalomyelitis
Venezuelan equine encephalitis virus	Central/South America, Caribbean	Cotton rat	Encephalomyelitis
Ross River virus[a]	Australia, Papua New Guinea	Marsupial and placental mammals	Systemic: hemolymphatic Neurologic: ataxia
Semliki Forest virus[a]	East and West Africa	Unknown	Encephalomyelitis
Flavivirus			
Japanese encephalitis	Asia, India, Russia, Western Pacific	Birds, swine	Encephalomyelitis
Murray Valley	Australia, Papua New Guinea	Birds, horses, cattle, marsupials, and foxes	Encephalomyelitis
Kunjin virus	Australia	Water birds: herons and ibis	Encephalomyelitis
St. Louis encephalitis[a]	North, Central, and South America	Birds	Serologic only recorded
Usutu[a]	Europe, Africa	Birds	Serologic only recorded
West Nile	Africa; Middle East; Europe; North, Central, and South America; Australia	Passerine birds (crows, sparrows, robins)	Encephalomyelitis
Louping ill[a]	Iberian Peninsula, United Kingdom	Sheep, grouse	Encephalomyelitis
Powassan[a]	North America, Russia	Lagomorphs, rodents, mice, skunks, dogs, birds	Encephalomyelitis
Tick-borne encephalitis[a]	Asia, Europe, Finland, Russia	Small rodents	Encephalomyelitis
Bunyavirus[a]			
California serogroup: California encephalitis, Jamestown Canyon, La Crosse, Snowshoe hare	North America (United States and Canada), parts of eastern Asia	Rodents and lagomorphs	Encephalomyelitis

[a] Not discussed in body of text, but included here for completeness.

positive-sense ribonucleic acid (RNA) viruses measuring 60 to 70 nm in diameter. Within the envelope there is a nucleocapsid with icosahedral symmetry composed of peplomers arranged as trimers. The glycoproteins E1 and E2 are immunodominant proteins that induce neutralizing antibody.

Epidemiology

Eastern equine encephalitis has primarily a mosquito-bird life cycle, the latter being the major reservoir. Horses and humans are incidental and dead-end hosts, meaning that although there may be a short viremia, it is not high enough to transmit virus to a mosquito vector. Recent work in Alabama indicates that the northern cardinal is the primary target for the primary mosquito vector, *Culiseta melanura*, but other mosquitoes (*Culex erraticus*) are often infected and capable of feeding on a wider variety of birds, including robins, chickadees, owls, and mockingbirds, in addition to bridging to mammals.[4–6] In Central and South America, the principal vectors of EEE virus (EEEV) belong to the *Culex* (Melanoconion) spp. These vectors feed on birds, rodents, marsupials, and reptiles, with South American (SA) EEEV having high viral loads in the cotton rat (also a possible reservoir for the North American [NA] VEE virus [VEEV] strain, called Everglades virus) compared with NA EEEV.[7] Before 2000, comparatively few epidemics of EEEV in horses were recorded in South America, with minimal disease reported in humans due to the notable divergence of NA and SA strains. More recently, in 2008 and 2009, larger outbreaks of higher morbidity and mortality have occurred in Central and South America.[8–12] In northeastern Brazil, 229 horses were affected, with a case-fatality rate of 73% with severity of disease similar to that of NA EEEV.[12] Recently, snakes have been identified as a possible reservoir.[13–15]

Habitat type is also associated with propensity for EEEV reemergence in northern latitudes and the uninterrupted transmission in the southern United States.[6,16–18] Freshwater hardwood swamps are the most associated ecological niche for EEEV. In Florida, disease within mammalian hosts occurs in "tree farms" that are associated with inland freshwater swamps where cultivated swamp edges allow comingling of susceptible domesticated species and humans with infected mosquitos.[6,18,19] In recent years, intense focal activity has been reported in Michigan, Wisconsin, Ohio, Massachusetts, and New Hampshire.[20–23] In 2005, Massachusetts experienced an outbreak with a high case-fatality rate demonstrating affected people resided with one-half mile of a cranberry bog or swamp associated with forest habitat. During this time, there were clinically affected horses (9), alpacas (4), emus (2), and llamas (1).[23–25]

Clinical Signs

In Florida, many horses that succumb to EEEV are not vaccinated, are younger than 3 years old, and are stock-type horses (Maureen T. Long, unpublished data, 2008).[26] Clinical signs are progressive in nature and primarily result in rapid deterioration of mentation because of severe forebrain damage (**Fig. 1**). Nearly all horses with NA EEEV die. Previous data and literature suggested that SA EEEV was less virulent, but the latest published data demonstrate extremely low survivorship.[12]

Diagnosis

The major differential diagnoses for arboviruses include rabies, equine protozoal myeloencephalitis (EPM), equine herpesvirus (EHV)-1, verminous encephalitis (VE), hepatoencephalopathy, moldy corn poisoning, botulism, trauma, cervical vertebral myelopathy, neoplasia, and laminitis. Where present geographically, neuroborelliosis should be considered. The recent identification of expansion of *Angiostrongylus cantonensis* in the south many also confound diagnosis.[27,28]

One of the most diagnostically useful tools is cerebrospinal fluid (CSF) analysis (**Table 2**). Although frequently normal for many diseases, such as rabies and EPM, diseases such as EEEV, West Nile virus (WNV), EHV-1, and VE are frequently abnormal and the index of suspicion for an infectious etiology can be raised before any other

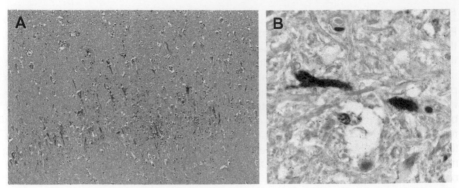

Fig. 1. (A) Photomicrograph of immunohistochemistry of a clinically affected horse with EEEV in which a typical intense amount of antigen is detected (*dark red*), indicating the high viral load. (B) Photomicrograph of immunohistochemistry of a clinically affected horse with WNV, demonstrating only one positive neuron in the field, consistent with low viral load. (*Courtesy of* [A] Gretchen Delcambre, DVM; University of Florida College of Veterinary Medicine; and [B] Carol Detrisac, DVM, University of Chicago, Chicago, IL.)

confirmatory test results are available. By comparison, in acute EEEV infection, the pleocytosis is predominately neutrophilic, whereas in acute WNV, if pleocytosis is present, mononuclear cells predominate (**Fig. 2**).

Antemortem confirmatory diagnostic testing now relies on the identification of immunoglobulin M (IgM) antibody at a single dilution of 1:400 for WNV, EEEV, and other arboviruses for which there are a set of established controls for validation.[29,30] Control antigen must be concurrently run to detect false-positive results that some horses have due to high nonspecific background. Neutralization testing can be performed, but paired sera must be used for interpretation. Interpretation of all formats must be performed in the light of vaccination history (**Box 1**).

CSF IgM can be detected, however the single dilution is more reliable at 1:10. Although CSF IgM testing is considered highly reliable in humans, it is less consistent than serum in horses.[31,32] However, CSF IgM levels are of value in the postmortem horse in lieu of antemortem serology.

Rapid real-time polymerase chain reaction (PCR) performed on clinical specimens can differentiate between the alphaviruses and flaviviruses.[33,34] For EEEV, a variety of antigen-detection methods on fresh and fixed tissues have a high yield of reliable results; these include reverse transcription PCR, immunohistochemistry (IHC), and viral isolation (**Fig. 3**). Even though EEEV is a disease of high viral load in the brains

Table 2
Summary of known cerebrospinal fluid findings for arbovirus diseases

	Protein	Cells	Cell Types	Color
Eastern equine encephalitis virus	▲ ▲	▲ ▲	Neutrophils Mononuclear	Normal to mildly turbid
Western equine encephalitis virus	▲	▲	Mononuclear	Normal
West Nile virus	N to ▲	N to ▲ ▲	Mononuclear	Mildly xanthochromic
Kunjin virus	▲	N to ▲ ▲	Mononuclear (some neutrophils)	Mildly xanthochromic

Abbreviations: ▲, elevated; N, normal.

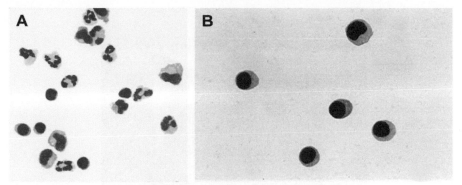

Fig. 2. (*A*) Photomicrograph of CSF from a horse with EEE. This horse was not vaccinated and exhibited clinical signs consistent with EEEV when the CSF was obtained. The CSF contains more than 70% nondegenerate neutrophils (Modified Giemsa Stain, original magnification ×400). (*B*) Photomicrograph of CSF from a horse with WNV encephalomyelitis. The CSF contains more than 90% macrophages and lymphocytes (Wright-Giemsa Stain, original magnification ×500). (Photomicrographs *courtesy of* Heather Wamsley, DVM, PhD, University of Florida).

of affected horses, culture of EEEV can be more difficult once tissues are frozen, even though the virus is still infectious. Viral culture is still the gold standard, but freezing of tissues substantially decreases the ability to isolate virus.

Pathologic Findings

In horses, brain lesions are thought to be the direct result of viral replication and are characterized by necrotizing encephalitis with neuronal dysfunction. EEEV infection is fairly easily differentiated even on light microscopy from flavivirus infections based on severity and location of the lesions. The meninges are very congested and there are frequent, focal areas of dark discoloration found in brain slices, most prominently in the gray matter of the cerebrum at the level of the corona radiata. Histologically,

---

Box 1
Crucial aspects of vaccination history for ruling-out arboviral disease

1. Lifelong vaccination history or at minimum past 3–5 years of vaccination history.

2. Frequency of vaccine history over at least the past 3–5 years.

3. Age-related questions:

   a. If younger than 3 years, did the horse receive primary vaccination as a foal?

   b. How many times overall per year has the horse been vaccinated?

   c. Was the dam vaccinated?

   d. If older, what is disease history? Neoplasia? Metabolic disease? Pituitary adenoma? Renal disease?

4. Travel-related questions:

   a. Is this horse a new arrival to an endemic area?

   b. If this horse is a new arrival, did the horse receive a booster vaccine before arrival if annually vaccinated?

   c. If this horse is a new arrival, did the horse receive a full series (at least 2 injections) of vaccine before arrival?

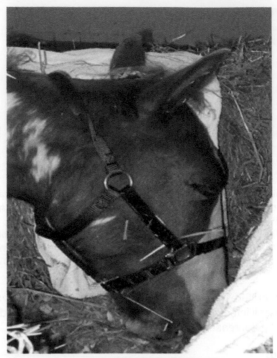

Fig. 3. Two-year-old American Paint horse profoundly affected with EEE virus. This horse had clinical signs for less than 48 hours. Initial signs consisted of fever and depression. The horse rapidly deteriorated, and by 72 hours after onset was not arousable. Note swelling over eyelids and disproportionate head. In addition to trauma, subcutaneous edema of the head developed due to obtunded mentation and standing for an extended period with his head lowered before becoming recumbent. (*Courtesy of* Michael B. Porter, DVM, PhD; PhD Veterinary Services, Gainesville, FL.)

neuronal necrosis with neurophagia, marked perivascular cuffing with both mononuclear and many polymorphonuclear leukocytes, and focal and diffuse microglial proliferation are evident. The lesions are more pronounced in the gray matter than in the white matter of the brain. Lesions are most marked in the cerebral cortex, thalamus, and hypothalamus, whereas the spinal cord is mildly affected. Severe lesions usually occur more often in the cervical spinal cord than in lumbar cord segments.

Therapeutic Strategies

No known antiviral medications demonstrate reliable activity against alphaviruses. In human patients, treatment with methylprednisolone (1000 mg/100-kg patient) has often been recommended; however, survivorship is still very low. Intravenous immunoglobulin therapy has been used in humans for both its proposed neutralization of virus and immunomodulatory effects.[35] Interferon-α (IFN-α) is a relatively common therapy, but no controlled studies support its use.[36–38] Model data support the suppression of type I interferons in the pathogenesis of EEEV infection, suggesting that IFN-α therapy could be of value. Recent reports indicate that aggressive control of cerebral edema and hypertension with seizure control is important.[39] Most patients require ventilatory support during clinically severe periods of seizure activity or when comatose. Long-term disability is common in survivors.

Control Strategies

EEE is 100% preventable in the horse with proper vaccination. Horses that reside in endemic areas and are aged *4 years or younger should receive alphavirus vaccines 3 times per year*. It is essential that all broodmares be vaccinated 1 month before foaling to ensure adequate passive transfer to foals. All foals should be tested for adequate passive transfer 24 hours after birth. In foals from vaccinated dams, vaccination should be performed at 6, 7, and 9 months. In foals whose dam has not been adequately vaccinated, vaccination should be performed at 4, 5, and 7 months. However, mare vaccine history is essential, because in our laboratory, we have detected little antibody response in foals suckling multiparous mares of known vaccination history (Maureen T. Long, unpublished data, 2008).[40] Foals should undergo a full 3 injection immunization series at 6, 7, and 9 months of age. Foals younger than 5 months should be vaccinated only if the mare has an unknown vaccination history. Even if foals receive a full round of vaccines, all yearlings should be vaccinated between January and March within the year after birth, and receive at least 2 more injections 4 months apart. This vaccination schedule should continue until horses are 4 years of age. All horses arriving in the south from northern states should be vaccinated 30 days before arrival and consideration of a second booster after arrival should be given. Imported horses that ship directly to southern states from countries in which the vaccine cannot be obtained before arrival are at risk for EEEV throughout the first 2 years of their arrival. It is imperative that these horses receive 3 initial injections and then continue 3 times a year for at least 2 years after arriving in the southern United States.

The most important future need for EEEV prevention is development of new vaccines that rapidly induce complete immunity in naïve or young horses exposed to high levels of EEEV. Several new alphavirus constructs have been shown to provide complete protection against homologous challenge in mouse models.[41–49] There have been approximately a dozen vaccine constructs, but as of this writing, none have been tested in the horse.

WESTERN EQUINE ENCEPHALOMYELITIS
Etiology and Epidemiology

Western equine encephalitis virus (WEEV) is also an alphavirus. Phylogenetic analyses indicate that NA and SA WEE lineages appear to have evolved independently over several decades. A variant WEEV virus has been reported in several countries in South America (Argentina, Guyana, Ecuador, Brazil, and Uruguay). Over the past decade, reports of WEEV in horses have been limited and sporadic, likely reflecting vaccination and protective immunity gained by subclinical exposure.

Clinical Signs

Like its other neurotropic relatives, WEEV is more likely to cause clinical central nervous system (CNS) disease in children and young animals of all susceptible species. Most horses fully recover from WEEV and the case-fatality rate is 20% to 30%.

Diagnosis

Diagnosis is similar to that of EEEV, except that the CSF is composed of a mononuclear cell population primarily consisting of lymphocytes.

Treatment

In a hamster model of WEEV, treatment with IFN-α increased survivorship.[37] Other novel antiviral agents may be on the horizon.[50,51] These include a pyrazinecarboxamide derivative (T-705) that blocks viral polymerase enzymes and thieno[3,2-b] pyrrole-based "chiral" molecules that may affect viral assembly, respectively.

Prevention

Based on the lack of WEEV activity in NA and protection afforded in experimental challenge models, WEEV is 100% preventable using the vaccination protocols indicated for EEEV in this article. Even though the incidence of WEEV has dramatically declined in the United States, the utility of multivalent preparations containing both EEEV and WEEV for immunization is still important because WEEV disease occurs in Central and South America.[52]

VENEZUELAN EQUINE ENCEPHALITIS
Etiology and Epidemiology

VEEV is one of the most important human and veterinary pathogens in the New World.[53] Epidemics reveal the potential for VEEV to spread rapidly within an equine population, with a case-fatality rate approaching 90% in some areas. Outbreaks of VEEV continue to occur in Chiapas and Oaxaca, Mexico, and in Venezuela and Colombia.[54–56]

Key to understanding the epidemiology of VEEV is recognition of the differences in the basic biology of 2 transmission cycles, enzootic and epizootic, of this virus.[53] Three basic changes occur in enzootic to epizootic cycling: (1) the virus mutates closer to the more pathogenic strains, (2) there is a change in reservoir host, and (3) there is a change in mosquito vector.[57,58] The enzootic cycle centers around sylvatic rodents, such as spiny and cotton rats, and the epizootic cycle centers around equids as transmitting reservoir hosts, respectively.[58–60]

Clinical Findings

The clinical findings are similar to EEEV except that there can be a wider variation in mortality in horses, ranging from 40% to 90%. Diagnosis and pathologic findings also are similar to EEEV and WEEV.

Prevention

Immunization of horses has proved highly effective as an adjunct to other control measures, particularly in epidemics of VEEV because horses serve as a source of infection for mosquitoes. Because horses become the primary reservoir in VEEV epidemics, the distinct opportunity exists that these could be eliminated if sustained and widespread equine vaccination was performed in Central and South America.[61] Development of new formulations of VEE vaccines is an intense area of research.[41–43,46,48,62–67] Several experimental vaccines have been developed and these include subunit vaccines using various constructs and gene deletions, DNA vaccines, adenovirus-vectored vaccines, and encephalomyocarditis virus (internal ribosome entry site) vaccines.[41–43,46,48,62–67] Of all of these, the gene-deleted live mutant vaccine, V3526, has been tested in horses and has demonstrated 100% clinical efficacy against challenge with 10^4 pfu of live virus.[68] Importantly, this vaccine virus was shown to block all viremia in horses.

WEST NILE VIRUS
Etiology

Among the 53 species of *Flavivirus*, there are a number of historically significant and pathologically active viruses responsible for disease in horses, including Japanese encephalitis virus (JEV), WNV, Kunjin virus (KV), and Murray Valley encephalitis virus (MVEV).[31,69] Overall, the diseases caused by the JEV serogroup are similar and thus are discussed as a group, except where differences are notable. KV is actually a strain of WNV. Disease in horses caused by MVEV is geographically restricted to the South Pacific and is sporadic in occurrence.[70–72] Several other members of the flavivirus genus have also been detected serologically in horses, but with limited reports of clinical disease (see **Table 1**).

Flaviviruses are positive-sense, single-stranded RNA viruses measuring approximately 50 nm in external diameter.[31] The virions are spherical, enveloped, and contain a nucleocapsid.[73,74] Electron microscopy reveals an icosahedral symmetry of the envelope and capsid. An approximately 11-kilobase (kb) genome contains a single open reading frame that is translated in its entirety and cleaved into 10 viral proteins by both cell and viral proteases. There are 3 structural proteins, including capsid, pre-membrane and membrane, and envelope (E), and 7 nonstructural proteins.[75,76]

Epidemiology

WNV is part of the JEV serogroup of viruses that are vector-borne, with transmission occurring to avian and mammalian hosts by blood meal–seeking mosquitoes.[77–79] *Culex pipiens* is the most important mosquito transmitter and more recent publications still confirm this in other countries.[78,79] Although relatively little is known regarding the most important vector of transmission to the horse, *C pipiens* has demonstrated successful feeding on mammalian species, even though considered an avian feeder. For all of the known JEV serogroup viruses, horses are dead-end hosts as defined for EEEV and WEEV. In general, the overall transmission cycle is mosquito-avian with limited exceptions.

For this group of viruses, the past 5 years has demonstrated continued worldwide reemergence of WNV. Based on the latest phylogeny, WNV itself has 7 lineages, with lineages 1 and 2 affecting humans and horses.[80,81] Lineage 1 has 3 sublineages: 1a, 1b, and 1c.[82–85] Lineage 1a activity in the United States and Europe dominated much of the end of the 1990s until the mid-2000s, demonstrating widespread emergence usually with neuroinvasive infections in humans and horses in Africa, Europe, Australia, Asia, North and Central America, and the Middle East.[81,82,85–88] In the latter half of the past decade, 1a was most often associated with enzootics, and in 2012, a very large US epizootic reoccurred, with 5674 human and 690 horse cases reported.[89] New emergences have occurred in Greece and Serbia, and the first WNV L1a case in India was detected in 2012.[85,90] Lineage 1b viruses are primarily represented by KV found in Australia, some southeast Asian countries, and New Guinea. In 2011, Australia experienced the largest epidemic of arboviral disease in history, affecting approximately 900 horses. Although multiple pathogens were detected, including KV, MVEV, and Ross River virus (RRV), there was emergence of a new strain of KV.[91] The 1c viruses are fairly nonpathogenic and found in India. This sublineage may soon be designated as lineage 5.

The surge in neuroinvasive disease due to WNV lineage 2 (L2) is of note. Previously, WNV L2 was considered endemic in Africa, causing only flulike clinical disease; however, in the latter years of the first decade, L2 has dramatically increased in virulence and geographically, cropping up across Europe in Hungary, Austria, Italy, and Greece.[82,84,85,90,92] Greece has experienced at least 4 epidemic cycles, and several cases of neuroinvasive L2 have been identified in horses.[84,92]

Older people appear more susceptible to neuroinvasive disease from both JEV and WNV.[93] This age bias in reporting also appears true in horses, at least for WNV.[94] The risk factors associated with WNV disease in people deserve a second look in horses.

The 2 most common risk factors in people are hypertension and diabetes mellitus.[95–102] There are limited data on equine cases of older horses, with risk factors such as underlying cardiac disease, metabolic syndrome, and pituitary adenoma.

Although many pathogenesis studies in knockout mice indicate genetic relationships, there are limited studies that directly analyze genetic polymorphisms in humans and horses associated with WNV. By far the most work has been done with the antiviral pathway 2-5-oliogadenylate synthetase.[103–106] This important locus encodes for a family of type 1 IFN-inducible proteins, resulting in the destruction of intracellular "foreign" RNAs. Single nucleotide polymorphisms associated with the IFN-α pathways, including interferon response factor-3 and mixovirus-1 loci, also have been associated with increased risk for encephalitis and paralysis.[107]

Pathogenesis

There has been excellent work using mouse models to understand the pathogenesis of WNV infection and these can be reviewed elsewhere.[108–110] Transport of WNV into the brain and generation of bystander injury is the focus of this review, because these mechanisms have potential for generating therapeutics. Using murine models, 2 basic mechanisms of neuroinvasion are proposed: (1) via the blood brain barrier (BBB), and (2) via retrograde transaxonal movement of virus.[111–118] In BBB invasion, generalized disease would likely account for presentation with meningitis/encephalomyelitis, whereas transaxonal invasion would present as focal flaccid paralysis. Experimental data have supported both transcellular and paracellular pathways across the BBB.[112,115,117,119,120] Although demonstrated with viruslike particles experimentally and with virus in JEV, the acceptance of transcellular migration is equivocal.[113–115,120,121] One observation that does not support this pathway is the lack of antigen in the endothelium in WNV infection. Given the low viral load and the lack of data on very early infection, this route may be difficult to substantiate.[120] In vitro, WNV infects endothelial cells readily, although infection results in little cytopathic effect (CPE) and is highly variable in individual cells.[115] This may indicate that transendothelial infection is highly efficient, leading to CNS invasion without significant damage to the endothelium. With paracellular movement, if the BBB is disrupted, then virus or infected cells can traverse the obstacle because tight junctions are disrupted.[115,117,122] In mouse models and in vitro studies, tight junction protein mRNA expression is downregulated with disruption of these proteins due to cytokines, such as tumor necrosis factor-α, interleukin-6, macrophage migration inhibition factors, and metalloproteinases.[114,117] Virus also could enter the CNS via an infected cell.[113] Problematic is the lack of viral infection found in peripheral blood mononuclear cell (PBMCs) both in vivo and in vitro. In vitro, propagation in human PBMCs has been accomplished via ConA stimulation before infection; however, this could not be repeated in equine cells (Seino KS, unpublished data, 2008). For transaxonal infection, footpad WNV challenge models demonstrate localization to the olfactory bulb after infection.[120] Work in hamsters demonstrated that injection in the vicinity of the sciatic nerve results in transaxonal movement of virus into the spinal cord with resulting flaccid paralyais.[118]

In the horse, there is limited viral load in the CNS,[123] thus a component of pathogenesis is likely related to indirect injury. One mechanism is the release of excitatory neurotransmitters that can damage surrounding neurons through chronic signaling. Both in the horse and in the mouse model, almost all glutamate transporters and receptors are downregulated after infection. This observation is highly indicative of an excess of the excitatory neurotransmitters in the synaptic cleft.[124–128] Overexcitation, if calcium dependent, leads to apoptosis of neurons. Autonomic nervous system dysfunction likely accounts for the respiratory failure and gastrointestinal disturbances.[129]

Clinical Findings

A complete description of clinical signs for WNV is described elsewhere.[130–133] Because all of the flaviviruses are spreading globally, a comparative approach is provided herein. From a comparative standpoint, flaviviruses produce similar clinical signs, except that fatal JEV infection in horses usually results in blindness, coma, and death, whereas hindbrain clinical signs occur in equine WNV infection. Infection with JEV may result in severe clinical disease in naive horses, but great variation in virulence is actually seen. MVEV and KV are more similar to WNV; MVEV is more pathogenic, whereas KV appears less severe.[91] For all of these, subclinical infection is the primary syndrome in both people and horses. Overall, the combination, severity, and duration of clinical signs can be highly variable. The overall mortality rate for JEV is 10% to 30%, WNV is 35% to 45%, MVEV is 10%, and KV is 8% to 10%.[133,134]

Diagnosis and Pathologic Findings

No pathognomonic signs distinguish flavivirus infection in horses from other CNS diseases, and a full diagnostic evaluation should be performed. Confirmation of flavivirus infection with encephalitis in horses begins with assessment of (1) whether the horse meets the case definition based on clinical signs; (2) if the horse resides in an area in which flavivirus has been confirmed in the current calendar year in mosquitos, birds, humans, or horses; and (3) lack of appropriate vaccination. Antemortem, serologic testing is based on detection of the IgM antibody response that uniformly occurs in acutely infected horses and this has been found for most. Recent work indicates that this response is confounded by recent vaccination.[135–137] The most common neutralizing antibody test formats are the classic plaque-reduction neutralization test (PRNT), and a more recently developed microwell format.[138] Practical application of the microwell versus the PRNT indicates that the end point titer in the former can be several logs higher than the PRNT.

The latest work on diagnostic testing continues to confirm the unreliability of detection of virus, even by PCR, due to the low viral load in WNV infection.[139,140] IHC and PCR for EEEV and EHV-1 are relatively straightforward comparatively. In contrast, when tested by IHC, single neurons in single sections will yield positive virus staining in the horse (see Fig. 1B). When tested by PCR, the limited viral load dictates accurate testing of appropriate tissues consisting of several locations, including thalamus, hypothalamus, rostral colliculus, pons, medulla, and anatomically identified spinal cord. In our laboratory, real-time PCR will successfully detect WNV in most acute cases when testing these areas of the CNS; however, when complete localization or sequencing of the virus is necessary, nested PCR is more sensitive. Viral isolation is still important for pathogenesis work.

Therapy

No known antiviral medications are currently marketed for treatment of neuroinvasive flaviviruses. However, several compounds are under investigation for treatment.[141] One of the most intriguing is nitazoxanide (NTZ), developed and marketed for treatment of equine protozoal myeloencephalitis, which has been shown to inhibit replication of JEV in vitro. However, NTZ had no efficacy against hepatitis C virus (also a flavivirus).[142] Other compounds include T-705, discussed previously for WEEV treatment.[143] Controversy remains as to whether or not corticosteroids enhance peripheral and CNS viral load; in a canine model of WNV, viremia was increased 40 to 50 times with methylprednisolone therapy.[144]

The recommendation for IFN-α therapy is based on anecdotal reports in the human and veterinary literature.[145–147] Therapy with WNV-specific recombinant immunoglobulin also has been recommended, and a monoclonal antibody has been undergoing clinical trials.[141,148]

Prevention

Currently, several whole inactivated virion vaccines, one recombinant inactivated vaccine, and a canarypox vectored vaccine are licensed for prevention of WNV viremia in most of the Americas, including the United States and Canada, and Europe.[138,149–151] An inactivated virus vaccine is readily available against JEV.[135,152–154] The most recent work of note is evidence that the canarypox WNV L1 vaccine provides cross protection against WNV L2 infection.[155]

SUMMARY

Even with readily available vaccines, disease due to flaviviruses and alphaviruses will continue due to emergence of viruses in new locales and the appearance of new strains and viruses. Vaccination will remain a core component of annual or biannual vaccine regimens and it is hoped that widespread vaccination against VEEV with new vaccines will start to control epizootics in central and South America. Research into the mechanisms of viral invasion and antiviral effects of new compounds will lead to better treatment options in the future.

REFERENCES

1. Powers AM, Roehrig JT. Alphaviruses. Methods Mol Biol 2011;665:17–38.
2. Jacups SP, Whelan PI, Currie BJ. Ross River virus and Barmah Forest virus infections: a review of history, ecology, and predictive models, with implications for tropical northern Australia. Vector Borne Zoonotic Dis 2008;8(2):283–97.
3. Weaver SC. Host range, amplification and arboviral disease emergence. Arch Virol Suppl 2005;19:33–44.
4. Oliveira A, Katholi CR, Burkett-Cadena N, et al. Temporal analysis of feeding patterns of *Culex erraticus* in central Alabama. Vector Borne Zoonotic Dis 2011;11(4):413–21.
5. Estep LK, McClure CJ, Burkett-Cadena ND, et al. A multi-year study of mosquito feeding patterns on avian hosts in a southeastern focus of eastern equine encephalitis virus. Am J Trop Med Hyg 2011;84(5):718–26.
6. Estep LK, McClure CJ, Vander KP, et al. Risk of exposure to eastern equine encephalomyelitis virus increases with the density of northern cardinals. PLoS One 2013;8(2):e57879.
7. Arrigo NC, Adams AP, Watts DM, et al. Cotton rats and house sparrows as hosts for North and South American strains of eastern equine encephalitis virus. Emerg Infect Dis 2010;16(9):1373–80.
8. Aguilar PV, Robich RM, Turell MJ, et al. Endemic eastern equine encephalitis in the Amazon region of Peru. Am J Trop Med Hyg 2007;76(2):293–8.
9. Mendoza LP, Bronzoni RV, Takayanagui OM, et al. Viral infections of the central nervous system in Brazil. J Infect 2007;54(6):589–96.
10. Figueiredo LT. Emergent arboviruses in Brazil. Rev Soc Bras Med Trop 2007; 40(2):224–9.
11. Forshey BM, Guevara C, Laguna-Torres VA, et al. Arboviral etiologies of acute febrile illnesses in Western South America, 2000-2007. PLoS Negl Trop Dis 2010;4(8):e787.

12. Silva ML, Galiza GJ, Dantas AF, et al. Outbreaks of Eastern equine encephalitis in northeastern Brazil. J Vet Diagn Invest 2011;23(3):570–5.
13. Bingham AM, Graham SP, Burkett-Cadena ND, et al. Detection of eastern equine encephalomyelitis virus RNA in North American snakes. Am J Trop Med Hyg 2012;87(6):1140–4.
14. Graham SP, Hassan HK, Chapman T, et al. Serosurveillance of eastern equine encephalitis virus in amphibians and reptiles from Alabama, USA. Am J Trop Med Hyg 2012;86(3):540–4.
15. White G, Ottendorfer C, Graham S, et al. Competency of reptiles and amphibians for eastern equine encephalitis virus. Am J Trop Med Hyg 2011;85(3):421–5.
16. Lubelczyk C, Mutebi JP, Robinson S, et al. An epizootic of eastern equine encephalitis virus, Maine, USA in 2009: outbreak description and entomological studies. Am J Trop Med Hyg 2013;88(1):95–102.
17. Bingham AM, Burkett-Cadena ND, Hassan HK, et al. Field investigations of winter transmission of eastern equine encephalitis virus in Florida. Am J Trop Med Hyg 2014. [Epub ahead of print].
18. Kelen PV, Downs JA, Unnasch T, et al. A risk index model for predicting eastern equine encephalitis virus transmission to horses in Florida. Appl Geogr 2014;48: 79–86.
19. Vander Kelen PT, Downs JA, Stark LM, et al. Spatial epidemiology of eastern equine encephalitis in Florida. Int J Health Geogr 2012;11:47.
20. Armstrong PM, Andreadis TG, Anderson JF, et al. Tracking eastern equine encephalitis virus perpetuation in the northeastern United States by phylogenetic analysis. Am J Trop Med Hyg 2008;79(2):291–6.
21. Centers for Disease Control and Prevention (CDC). West Nile virus disease and other arboviral diseases—United States, 2010. MMWR Morb Mortal Wkly Rep 2011;60(30):1009–13.
22. Centers for Disease Control and Prevention (CDC). West Nile virus disease and other arboviral diseases—United States, 2011. MMWR Morb Mortal Wkly Rep 2012;61(27):510–4.
23. Silverman MA, Misasi J, Smole S, et al. Eastern equine encephalitis in children, Massachusetts and New Hampshire, USA, 1970-2010. Emerg Infect Dis 2013; 19(2):194–201.
24. Centers for Disease Control and Prevention (CDC). Eastern equine encephalitis—New Hampshire and Massachusetts, August-September 2005. MMWR Morb Mortal Wkly Rep 2006;55(25):697–700.
25. Molaei G, Andreadis TG, Armstrong PM, et al. Vector-host interactions and epizootiology of eastern equine encephalitis virus in Massachusetts. Vector Borne Zoonotic Dis 2013;13:312–23.
26. Wilson JH, Rubin HL, Lane TJ, et al. Eastern equine encephalitis in Florida horses: prevalence, economic impact, and management practices, 1982-1983. Prev Vet Med 2006;4:261–71.
27. Emerson JA, Walden HS, Peters RK, et al. Eosinophilic meningoencephalomyelitis in an orangutan (Pongo pygmaeus) caused by Angiostrongylus cantonensis. Vet Q 2013;33(4):191–4.
28. Teem JL, Qvarnstrom Y, Bishop HS, et al. The occurrence of the rat lungworm, Angiostrongylus cantonensis, in nonindigenous snails in the Gulf of Mexico region of the United States. Hawaii J Med Public Health 2013;72(6 Suppl 2):11–4.
29. Long MT, Jeter W, Hernandez J, et al. Diagnostic performance of the equine IgM capture ELISA for serodiagnosis of West Nile virus infection. J Vet Intern Med 2006;20(3):608–13.

30. Wagner B, Glaser A, Hillegas JM, et al. Monoclonal antibodies to equine IgM improve the sensitivity of West Nile virus-specific IgM detection in horses. Vet Immunol Immunopathol 2008;122(1–2):46–56.
31. Petersen LR, Brault AC, Nasci RS. West Nile virus: review of the literature. JAMA 2013;310(3):308–15.
32. Racsa L, Gander R, Chung W, et al. Clinical features of West Nile virus epidemic in Dallas, Texas, 2012. Diagn Microbiol Infect Dis 2014;78(2):132–6.
33. Studdert MJ, Azuolas JK, Vasey JR, et al. Polymerase chain reaction tests for the identification of Ross River, Kunjin and Murray Valley encephalitis virus infections in horses. Aust Vet J 2003;81(1–2):76–80.
34. Wang E, Paessler S, Aguilar PV, et al. Reverse transcription-PCR-enzyme-linked immunosorbent assay for rapid detection and differentiation of alphavirus infections. J Clin Microbiol 2006;44(11):4000–8.
35. Hunt AR, Frederickson S, Hinkel C, et al. A humanized murine monoclonal antibody protects mice either before or after challenge with virulent Venezuelan equine encephalomyelitis virus. J Gen Virol 2006;87(Pt 9):2467–76.
36. Chikkanna-Gowda CP, McNally S, Sheahan BJ, et al. Inhibition of murine K-BALB and CT26 tumour growth using a Semliki Forest virus vector with enhanced expression of IL-18. Oncol Rep 2006;16(4):713–9.
37. Julander JG, Siddharthan V, Blatt LM, et al. Effect of exogenous interferon and an interferon inducer on western equine encephalitis virus disease in a hamster model. Virology 2007;360(2):454–60.
38. Sentsui H, Wu D, Murakami K, et al. Antiviral effect of recombinant equine interferon-gamma on several equine viruses. Vet Immunol Immunopathol 2010;135(1–2):93–9.
39. Wendell LC, Potter NS, Roth JL, et al. Successful management of severe neuro-invasive eastern equine encephalitis. Neurocrit Care 2013;19(1):111–5.
40. Wilkins PA, Glaser AL, McDonnell SM. Passive transfer of naturally acquired specific immunity against West Nile Virus to foals in a semi-feral pony herd. J Vet Intern Med 2006;20(4):1045–7.
41. Geall AJ, Verma A, Otten GR, et al. Nonviral delivery of self-amplifying RNA vaccines. Proc Natl Acad Sci U S A 2012;109(36):14604–9.
42. Pandya J, Gorchakov R, Wang E, et al. A vaccine candidate for eastern equine encephalitis virus based on IRES-mediated attenuation. Vaccine 2012;30(7):1276–82.
43. Atasheva S, Kim DY, Akhrymuk M, et al. Pseudoinfectious Venezuelan equine encephalitis virus: a new means of alphavirus attenuation. J Virol 2013;87(4):2023–35.
44. Roy CJ, Adams AP, Wang E, et al. A chimeric Sindbis-based vaccine protects cynomolgus macaques against a lethal aerosol challenge of eastern equine encephalitis virus. Vaccine 2013;31(11):1464–70.
45. Slovin SF, Kehoe M, Durso R, et al. A phase I dose escalation trial of vaccine replicon particles (VRP) expressing prostate-specific membrane antigen (PSMA) in subjects with prostate cancer. Vaccine 2013;31(6):943–9.
46. Tretyakova I, Lukashevich IS, Glass P, et al. Novel vaccine against Venezuelan equine encephalitis combines advantages of DNA immunization and a live attenuated vaccine. Vaccine 2013;31(7):1019–25.
47. Wu Q, Xu F, Fang L, et al. Enhanced immunogenicity induced by an alphavirus replicon-based pseudotyped baculovirus vaccine against porcine reproductive and respiratory syndrome virus. J Virol Methods 2013;187(2):251–8.
48. Trobaugh DW, Ryman KD, Klimstra WB. Can understanding the virulence mechanisms of RNA viruses lead us to a vaccine against eastern equine

encephalitis virus and other alphaviruses? Expert Rev Vaccines 2014;1–3 [Epub ahead of print].

49. Phillips AT, Schountz T, Toth AM, et al. Liposome-antigen-nucleic acid complexes protect mice from lethal challenge with western and eastern equine encephalitis viruses. J Virol 2014;88(3):1771–80.

50. Julander JG, Smee DF, Morrey JD, et al. Effect of T-705 treatment on western equine encephalitis in a mouse model. Antiviral Res 2009;82(3):169–71.

51. Sindac JA, Yestrepsky BD, Barraza SJ, et al. Novel inhibitors of neurotropic alphavirus replication that improve host survival in a mouse model of acute viral encephalitis. J Med Chem 2012;55(7):3535–45.

52. Delfraro A, Burgueno A, Morel N, et al. Fatal human case of Western equine encephalitis, Uruguay. Emerg Infect Dis 2011;17(5):952–4.

53. Weaver SC, Barrett AD. Transmission cycles, host range, evolution and emergence of arboviral disease. Nat Rev Microbiol 2004;2(10):789–801.

54. Quiroz E, Aguilar PV, Cisneros J, et al. Venezuelan equine encephalitis in Panama: fatal endemic disease and genetic diversity of etiologic viral strains. PLoS Negl Trop Dis 2009;3(6):e472.

55. Pisano MB, Re VE, Diaz LA, et al. Enzootic activity of pixuna and Rio Negro viruses (Venezuelan equine encephalitis complex) in a neotropical region of Argentina. Vector Borne Zoonotic Dis 2010;10(2):199–201.

56. Pisano MB, Spinsanti LI, Diaz LA, et al. First detection of Rio Negro virus (Venezuelan equine encephalitis complex subtype VI) in Cordoba, Argentina. Mem Inst Oswaldo Cruz 2012;107(1):125–8.

57. Greene IP, Paessler S, Austgen L, et al. Envelope glycoprotein mutations mediate equine amplification and virulence of epizootic Venezuelan equine encephalitis virus. J Virol 2005;79(14):9128–33.

58. Smith DR, Carrara AS, Aguilar PV, et al. Evaluation of methods to assess transmission potential of Venezuelan equine encephalitis virus by mosquitoes and estimation of mosquito saliva titers. Am J Trop Med Hyg 2005;73(1): 33–9.

59. Carrara AS, Gonzales G, Ferro C, et al. Venezuelan equine encephalitis virus infection of spiny rats. Emerg Infect Dis 2005;11(5):663–9.

60. Carrara AS, Coffey LL, Aguilar PV, et al. Venezuelan equine encephalitis virus infection of cotton rats. Emerg Infect Dis 2007;13(8):1158–65.

61. Weaver SC, Ferro C, Barrera R, et al. Venezuelan equine encephalitis. Annu Rev Entomol 2004;49:141–74.

62. Erwin-Cohen R, Porter A, Pittman P, et al. Host responses to live-attenuated Venezuelan equine encephalitis virus (TC-83): comparison of naive, vaccine responder and nonresponder to TC-83 challenge in human peripheral blood mononuclear cells. Hum Vaccin Immunother 2012;8(8):1053–65.

63. Osada T, Berglund P, Morse MA, et al. Co-delivery of antigen and IL-12 by Venezuelan equine encephalitis virus replicon particles enhances antigen-specific immune responses and antitumor effects. Cancer Immunol Immunother 2012; 61(11):1941–51.

64. Vander Veen RL, Harris DL, Kamrud KI. Alphavirus replicon vaccines. Anim Health Res Rev 2012;13(1):1–9.

65. Dupuy LC, Richards MJ, Ellefsen B, et al. A DNA vaccine for Venezuelan equine encephalitis virus delivered by intramuscular electroporation elicits high levels of neutralizing antibodies in multiple animal models and provides protective immunity to mice and nonhuman primates. Clin Vaccine Immunol 2011;18(5): 707–16.

66. Sharma A, Gupta P, Glass PJ, et al. Safety and protective efficacy of INA-inactivated Venezuelan equine encephalitis virus: implication in vaccine development. Vaccine 2011;29(5):953–9.
67. Dupuy LC, Richards MJ, Reed DS, et al. Immunogenicity and protective efficacy of a DNA vaccine against Venezuelan equine encephalitis virus aerosol challenge in nonhuman primates. Vaccine 2010;28(46):7345–50.
68. Fine DL, Roberts BA, Teehee ML, et al. Venezuelan equine encephalitis virus vaccine candidate (V3526) safety, immunogenicity and efficacy in horses. Vaccine 2007;25(10):1868–76.
69. Gould EA, Solomon T. Pathogenic flaviviruses. Lancet 2008;371(9611):500–9.
70. Evans IA, Hueston L, Doggett SL. Murray Valley encephalitis virus. N S W Public Health Bull 2009;20(11–12):195–6.
71. Williams CR, Fricker SR, Kokkinn MJ. Environmental and entomological factors determining Ross River virus activity in the River Murray Valley of South Australia. Aust N Z J Public Health 2009;33(3):284–8.
72. Factsheet: Murray Valley encephalitis. N S W Public Health Bull 2010;21(5–6):148–9.
73. Roosendaal J, Westaway EG, Khromykh A, et al. Regulated cleavages at the West Nile virus NS4A-2K-NS4B junctions play a major role in rearranging cytoplasmic membranes and Golgi trafficking of the NS4A protein. J Virol 2006;80(9):4623–32.
74. Heinz FX, Stiasny K. Flaviviruses and their antigenic structure. J Clin Virol 2012;55(4):289–95.
75. Mukhopadhyay S, Kuhn RJ, Rossmann MG. A structural perspective of the flavivirus life cycle. Nat Rev Microbiol 2005;3(1):13–22.
76. Mukhopadhyay S, Kim BS, Chipman PR, et al. Structure of West Nile virus. Science 2003;302(5643):248.
77. Amraoui F, Krida G, Bouattour A, et al. *Culex pipiens*, an experimental efficient vector of West Nile and Rift Valley fever viruses in the Maghreb region. PLoS One 2012;7(5):e36757.
78. Andreadis TG. The contribution of *Culex pipiens* complex mosquitoes to transmission and persistence of West Nile virus in North America. J Am Mosq Control Assoc 2012;28(Suppl 4):137–51.
79. Balenghien T, Fouque F, Sabatier P, et al. Theoretical formulation for mosquito host-feeding patterns: application to a West Nile virus focus of southern France. J Med Entomol 2011;48(5):1076–90.
80. Singha H, Gulati BR, Kumar P, et al. Complete genome sequence analysis of Japanese encephalitis virus isolated from a horse in India. Arch Virol 2013;158(1):113–22.
81. Mann BR, McMullen AR, Swetnam DM, et al. Continued evolution of West Nile virus, Houston, Texas, USA, 2002-2012. Emerg Infect Dis 2013;19(9):1418–27.
82. Barzon L, Pacenti M, Franchin E, et al. Whole genome sequencing and phylogenetic analysis of West Nile virus lineage 1 and lineage 2 from human cases of infection, Italy, August 2013. Euro Surveill 2013;18:1–8.
83. Anez G, Grinev A, Chancey C, et al. Evolutionary dynamics of West Nile virus in the United States, 1999-2011: phylogeny, selection pressure and evolutionary time-scale analysis. PLoS Negl Trop Dis 2013;7(5):e2245.
84. Ciccozzi M, Peletto S, Cella E, et al. Epidemiological history and phylogeography of West Nile virus lineage 2. Infect Genet Evol 2013;17:46–50.
85. McMullen AR, Albayrak H, May FJ, et al. Molecular evolution of lineage 2 West Nile virus. J Gen Virol 2013;94(Pt 2):318–25.

86. Iyer AV, Boudreaux MJ, Wakamatsu N, et al. Complete genome analysis and virulence characteristics of the Louisiana West Nile virus strain LSU-AR01. Virus Genes 2009;38(2):204–14.
87. Barzon L, Squarzon L, Cattai M, et al. West Nile virus infection in Veneto region, Italy, 2008-2009. Euro Surveill 2009;14(31).
88. Sambri V, Capobianchi M, Charrel R, et al. West Nile virus in Europe: emergence, epidemiology, diagnosis, treatment, and prevention. Clin Microbiol Infect 2013;19(8):699–704.
89. Centers for Disease Control and Prevention (CDC). West Nile virus and other arboviral diseases—United States, 2012. MMWR Morb Mortal Wkly Rep 2013; 62(25):513–7.
90. Chaintoutis SC, Chaskopoulou A, Chassalevris T, et al. West Nile virus lineage 2 strain in Greece, 2012. Emerg Infect Dis 2013;19(5):827–9.
91. Roche SE, Wicks R, Garner MG, et al. Descriptive overview of the 2011 epidemic of arboviral disease in horses in Australia. Aust Vet J 2013;91(1–2):5–13.
92. Kutasi O, Bakonyi T, Lecollinet S, et al. Equine encephalomyelitis outbreak caused by a genetic lineage 2 West Nile virus in Hungary. J Vet Intern Med 2011;25(3):586–91.
93. Hayes CG. West Nile virus: Uganda, 1937, to New York City, 1999. Ann N Y Acad Sci 2001;951:25–37.
94. Schuler LA, Khaitsa ML, Dyer NW, et al. Evaluation of an outbreak of West Nile virus infection in horses: 569 cases (2002). J Am Vet Med Assoc 2004;225(7): 1084–9.
95. Murray K, Baraniuk S, Resnick M, et al. Risk factors for encephalitis and death from West Nile virus infection. Epidemiol Infect 2006;134(6):1325–32.
96. Jean CM, Honarmand S, Louie JK, et al. Risk factors for West Nile virus neuroinvasive disease, California, 2005. Emerg Infect Dis 2007;13(12):1918–20.
97. Murray KO, Koers E, Baraniuk S, et al. Risk factors for encephalitis from West Nile Virus: a matched case-control study using hospitalized controls. Zoonoses Public Health 2009;56(6–7):370–5.
98. Cook RL, Xu X, Yablonsky EJ, et al. Demographic and clinical factors associated with persistent symptoms after West Nile virus infection. Am J Trop Med Hyg 2010;83(5):1133–6.
99. Sejvar JJ, Lindsey NP, Campbell GL. Primary causes of death in reported cases of fatal West Nile Fever, United States, 2002-2006. Vector Borne Zoonotic Dis 2011;11(2):161–4.
100. Lindsey NP, Staples JE, Lehman JA, et al. Medical risk factors for severe West Nile Virus disease, United States, 2008-2010. Am J Trop Med Hyg 2012;87(1): 179–84.
101. Vyas JM, Gonzalez RG, Pierce VM. Case records of the Massachusetts General Hospital. Case 15-2013. A 76-year-old man with fever, worsening renal function, and altered mental status. N Engl J Med 2013;368(20):1919–27.
102. Hoffman JE, Paschal KA. Functional outcomes of adult patients with West Nile virus admitted to a rehabilitation hospital. J Geriatr Phys Ther 2013; 36(2):55–62.
103. Lim JK, Lisco A, McDermott DH, et al. Genetic variation in OAS1 is a risk factor for initial infection with West Nile virus in man. PLoS Pathog 2009;5(2):e1000321.
104. Moritoh K, Yamauchi H, Asano A, et al. Generation of congenic mouse strains by introducing the virus-resistant genes, Mx1 and Oas1b, of feral mouse-derived inbred strain MSM/Ms into the common strain C57BL/6J. Jpn J Vet Res 2009; 57(2):89–99.

105. Rios JJ, Fleming JG, Bryant UK, et al. OAS1 polymorphisms are associated with susceptibility to West Nile encephalitis in horses. PLoS One 2010;5(5):e10537.
106. Courtney SC, Di H, Stockman BM, et al. Identification of novel host cell binding partners of Oas1b, the protein conferring resistance to flavivirus-induced disease in mice. J Virol 2012;86(15):7953–63.
107. Bigham AW, Buckingham KJ, Husain S, et al. Host genetic risk factors for West Nile virus infection and disease progression. PLoS One 2011;6(9):e24745.
108. Cho H, Diamond MS. Immune responses to West Nile virus infection in the central nervous system. Viruses 2012;4(12):3812–30.
109. Diamond MS, Gale M Jr. Cell-intrinsic innate immune control of West Nile virus infection. Trends Immunol 2012;33(10):522–30.
110. Suthar MS, Diamond MS, Gale M Jr. West Nile virus infection and immunity. Nat Rev Microbiol 2013;11(2):115–28.
111. Diamond MS, Klein RS. West Nile virus: crossing the blood-brain barrier. Nat Med 2004;10(12):1294–5.
112. Olsen AL, Morrey JD, Smee DF, et al. Correlation between breakdown of the blood-brain barrier and disease outcome of viral encephalitis in mice. Antiviral Res 2007;75(2):104–12.
113. Sitati E, McCandless EE, Klein RS, et al. CD40-CD40 ligand interactions promote trafficking of CD8+ T cells into the brain and protection against West Nile virus encephalitis. J Virol 2007;81(18):9801–11.
114. Morrey JD, Olsen AL, Siddharthan V, et al. Increased blood-brain barrier permeability is not a primary determinant for lethality of West Nile virus infection in rodents. J Gen Virol 2008;89(Pt 2):467–73.
115. Verma S, Lo Y, Chapagain M, et al. West Nile virus infection modulates human brain microvascular endothelial cells tight junction proteins and cell adhesion molecules: transmigration across the in vitro blood-brain barrier. Virology 2009;385(2):425–33.
116. Sultana H, Foellmer HG, Neelakanta G, et al. Fusion loop peptide of the West Nile virus envelope protein is essential for pathogenesis and is recognized by a therapeutic cross-reactive human monoclonal antibody. J Immunol 2009; 183(1):650–60.
117. Roe K, Kumar M, Lum S, et al. West Nile virus-induced disruption of the blood-brain barrier in mice is characterized by the degradation of the junctional complex proteins and increase in multiple matrix metalloproteinases. J Gen Virol 2012; 93(Pt 6):1193–203.
118. Wang H, Siddharthan V, Hall JO, et al. West Nile virus preferentially transports along motor neuron axons after sciatic nerve injection of hamsters. J Neurovirol 2009;15(4):293–9.
119. Morrey JD, Siddharthan V, Olsen AL, et al. Humanized monoclonal antibody against West Nile virus envelope protein administered after neuronal infection protects against lethal encephalitis in hamsters. J Infect Dis 2006;194(9): 1300–8.
120. Suen WW, Prow NA, Hall RA, et al. Mechanism of West Nile virus neuroinvasion: a critical appraisal. Viruses 2014;6(7):2796–825.
121. McCandless EE, Zhang B, Diamond MS, et al. CXCR4 antagonism increases T cell trafficking in the central nervous system and improves survival from West Nile virus encephalitis. Proc Natl Acad Sci U S A 2008;105(32):11270–5.
122. Schuessler A, Funk A, Lazear HM, et al. West Nile virus noncoding subgenomic RNA contributes to viral evasion of the type I interferon-mediated antiviral response. J Virol 2012;86(10):5708–18.

123. Bunning ML, Bowen RA, Cropp CB, et al. Experimental infection of horses with West Nile virus. Emerg Infect Dis 2002;8(4):380–6.
124. Durso RJ, Andjelic S, Gardner JP, et al. A novel alphavirus vaccine encoding prostate-specific membrane antigen elicits potent cellular and humoral immune responses. Clin Cancer Res 2007;13(13):3999–4008.
125. Blakely PK, Kleinschmidt-DeMasters BK, Tyler KL, et al. Disrupted glutamate transporter expression in the spinal cord with acute flaccid paralysis caused by West Nile virus infection. J Neuropathol Exp Neurol 2009;68(10):1061–72.
126. Bourgeois MA, Denslow ND, Seino KS, et al. Gene expression analysis in the thalamus and cerebrum of horses experimentally infected with West Nile virus. PLoS One 2011;6(10):e24371.
127. Wang H, Rascoe AM, Holley DC, et al. Novel dicarboxylate selectivity in an insect glutamate transporter homolog. PLoS One 2013;8(8):e70947.
128. Clarke P, Leser JS, Bowen RA, et al. Virus-induced transcriptional changes in the brain include the differential expression of genes associated with interferon, apoptosis, interleukin 17 receptor A, and glutamate signaling as well as flavivirus-specific upregulation of tRNA synthetases. MBio 2014;5(2):e00902–14.
129. Wang H, Siddharthan V, Hall JO, et al. Autonomic nervous dysfunction in hamsters infected with West Nile virus. PLoS One 2011;6(5):e19575.
130. Cantile C, Di GG, Eleni C, et al. Clinical and neuropathological features of West Nile virus equine encephalomyelitis in Italy. Equine Vet J 2000;32(1):31–5.
131. Ostlund EN, Crom RL, Pedersen DD, et al. Equine West Nile encephalitis, United States. Emerg Infect Dis 2001;7(4):665–9.
132. Snook CS, Hyman SS, Del PF, et al. West Nile virus encephalomyelitis in eight horses. J Am Vet Med Assoc 2001;218(10):1576–9.
133. Porter MB, Long MT, Getman LM, et al. West Nile virus encephalomyelitis in horses: 46 cases (2001). J Am Vet Med Assoc 2003;222(9):1241–7.
134. Epp T, Waldner C, West K, et al. Factors associated with West Nile virus disease fatalities in horses. Can Vet J 2007;48(11):1137–45.
135. Kitai Y, Shirafuji H, Kanehira K, et al. Specific antibody responses to West Nile virus infections in horses preimmunized with inactivated Japanese encephalitis vaccine: evaluation of blocking enzyme-linked immunosorbent assay and complement-dependent cytotoxicity assay. Vector Borne Zoonotic Dis 2011; 11(8):1093–8.
136. Yeh JY, Lee JH, Park JY, et al. A diagnostic algorithm to serologically differentiate West Nile virus from Japanese encephalitis virus infections and its validation in field surveillance of poultry and horses. Vector Borne Zoonotic Dis 2012; 12(5):372–9.
137. De FM, Ulbert S, Diamond M, et al. Recent progress in West Nile virus diagnosis and vaccination. Vet Res 2012;43(1):16.
138. Davidson AH, Traub-Dargatz JL, Rodeheaver RM, et al. Immunologic responses to West Nile virus in vaccinated and clinically affected horses. J Am Vet Med Assoc 2005;226(2):240–5.
139. Pennick KE, McKnight CA, Patterson JS, et al. Diagnostic sensitivity and specificity of in situ hybridization and immunohistochemistry for Eastern equine encephalitis virus and West Nile virus in formalin-fixed, paraffin-embedded brain tissue of horses. J Vet Diagn Invest 2012;24(2):333–8.
140. Hatanpaa KJ, Kim JH. Neuropathology of viral infections. Handb Clin Neurol 2014;123:193–214.
141. Nath A, Tyler KL. Novel approaches and challenges to treatment of CNS viral infections. Ann Neurol 2013;74:412–22.

142. Shi Z, Wei J, Deng X, et al. Nitazoxanide inhibits the replication of Japanese encephalitis virus in cultured cells and in a mouse model. Virol J 2014;11:10.

143. Morrey JD, Taro BS, Siddharthan V, et al. Efficacy of orally administered T-705 pyrazine analog on lethal West Nile virus infection in rodents. Antiviral Res 2008;80(3):377–9.

144. Bowen RA, Rouge MM, Siger L, et al. Pathogenesis of West Nile virus infection in dogs treated with glucocorticoids. Am J Trop Med Hyg 2006;74(4):670–3.

145. Chan-Tack KM, Forrest G. Failure of interferon alpha-2b in a patient with West Nile virus meningoencephalitis and acute flaccid paralysis. Scand J Infect Dis 2005;37(11–12):944–6.

146. Chan-Tack KM, Forrest G. West Nile virus meningoencephalitis and acute flaccid paralysis after infliximab treatment. J Rheumatol 2006;33(1):191–2.

147. Lewis M, Amsden JR. Successful treatment of West Nile virus infection after approximately 3 weeks into the disease course. Pharmacotherapy 2007;27(3):455–8.

148. Diamond MS. Development of effective therapies against West Nile virus infection. Expert Rev Anti Infect Ther 2005;3(6):931–44.

149. Siger L, Bowen R, Karaca K, et al. Evaluation of the efficacy provided by a recombinant canarypox-vectored equine West Nile Virus vaccine against an experimental West Nile Virus intrathecal challenge in horses. Vet Ther 2006;7(3):249–56.

150. Long MT, Gibbs EP, Mellencamp MW, et al. Efficacy, duration, and onset of immunogenicity of a West Nile virus vaccine, live Flavivirus chimera, in horses with a clinical disease challenge model. Equine Vet J 2007;39(6):491–7.

151. El GH, Minke JM, Rehder J, et al. A West Nile virus (WNV) recombinant canarypox virus vaccine elicits WNV-specific neutralizing antibodies and cell-mediated immune responses in the horse. Vet Immunol Immunopathol 2008;123(3–4):230–9.

152. Lam KH, Ellis TM, Williams DT, et al. Japanese encephalitis in a racing thoroughbred gelding in Hong Kong. Vet Rec 2005;157(6):168–73.

153. Konishi E, Shoda M, Kondo T. Analysis of yearly changes in levels of antibodies to Japanese encephalitis virus nonstructural 1 protein in racehorses in central Japan shows high levels of natural virus activity still exist. Vaccine 2006;24(4):516–24.

154. Satou K, Nishiura H. Evidence of the partial effects of inactivated Japanese encephalitis vaccination: analysis of previous outbreaks in Japan from 1953 to 1960. Ann Epidemiol 2007;17(4):271–7.

155. Minke JM, Siger L, Cupillard L, et al. Protection provided by a recombinant ALVAC((R))-WNV vaccine expressing the prM/E genes of a lineage 1 strain of WNV against a virulent challenge with a lineage 2 strain. Vaccine 2011;29(28):4608–12.

Equine Viral Arteritis

Udeni B.R. Balasuriya, BVSc, MS, PhD

KEYWORDS

- Equine viral arteritis • Equine arteritis virus • EAV • EVA

KEY POINTS

- Equine arteritis virus (EAV) is the causative agent of equine viral arteritis (EVA).
- EVA is a respiratory and reproductive disease of the horse that occurs throughout the world.
- Most EAV infections are inapparent (or subclinical); however, acutely infected animals may develop a wide range of clinical signs.
- Virus causes abortion in pregnant mares and a high proportion of acutely infected stallions become persistently infected and shed the virus in semen.
- EAV infection can cause a severe fulminating interstitial pneumonia and a progressive pneumoenteric syndrome in young foals.

VIRUS

EAV was first isolated from the lung of an aborted fetus after an extensive outbreak of respiratory disease and abortion on a Standardbred breeding farm near Bucyrus, Ohio, in 1953.[1,2] After isolation of the causative virus (EAV) and description of characteristic vascular lesions, EVA was identified as an etiologically distinct disease of the horse.[1] EAV is a small enveloped, positive-sense, single-stranded RNA virus that is the prototype virus in the family *Arteriviridae* (genus *Arterivirus*), order *Nidovirales*, a taxonomic grouping that includes porcine reproductive and respiratory syndrome virus, simian hemorrhagic fever virus, lactate dehydrogenase-elevating virus of mice, and recently identified wobbly possum disease virus of free-ranging Australian brushtail possums (*Trichosurus vulpecula*) in New Zealand.[3,4]

The molecular properties of EAV were reviewed by Balasuriya and colleagues[5,6] (2013 and 2014). Briefly, the EAV genome length varies between 12,704 and 12,731 base pair among different viral strains and includes a 5′ leader sequence (224 nucleotides) and at least 10 open reading frames (ORFs).[5] The 2 most 5′-proximal ORFs (1a and 1b) occupy approximately three-fourths of the genome and encode

This work was partially supported by Agriculture and Food Research Initiative competitive grant no. 2013-68004-20360 from the USDA National Institute of Food and Agriculture.
Department of Veterinary Science, Maxwell H. Gluck Equine Research Center, College of Agriculture, Food and Environment, University of Kentucky, Lexington, KY 40546-0099, USA
E-mail address: ubalasuriya@uky.edu

2 replicase polyproteins (pp1a and pp1ab). These precursor proteins are extensively processed after translation into at least 13 nonstructural proteins (nsp1–12, including nsp7 α/β) by 3 viral proteases (nsp1, 2, and 4).[5] The structural proteins of EAV include seven envelope proteins (E, GP2, GP3, GP4, ORF5a protein, GP5, and M [encoded by ORFs 2a, 2b, 3-4, 5a, 5b, and 6]) and a nucleocapsid protein (N [encoded by ORF7]). All the structural protein encoding ORFs are located at the 3 proximal quarter of the genome (**Fig. 1**).[5,7] Three of the minor envelope glycoproteins (GP2, GP3, and GP4) form a heterotrimer in the EAV particle, and the M (nonglycosylated) and GP5 (glycosylated) proteins form a disulfide-linked heterodimer.[5,7]

Organ samples and tissue culture fluid containing EAV can be stored frozen (−70°C to −80°C) for decades without significant loss of virus infectivity. The virus also survives in cryopreserved semen samples and embryos for many years. EAV remain infectious 75 days at 4°C, between 2 to 3 days at 37°C, and 20 to 30 minutes at 56°C. EAV is readily inactivated by lipid solvents (ether and chloroform) and by common disinfectants and detergents.

CLINICAL SIGNS

The clinical signs displayed by EAV-infected horses depend on a variety of factors, including the genetics, age, and physical condition of the horses; challenge dose; route of infection; strain of virus; and environmental conditions.[8–11] Although there is only 1 known serotype of EAV, there is significant variation in virulence phenotype between EAV field strains.[5,11] Based on the clinical severity of the disease during natural outbreaks, EAV field strains could be segregated into viruses that cause moderate to severe disease (eg, EAV KY84, EAV AZ87, EAV IL93, and EAV PA96), mild disease (eg, EAV SWZ 64, EAV AUT68, EAV IL94, and EAV CA97) and asymptomatic infection (EAV KY63, EAV PA76, EAV KY77, and EAV CA95; Moore and colleagues,[12] 2002). Similarly, laboratory and vaccine strains differ significantly in their virulence phenotype from the highly virulent, horse-adapted Bucyrus strain (virulent Bucyrus

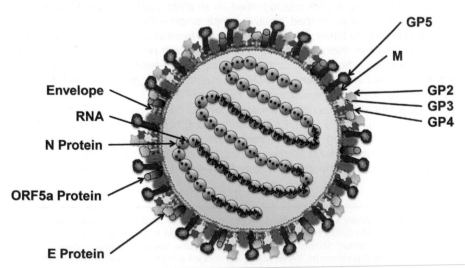

Fig. 1. Virion architecture. EAV particle consists of a nucleocapsid (N) and 7 envelope proteins, which include 2 major envelope proteins (GP5 and M form a dimer), 3 minor envelope glycoproteins (GP2, GP3, and GP4 form a trimer), and 2 other minor envelope proteins (E and ORF5a protein).

strain [VBS] of EAV; ATCC VR-796) of EAV, and the highly attenuated modified live virus (MLV) vaccine derived from it, to the highly attenuated recombinant EAV 030 strain derived from an infectious cDNA clone of the virus.[6] With the sole and notable exception of the experimentally derived and highly horse-adapted EAV VBS, other strains and field isolates of EAV very rarely cause fatal infection in adult horses.[11,13]

Most EAV infections are inapparent, especially those that occur in mares bred to persistently infected stallions.[8,14,15] The incubation period of 2 to 14 days (usually 6 to 8 days following venereal exposure) is followed by fever of up to 41°C that may persist for 2 to 9 days (**Fig. 2**).[5,6] Very young, old, debilitated, and immunosuppressed horses are predisposed to severe EVA and may develop a wide range of clinical signs, including fever, depression, anorexia, dependent edema (scrotum, ventral trunk, and limbs), stiffness of gait, conjunctivitis, lacrimation, periorbital and supraorbital edema, respiratory distress, urticaria (that may be localized to sides of the neck or face or may be generalized over most of the body), and leukopenia.[5,8] The most consistent clinical features of EAV infection are pyrexia and leukopenia.[16–18] Less frequently observed signs include icterus; photophobia; corneal opacity; coughing and dyspnea; abdominal pain and diarrhea; ataxia; petechiation of the nasal mucosa, conjunctiva, and oral mucous membranes; submaxillary and submandibular lymphadenopathy; and adventitious edema in the intermandibular space, beneath the sternum, or in the shoulder region.[1,2,19–25]

The virus causes abortion in pregnant mares. Abortion rates during natural outbreaks of EVA can vary from less than 10% to 71% of infected mares.[8,22] EAV-induced abortions can occur at any time between 3 and 10 months of gestation. The abortigenic potential of different strains of EAV has not been adequately compared but it seems that strains differ in their abortigenic potential as they do in their virulence characteristics. EAV infection can cause a severe fulminating interstitial pneumonia in neonatal foals and a progressive pneumoenteric syndrome in older foals.[9] A high proportion of acutely infected stallions (10%–70%) become persistently infected and shed the virus in semen; however, there is no evidence of any analogous persistent infection in mares, geldings, or foals (**Fig. 3**).[8,15,26] With the exception of persistently infected stallions, EAV is cleared from the tissues of infected horses by 28 days after the exposure. The virus persists in the ampulla and the accessory sex glands of the male reproductive tract and the establishment and maintenance of the

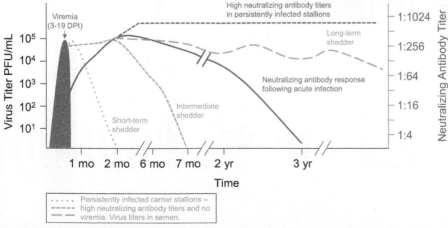

Fig. 2. Outcome of EAV infection.

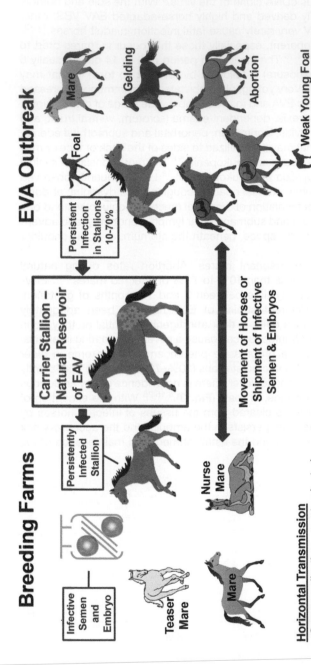

Fig. 3. Transmission of EAV between horses and the central role of carrier stallion in maintenance and perpetuation of the virus in equine populations.

carrier state in stallions is testosterone-dependent.[8] Stallions may undergo a period of temporary subfertility associated with decreased libido, sperm motility, and concentration, and an increased percentage of morphologically abnormal sperm in ejaculates during acute EAV infection. These changes can persist for up to 6 to 7 weeks after experimental EAV infection of stallions.[8,27] During acute infection, scrotal edema and fever could exert independent effects on all the semen quality parameters, including total motile (TMOT) and progressively motile (PMOT) sperm cells, total number of spermatozoa (TNS), curvilinear velocity (VCL), percentage of live spermatozoa (LS), and percentage of morphologically normal spermatozoa (MNS). It has been shown that following experimental infection, there is significant decrease in all parameters evaluated for semen quality (TMOT and PMOT, TNS, LS, MNS, VCL) between 9 to 76 days postinfection (DPI).[28] The common sperm abnormalities include detached heads, head and proximal droplet defects, and tail, midpiece, and acrosome defects. Semen quality is apparently normal in persistently infected stallions, despite high titer virus shedding in the semen. Because virus titers remained high long after semen quality returned to baseline, the virus seems to exert little to no direct effect (see **Fig. 2**).[28] Venereal infection of mares by persistently infected carrier stallions does not seem to result in subsequent fertility problems.[8]

EPIDEMIOLOGY

EAV is distributed throughout the world, although the seroprevalence of EAV infection varies between countries and horses of different breeds and age in the same country. Serologic surveys have shown that EAV infection has occurred among horses in North and South America, Europe, Australia, Africa, and Asia.[8,29] Other countries, such as Iceland and Japan, are apparently free of the virus. Recent studies have shown that New Zealand is also free of EAV.[30] In the United States, a very high percentage of adult Standardbred and Saddlebred horses are seropositive (70%–90% and 8%–25%, respectively) for EAV, compared with the Thoroughbred population where seroprevalence is very low (<5.4%). The 1998 National Animal Health Monitoring System equine survey showed that only 0.6% of the US American Quarter Horse (AQH) population was seropositive to EAV.[31] However, the extensive US outbreak of EVA in 2006 to 2007 mainly involved AQHs and this probably significantly increased the seroprevalence of EAV within this breed. The seroprevalence of EAV infection of Warmblood stallions is also very high in several European countries, with some 55% to 93% of Austrian Warmblood stallions being seropositive to EAV.[32] Similarly, there is high seroprevalence among mares and stallions of Hucul horses in Poland, 53.2% and 68.2%, respectively.[33] Seroprevalence of EAV increases with age, indicating that horses may be repeatedly exposed to the virus as they age.

Transmission of EAV between horses occurs through either respiratory or venereal routes (see **Fig. 3**).[2,8,14,15,22,34] Horizontal respiratory transmission of EAV occurs after aerosolization of infected respiratory tract secretions from acutely infected horses; high titers of EAV are present in respiratory secretions for 7 to 14 days during acute infection.[34] However, direct and close contact is necessary for aerosol transmission of EAV between horses.[21,35] EAV can also be transmitted by aerosol from urine and other body secretions of acutely infected horses, aborted fetuses and their membranes, and the masturbates of acutely or chronically infected stallions.[10,32,34,36–39]

Venereal transmission of EAV contained in the semen of stallions that are either acutely or chronically infected with EAV is the other important route of natural transmission of the virus.[14,15] Persistently infected carrier stallions are the essential reservoir responsible for perpetuation and maintenance of EAV in equine populations; thus,

85% to 100% of seronegative mares bred to long-term carrier stallions become infected with the virus and seroconvert within 28 days. Mares are also readily infected by artificial insemination with semen collected from shedding stallions.[40] Mares that become infected following natural or artificial insemination develop clinical signs of EAV and can readily transmit the virus by the respiratory route to susceptible cohorts in close proximity.[22] Virus can be transmitted to a naïve recipient mare via embryo transfer from a donor mares inseminated with EAV-infective semen.[41] Furthermore, congenital infection of foals after transplacental transmission of the virus in mares infected in late gestation can occur.[9] The congenitally infected foals frequently develop a rapidly progressive, fulminating interstitial pneumonia and fibronecrotic enteritis.[9,42–45] Lateral dissemination of EAV also can occur through contaminated fomites (eg, personnel, clothing, vehicles, and equipment such as artificial vaginas).[8,10,21,35]

PATHOGENESIS AND PATHOLOGIC CONDITION

The pathogenesis of EVA has been studied by both the experimental inoculation (intranasal, intramuscular, and intravenous) of horses with strains of EAV of different virulence and the careful evaluation of natural outbreaks of EVA.[11,17,18,22,24,34,38,46–49] Quantitative distribution of EAV has differed greatly between individual experiments, which likely reflects the inherent differences in the route of infection, virus dose, strain of virus, and quality of the specimens used for virus isolation (VI).[50] It is to be stressed that, with the notable exception of fetal and neonatal infections, EAV infection of horses is seldom fatal.[13] The numerous publications describing lesions caused by the highly virulent horse-adapted VBS of EAV reflect a severe fatal infection that is not representative of the disease caused by field strains of the virus.

Following respiratory infection, initial multiplication of the virus takes place in the upper respiratory tract epithelium and alveolar macrophages in the lung. The virus soon appears in the regional lymph nodes, especially the bronchial nodes. Within 3 days, the virus is present in blood (viremia lasts for 3–19 DPI; see **Fig. 2**) and virtually all organs and tissues, where it replicates in macrophages and endothelial cells. The clinical manifestations of EVA reflect endothelial cell injury and increased vascular permeability.[5] In vitro and in vivo studies have demonstrated increased transcription of genes encoding proinflammatory mediators (interleukin [IL]-1β, II-6, IL-8, and tumor necrosis factor α) following EAV infection, suggesting that these cytokine mediators are critical in determining the outcome of infection and severity of the disease.[51,52]

EAV infection of pregnant mares can result in the abortion of fetuses, which are usually partially autolyzed at the time of expulsion. Aborted fetuses may exhibit interlobular pulmonary edema, pleural and pericardial effusion, and petechial and ecchymotic hemorrhages on the serosal and mucosal surfaces of the small intestine. The characteristic histologic feature of EVA is a severe necrotizing panvasculitis of small vessels. Affected muscular arteries show foci of intimal, subintimal, and medial necrosis, with edema and infiltration of lymphocytes and neutrophils. Prominent vascular lesions are also seen in the placenta, brain, liver, and spleen of the aborted fetuses. Lungs of affected neonatal foals have severe interstitial pneumonia.

Recent studies have demonstrated that clinical outcome of EAV infection is determined by host genetic factors.[52,53] Specifically, based on the in vitro susceptibility of CD3+ T lymphocytes to EAV infection, horses were divided into susceptible and resistant groups. Subsequently, a genome wide association study identified a common, genetically dominant haplotype associated with the in vitro susceptible phenotype in the region of equine chromosome 11 (ECA11; 49572804–49643932). Experimental inoculation with EAV into horses with in vitro CD3+ susceptibility or resistance showed a significant difference between the 2 groups of horses in terms of proinflammatory and immunomodulatory cytokine mRNA expression and evidence of increased clinical signs in horses possessing the in vitro CD3+ T cell resistant phenotype.[52] The studies have shown that stallions with EAV-susceptible CD3+ T lymphocytes are at a higher risk of becoming persistently infected compared with stallions that lack this phenotype.[54]

IMMUNE RESPONSE

Natural and experimental infection induces a solid protective immune response in horses that protects against subsequent infection with EAV. All 3 arms of the immune system (innate, humoral, and cell-mediated) are involved in providing protection against EAV. The innate immune response to EAV is not well studied. Recently, it has been shown that EAV inhibits type I interferon (IFN) production in infected equine endothelial cells and 3 of the viral nonstructural proteins (nsp1, 2, and 11) are capable of inhibiting type I IFN activity. Of these 3, nsp1 has the strongest inhibitory effect on IFN synthesis. Clearly, failure to induce type I IFN in EAV infected cells may allow the virus to subvert the equine innate immune response.

Following natural and experimental infection with EAV, horses develop both complement-fixing and virus-specific neutralizing (VN) antibodies.[55,56] Complement-fixing antibodies develop 1 to 2 weeks after infection, peak after 2 to 3 weeks, and steadily decline to disappear by 8 months, whereas VN antibodies are detected within 1 to 2 weeks after exposure, peak at 2 to 4 months, and persist 3 years or more.[8,17,18,56,57] Recent studies have shown that horses develop IgM antibodies to EAV at 6 DPI that peak after 10 DPI, and decline rapidly by 21 to 49 DPI (Chelvarajan RL, Edwards C, Eastes A, et al. Detection of early anti-EAV immunoglobulin M (IgM) and immunoglobulin G (IgG) in equine serum by capture enzyme-linked immunosorbent assays (ELISAs). Comparative Immunology, Microbiology & Infectious Diseases. Submitted for publication). Horses that are exposed to EAV mount an immune response to GP5, N, and M structural proteins, as well as nsp2, 4, 5, and 12.[58,59] Appearance of VN antibodies coincides with the disappearance of virus from the circulation of acutely infected horses.[46,60] However, virus persists in the reproductive tract of the carrier stallion for a variable period despite the presence of high titers of VN antibodies in serum (see **Fig. 2**).[8]

Foals born to immune mares are protected against clinical EVA by passive transfer of VN antibodies in the colostrum.[61,62] VN antibodies appear a few hours after colostrum feeding, peak at 1 week of age, and gradually decline to extinction between 2 to 6, rarely 7, months of age. The mean biological half-life of maternal antibodies in serum from foals is 32 days.[62]

There are no comprehensive studies to date that describe cell-mediated immune (CMI) response to EAV in horses. Castillo-Olivares and colleagues[63] (2003) showed that cytotoxicity induced by EAV-stimulated peripheral blood mononucleated cells was virus-specific, genetically restricted, and mediated by CD8+ T cells; and that EAV-specific cytotoxic T lymphocytes precursors persist for at least 1 year after experimental infection in ponies.

DIAGNOSIS

Clinical signs of EVA resemble many other infectious and noninfectious diseases of horses. Therefore, differential diagnoses should include other infectious diseases of horses that can result in similar clinical signs (depending on geographic location these could include equine herpesviruses (EHVs) 1 and 4, equine influenza virus, equine rhinitis

A and B viruses, equine adenovirus, Getah virus, equine infectious anemia virus, African horse sickness virus, Hendra virus, and bacterial diseases such as leptospira), as well as noninfectious diseases (purpura hemorrhagica, urticaria, and toxicosis due to hoary alyssum [Berteroa incana]). Abortion from EVA can also present a diagnostic dilemma and must be distinguished from EHV-1 (or rarely EHV-4) abortions. Thus, the clinical diagnosis of EAV should be further confirmed by laboratory diagnosis.

Laboratory diagnosis of EVA is currently based on any combination of the following techniques: VI, viral nucleic acid or antigen detection, and serology. The following clinical materials should be collected for laboratory testing for EAV infection during acute infections of adult horses and young foals: nasopharyngeal swab or nasal washing or swab, conjunctival swab, whole blood (in EDTA or citrate), and paired serum samples (21–28 days apart). Whole blood collected in heparin tubes is not suitable for laboratory testing of EAV. Lung, spleen, and lymphoid tissues (eg, thymus, mesenteric, and bronchial lymph nodes) from foals that died of pneumoenteric syndrome should be collected for laboratory testing. The following clinical materials should be collected from equine abortions: placenta, fetal fluids, lung, spleen, and lymphoid tissues from the fetus. For testing of stallions for EAV carrier state the following samples should be submitted to the laboratory: semen (sperm-rich fraction of the ejaculate) and a serum sample. All clinical samples for laboratory testing should be stored and shipped at 4°C by overnight delivery. Tissues (eg, thymus, placenta, lung, liver, lymph nodes) for histopathologic examination and immunohistochemical staining could be collected in 10% buffered formalin.

The VI and virus neutralization test (VNT) are the current World Organization for Animal Health (OIE) prescribed standard tests for EVA (OIE Manual of Diagnostic Tests and Vaccines for Terrestrial Animals[64]). EAV can be isolated from nasal swabs or buffy coat cells separated from anticoagulated blood collected from horses with clinical signs of EVA, or the tissues of aborted equine fetuses and foals that died of pneumonia. Serologic diagnosis of EVA is based on the VNT and demonstration of rising neutralizing antibody titers (4-fold or greater) in paired serum samples taken at a 21 to 28 day interval. Carrier stallions are first identified by serology because they are always seropositive, and persistent infection is confirmed by VI from semen in cell culture, by test-breeding using seronegative mares (and monitoring these for seroconversion to EAV after breeding), or by standard reverse transcription polymerase chain reaction (RT-PCR) or real-time RT-PCR (rRT-PCR) to identify viral nucleic acid in semen.

VI is currently the OIE-approved gold standard for the detection of EAV in semen and is the prescribed test for international trade. However, it has been demonstrated that at least 1 rRT-PCR assay described in the literature has equal to or higher sensitivity than VI for the detection of EAV nucleic acid in semen samples.[65–67] Very clearly, rRT-PCR has significant advantages compared with VI in terms of reproducibility between laboratories, ease and speed of completion, and cost.

Several ELISAs and a microsphere immunoassay (Luminex) to detect antibodies to EAV have been described.[5] Recently, a new commercial competitive ELISA (cELISA; VMRD Pullman, WA, USA) has become available on the market.[68] Histopathologic examination coupled with immunohistochemical (immunoperoxidase) staining is also useful for the detection of viral antigens in formalin-fixed paraffin-embedded samples, as well as in frozen tissue sections.[69,70]

TREATMENT

There is no specific antiviral treatment of horses infected with EAV. Almost all naturally infected horses recover from EVA without any complications, although horses with severe clinical signs should be treated symptomatically with nonsteroidal anti-inflammatory drugs, antipyretics to control fever, and diuretics and support wraps to reduce edema.[8,10] Breeding stallions and horses in training should be rested. There is no effective treatment of young foals with EAV-induced interstitial pneumonia or pneumoenteritis other than administration of antibiotics to treat possible secondary bacterial infections.

The EAV carrier state is testosterone-dependent and currently there are no means available of eliminating the carrier state in stallions persistently infected with EAV other than surgical castration. However, transient suppression of testosterone production in carrier stallions may offer therapeutic promise in the elimination of EAV infection.[8,10,71,72] Some studies support that antagonists of gonadotropin-releasing hormone (Gn-RH) or anti–Gn-RH vaccines can temporarily limit the shedding of virus in the semen of carrier stallions.[5,73] However, these studies need to be repeated with a significantly larger number of known EAV carrier stallions with careful evaluation of sperm quality following treatment.

It has been shown that a peptide-conjugated phosphorodiamidate morpholino oligomer (PPMO) targeting the genomic 5′ terminus of EAV is capable of curing HeLa cells persistently infected with EAV under in vitro conditions.[74] However, in vivo application of PPMO and other antiviral agents and therapy may be limited due to the large mass of horses and the inherent costs involved.

VACCINATION

An attenuated MLV vaccine, ARVAC (Zoetis Animal Health Inc, Kalamazoo, MI, USA), is licensed for use in the United States and Canada for prevention of EAV infection in horses.[8,38,75] The MLV vaccine is not licensed in either Europe or Japan, and an inactivated (killed) EAV vaccine containing an adjuvant, Artervac (Zoetis Animal Health Inc, Kalamazoo, MI, USA), is licensed for use in the United Kingdom, Ireland, France, Hungary, and Denmark.[76] The MLV vaccine is administered intramuscularly to horses and has been used for more than 30 years in the United States to prevent and control EVA. The MLV vaccine is generally very safe, efficacious, and induces protective immunity in vaccinated horses. A small minority of horses vaccinated with this MLV vaccine develops mild febrile reactions and transient lymphopenia.[77–80] Vaccine virus may be sporadically isolated from the nasopharynx and buffy coat, usually for only about 7 days but rarely up to 32 days after vaccination.[8,38,75] Vaccinated stallions usually do not shed virus in either semen or urine. However, a very low level of virus in the semen of 1 vaccinated stallion has been recently reported (<1 plaque-forming units/mL virus at 4 and 6 days postvaccination [DPV]).[79] Therefore, it is recommended not to breed or use semen from first-time vaccinated stallions for artificial insemination purposes before 28 DPV.

- There is no evidence that a vaccinated stallion will develop the carrier state with the MLV vaccine strain.
- The MLV vaccine is not recommended for use in pregnant mares, especially during the last 2 months of gestation, or in foals less than 6 weeks of age. Apparent fetal infections with MLV after vaccination of pregnant mares have been rarely documented.[81,82]
- If mares with foals are to be vaccinated with the MLV vaccine, the foals should be healthy and at least 6 weeks of age before its dam is vaccinated.
- It is recommended that foals be vaccinated at 6 months of age after disappearance of maternal antibodies (passive antibodies can neutralize the vaccine virus) but before the onset of puberty.[61,62] Foals can be vaccinated before 6 months of

age in high-risk situations but they should also be revaccinated after 6 months of age. Vaccinated colts are resistant to development of the persistently infected carrier state after subsequent exposure to EAV. The protective immunization of prepubertal colts is, therefore, central to effective control of the spread of EAV infection. However, vaccination has no impact on viral clearance in already persistently infected stallions.

- Virus-neutralizing antibodies are induced within 5 to 8 days after MLV vaccination and peak antibody titers are achieved by 7 to 14 DPV (maximum mean titer varies between 1:32 and 1:256 occurring during 13–14 DPV). Following vaccination, neutralizing antibodies will last for at least 2 years.[8,35] Revaccination greatly increases the serologic response of horses, providing protective immunity that persists for several breeding seasons.

- Although MLV vaccination provides sustained protection against clinical EVA, it does not always prevent reinfection of vaccinated horses or subsequent limited replication of field strains of the virus.[83]

- Vaccinated mares inseminated with semen from carrier stallions can become infected, evidenced by the transient isolation of virus from buffy coat and nasopharynx, but they will not develop EVA. Furthermore, a contact seronegative mare also became infected, indicating that infectious virus was shed by the vaccinated mares.

- The killed vaccine is administered intramuscularly and a booster immunization is recommended after 3 to 4 weeks and semiannually thereafter. Although this vaccine induces neutralizing antibodies, its ability to prevent EVA and persistent infection of stallions is less characterized than that of the MLV vaccine.

- Experimental EAV vaccines have also been recently developed using recombinant DNA technology but none of these vaccines have reached the market.[17,84]

PREVENTION AND CONTROL MEASURES

Spread of EAV could be prevented by implementing proper biosecurity or infection control programs on farms, racetracks, horse shows, and veterinary clinics and hospitals. It is imperative to identify and isolate the index case and horses that come in contact, thereby minimizing or eliminating direct or indirect contact of susceptible horses with the secretions and excretions of EAV-infected horses. If an outbreak of EVA on a farm is suspected based on clinical signs and history, the state veterinarian should be notified, affected and in-contact horses isolated, movement of horses on and off the farm discontinued (quarantine), at-risk horses vaccinated, and breeding activity stopped to prevent further spread of the virus. Stalls and equipment on the affected premises should be decontaminated with disinfectants (phenolic, chlorine, iodine, and quaternary ammonium compounds). Quarantine is discontinued when no additional clinical cases of EVA or serologic evidence of infection are observed for 3 to 4 weeks.

The EAV carrier stallion plays a pivotal role in the transmission and maintenance of EAV infection in horse populations (see **Fig. 3**).[8,14] Therefore, outbreaks of EVA can be prevented by the identification of persistently infected stallions and the institution of management practices to prevent the introduction of EAV-infected horses. The US Department of Agriculture Animal and Plant Health Inspection Service, *Equine Viral Arteritis: Uniform Methods and Rules*,[85] describes the minimum standards for detecting, controlling, and preventing EVA, as well as minimum EVA requirements for the interstate and intrastate movement of horses.

Guidelines for the Prevention and Control of Equine Arteritis Virus in Breeding Stallions

- All stallions should be tested for neutralizing antibodies to EAV before they are vaccinated with the MLV or inactivated EVA vaccines. The testing should be done at least 60 days before breeding.
- A neutralization antibody titer of 1:4 or greater (VNT titer ≥1:4) is regarded as positive. The owners of stallions that are seropositive should provide a valid vaccination certificate (the stallion should have been confirmed seronegative before the first vaccination against EVA).
- Nonvaccinated seropositive stallions (no vaccination history) for EAV (VNT titer ≥1:4) should be tested for the carrier state by test breeding or testing semen samples for the presence of EAV.
  1. Test breed 2 seronegative mares twice each on 2 consecutive days (4 covers). After 14 and 28 days after breeding, test the serum from both mares for neutralizing antibodies to EAV. There could be 2 outcomes:
     ○ If both mares seroconvert, the stallion is a carrier of EAV and should be reported to the state veterinarian (see later discussion for guidelines to breed EAV carrier stallion to a seropositive mare).
     ○ If both mares remain seronegative, identify the stallion as a seropositive nonshedding stallion or seropositive noncarrier. The stallion is qualified for breeding but needs to be vaccinated annually.
     OR
  2. Test 2 separate semen samples (2 separate collections) by VI in cell culture. If semen samples are positive for EAV by VI, identify the stallions as EAV carriers. If semen samples are negative for EAV by VI, identify the stallions as EAV noncarriers.
- Management of EAV carrier stallions
  ○ Carrier stallions must be housed, handled, and bred in a facility isolated from noncarrier stallions and mares.
  ○ Carrier stallions should be approved by the state veterinarian for breeding.
  ○ Carrier stallions should be bred only to mares that are seropositive either by natural exposure or by vaccination.
- If seronegative (titer <1:4), stallions should be vaccinated with the MLV vaccine after collecting a serum sample as proof. Record the vaccination (eg, date, vaccine type).
- Stallions should be vaccinated and isolated 28 days before the breeding season or semen collection. First-time vaccinated stallions should be isolated for 28 days after vaccination and receive boosters annually.

Guidelines for Breeding a Mare to an Equine Arteritis Virus–Shedding Stallion or Insemination with Equine Arteritis Virus–Contaminated Semen

- Stallions that are confirmed semen shedders and carriers of EAV can be used for breeding purposes provided that stringent requirements are met.[8,14,86–88]
- Carrier stallions should be kept physically isolated and bred only to mares that are seropositive from either previous natural exposure or vaccination (no <3 weeks previously). It is also critical that carrier stallions be isolated and collected separately to prevent contamination of collection equipment, teasers, and premises with ejaculate because EAV can be transmitted to susceptible horses by indirect aerosol contact. When embryo transfer is used for breeding, it is highly recommended that both donor and recipient mares be vaccinated against EVA if the former are to be bred with EAV-infective semen.[41]

- The mares to be bred to EAV carrier stallions should be tested for neutralizing antibodies at least 30 days before breeding.
- Neutralizing antibody titer greater than or equal to 1:64 is regarded as protective against EAV and, therefore, these mares can be bred to an EAV-shedding carrier stallion (natural breeding) or insemination with EAV infective semen (artificial breeding) without being vaccinated.
- The mares that are seronegative to EAV should be vaccinated with the MLV vaccine and the vaccination recorded. Vaccinated mares should be isolated for 21 days and should not be bred during this period. After 21 days, breed the shedding stallion (natural breeding) or inseminate with EAV infective semen (artificial breeding).
- Mares should be kept isolated from other nonvaccinated or seronegative horses for 3 weeks (21 days) after being bred to a shedding stallion or after insemination with infective semen.
- Management of mares after annual booster vaccination consists of an annual booster vaccination 21 days before breeding is required and no isolation necessary following booster vaccination. There is no need for isolation of mares after breeding to a carrier stallion for the second time.

Guidelines for the Movement of Horses

- Horses that travel for competitions or comingle with horses coming from outside the farm should be vaccinated.
- Stallions that are shuttled between Northern and Southern Hemispheres should be tested for EAV (neutralizing antibodies and carrier state) by an accredited laboratory.
- More widespread screening of stallion populations for EAV, as well as harmonization of various diagnostic tests (eg, VI, rRT-PCR, VNT, and ELISA) among laboratories with higher quality control measures, would increase detection of carrier stallions.

RECENT ADVANCES IN EQUINE ARTERITIS VIRUS RESEARCH

During last 20 years, there have been significant advances in molecular characterization of EAV and understanding of the pathogenesis of EVA. Major advances in understanding of EAV virion architecture; replication; reverse genetics; evolution; molecular epidemiology and genetic variation; pathogenesis, including the influence of host genetics on disease susceptibility; host immune response; and potential vaccination and treatment strategies have been recently published in 3 review articles.[4–6]

FUTURE DIRECTIONS

In contrast to equine serum raised against the VBS of EAV, equine serum from MLV-vaccinated horses fails to neutralize some of the field isolates of EAV.[5,89,90] Furthermore, horses vaccinated with the current inactivated vaccine do not consistently mount a strong neutralizing antibody response to the virus. Thus, the development of improved vaccines against currently circulating EAV strains should be a high priority.

- Current OIE-approved diagnostic assays are largely based on outdated classic virology techniques that should quickly be replaced with more appropriate contemporary assays.
  - It has been shown that the rRT-PCR assay and the insulated isothermal RT-PCR (iiRT-PCR) have equal or higher sensitivity than VI in RK-13 cells for the detection of EAV nucleic acid in semen samples.

- The rRT-PCR and iiRT-PCR have an enormous advantage in terms of assay standardization between laboratories as well as in operational time and cost.
- The results of the VNT can vary markedly among laboratories when insufficient attention is paid to standardization of both test reagents and procedures, thus there is an urgent need to adopt a highly specific and sensitive ELISA or cELISA or microsphere immunoassay (Luminex) for the detection of EAV antibodies in serum samples by regulatory bodies as the official test for national and international movement of horses.
- Identify the host genetic factors associated with the establishment of the carrier state.
- Characterize the CMI response to EAV and identify the T-cell epitopes of the virus.

ACKNOWLEDGMENTS

The author gratefully acknowledges the intellectual and creative input of Dr N. James MacLachlan (Department of Veterinary Pathology, Microbiology and Immunology, University of California, Davis, USA), Dr Peter Timoney, and the late Dr William H. McCollum (Maxwell H. Gluck Equine Research Center, Department of Veterinary Science, Lexington, KY, USA) included in this review article. The author would like to thank Ms Bora Nam and Ms Diane Furry for their help with figures and Ms Kathleen M. Shuck for critical reading of the article.

REFERENCES

1. Doll ER, Bryans JT, McCollum WH, et al. Isolation of a filterable agent causing arteritis of horses and abortion by mares; its differentiation from the equine abortion (influenza) virus. Cornell Vet 1957;47:3–41.
2. Doll ER, Knappenberger RE, Bryans JT. An outbreak of abortion caused by the equine arteritis virus. Cornell Vet 1957;47:69–75.
3. Dunowska M, Biggs PJ, Zheng T, et al. Identification of a novel nidovirus associated with a neurological disease of the Australian brushtail possum (*Trichosurus vulpecula*). Vet Microbiol 2012;156:418–24.
4. Snijder EJ, Kikkert M, Fang Y. Arterivirus molecular biology and pathogenesis. J Gen Virol 2013;94:2141–63.
5. Balasuriya UB, Go YY, Maclachlan NJ. Equine arteritis virus. Vet Microbiol 2013; 167:93–122.
6. Balasuriya UB, Zhang J, Go YY, et al. Experiences with infectious cDNA clones of equine arteritis virus: lessons learned and insights gained. Virology 2014; 462-463C:388–403.
7. Firth AE, Zevenhoven-Dobbe JC, Wills NM, et al. Discovery of a small arterivirus gene that overlaps the GP5 coding sequence and is important for virus production. J Gen Virol 2011;92:1097–106.
8. Timoney PJ, McCollum WH. Equine viral arteritis. Vet Clin North Am Equine Pract 1993;9:295–309.
9. Vaala WE, Hamir AN, Dubovi EJ, et al. Fatal, congenitally acquired infection with equine arteritis virus in a neonatal thoroughbred. Equine Vet J 1992;24:155–8.
10. Glaser AL, de Vries AA, Rottier PJ, et al. Equine arteritis virus: a review of clinical features and management aspects. Vet Q 1996;18:95–9.
11. McCollum WH, Timoney PJ. Experimental observations on the virulence of isolates of equine arteritis virus. In: Wernery U, Wade JF, Mumford JA, et al, editors. Proceedings of the 8th International Conference Equine Infectious Diseases. Suffolk(UK): R & W Publications (Newmarket) Ltd; 1999. p. 558–9.

12. Moore BD, Balasuriya UB, Hedges JF, et al. Growth characteristics of a highly virulent, a moderately virulent, and an avirulent strain of equine arteritis virus in primary equine endothelial cells are predictive of their virulence to horses. Virology 2002;298:39–44.

13. Pronost S, Pitel PH, Miszczak F, et al. Description of the first recorded major occurrence of equine viral arteritis in France. Equine Vet J 2010;42:713–20.

14. Timoney PJ, McCollum WH, Murphy TW, et al. The carrier state in equine arteritis virus infection in the stallion with specific emphasis on the venereal mode of virus transmission. J Reprod Fertil Suppl 1987;35:95–102.

15. Timoney PJ, McCollum WH, Roberts AW, et al. Demonstration of the carrier state in naturally acquired equine arteritis virus infection in the stallion. Res Vet Sci 1986;41:279–80.

16. Bryans JT, Crowe ME, Doll ER, et al. The blood picture and thermal reaction in experimental viral arteritis of horses. Cornell Vet 1957;47:42–52.

17. Balasuriya UB, Heidner HW, Davis NL, et al. Alphavirus replicon particles expressing the two major envelope proteins of equine arteritis virus induce high level protection against challenge with virulent virus in vaccinated horses. Vaccine 2002;20:1609–17.

18. Balasuriya UB, Snijder EJ, Heidner HW, et al. Development and characterization of an infectious cDNA clone of the virulent Bucyrus strain of equine arteritis virus. J Gen Virol 2007;88:918–24.

19. Doll ER, Bryans JT, Wilson JC, et al. Immunization against equine viral arteritis using modified live virus propagated in cell cultures of rabbit kidney. Cornell Vet 1968;48:497–524.

20. Clayton H. 1986 outbreak of EAV in Alberta, Canada. J Equine Vet Sci 1987;7: 101.

21. Collins JK, Kari S, Ralston SL, et al. Equine viral arteritis in a veterinary teaching hospital. Prev Vet Med 1987;4:389–97.

22. Cole JR, Hall RF, Gosser HS, et al. Transmissibility and abortogenic effect of equine viral arteritis in mares. J Am Vet Med Assoc 1986;189:769–71.

23. Gerber H, Steck F, Hofer B, et al. Clinical and serological investigation on equine viral arteritis. In: Bryans John T, Heinz Gerber, editors. Proceedings of the 4th International Conference on Equine Infectious Diseases. Princeton (NJ): Veterinary Publications, Inc; 1978. p. 461–5.

24. Jones TC. Clinical and pathologic features of equine viral arteritis. J Am Vet Med Assoc 1969;155:315–7.

25. Swerczek TW, Crowe MW, Prickett ME, et al. Focal bacterial hepatitis in foals: preliminary report. Mod Vet Pract 1973;54:66–7.

26. Holyoak GR, Balasuriya UB, Broaddus CC, et al. Equine viral arteritis: current status and prevention. Theriogenology 2008;70:403–14.

27. Neu SM, Timoney PJ, Lowry SR. Changes in semen quality following experimental equine arteritis virus infection in the stallion. Theriogenology 1992;37: 407–31.

28. Campos JR, Breheny P, Araujo RR, et al. Evaluation of semen quality of stallions challenged with the Kentucky 84 (KY84) strain of equine arteritis virus (EAV). Theriogenology 82(8):1068–79.

29. Echeverria MG, Pecoraro MR, Galosi CM, et al. The first isolation of equine arteritis virus in Argentina. Rev Sci Tech 2003;22:1029–33.

30. McFadden AM, Pearce PV, Orr D, et al. Evidence for absence of equine arteritis virus in the horse population of New Zealand. N Z Vet J 2013; 61(5):300–4.

31. Anonymous, NAHMS. Equine viral arteritis (EVA) and the US horse industry. Fort Collins (CO): USDA: APHIS:VS, CEAH, National Animal Health Monitoring System; 2000.
32. Burki F, Hofer A, Nowotny N. Objective data plead to suspend import-bans for seroreactors against equine arteritis virus except for breeder stallions. J Appl Anim Res 1992;1:31–42.
33. Rola J, Larska M, Rola JG, et al. Epizotiology and phylogeny of equine arteritis virus in hucul horses. Vet Microbiol 2011;148:402–7.
34. McCollum WH, Prickett ME, Bryans JT. Temporal distribution of equine arteritis virus in respiratory mucosa, tissues and body fluids of horses infected by inhalation. Res Vet Sci 1971;12:459–64.
35. Timoney PJ. Equine viral arteritis: epidemiology and control. J Equine Vet Sci 1988;8:54–9.
36. Guthrie AJ, Howell PG, Hedges JF, et al. Lateral transmission of equine arteritis virus among Lipizzaner stallions in South Africa. Equine Vet J 2003;35: 596–600.
37. McCollum WH, Timoney PJ, Tengelsen LA. Clinical, virological and serological responses of donkeys to intranasal inoculation with the KY-84 strain of equine arteritis virus. J Comp Pathol 1995;112:207–11.
38. McCollum WH. Pathologic features of horses given avirulent equine arteritis virus intramuscularly. Am J Vet Res 1981;42:1218–20.
39. Glaser AL, de Vries AA, Rottier PJ, et al. Equine arteritis virus: clinical symptoms and prevention. Tijdschr Diergeneeskd 1997;122:2–7 [in Dutch].
40. Balasuriya UB, Evermann JF, Hedges JF, et al. Serologic and molecular characterization of an abortigenic strain of equine arteritis virus isolated from infective frozen semen and an aborted equine fetus. J Am Vet Med Assoc 1998;213:1586–9, 1570.
41. Broaddus CC, Balasuriya UB, Timoney PJ, et al. Infection of embryos following insemination of donor mares with equine arteritis virus infective semen. Theriogenology 2011;76:47–60.
42. Del Piero F, Wilkins PA, Lopez JW, et al. Equine viral arteritis in newborn foals: clinical, pathological, serological, microbiological and immunohistochemical observations. Equine Vet J 1997;29:178–85.
43. Carman S, Rae C, Dubovi E. Equine arteritis virus isolated from a Standardbred foal with pneumonia. Can Vet J 1988;29:937.
44. Golnik W, Michalska Z, Michalak T. Natural equine viral arteritis in foals. Schweiz Arch Tierheilkd 1981;123:523–33.
45. Wilkins PA, Del Piero F, Lopez J, et al. Recognition of bronchopulmonary dysplasia in a newborn foal. Equine Vet J 1995;27:398.
46. Fukunaga Y, Imagawa H, Tabuchi E, et al. Clinical and virological findings on experimental equine viral arteritis in horses. Bull Equine Res Inst 1981;18:110–8.
47. MacLachlan NJ, Balasuriya UB, Rossitto PV, et al. Fatal experimental equine arteritis virus infection of a pregnant mare: immunohistochemical staining of viral antigens. J Vet Diagn Invest 1996;8:367–74.
48. McCollum WH. Responses of horses vaccinated with avirulent modified-live equine arteritis virus propagated in the E. Derm (NBL-6) cell line to nasal inoculation with virulent virus. Am J Vet Res 1986;47:1931–4.
49. McCollum WH, Timoney PJ, Lee JW Jr, et al. Features of an outbreak of equine viral arteritis on a breeding farm associated with abortion and fatal interstitial pneumonia in neonatal foals. In: Wernery U, Wade JF, Mumford JA, et al, editors. Proceeding of the 8th International Conference on Equine Infectious Diseases. Suffolk (UK): R & W Publications (Newmarket) Ltd; 1999. p. 559–60.

50. Snijder EJ, Spann WJ. Arteriviruses. In: Knipe DM, Howley PM, Griffin DE, et al, editors. Fields virology. 5th edition. Philadelphia: Lippincott Williams & Wilkins; 2007. p. 1337–55.

51. Moore BD, Balasuriya UB, Watson JL, et al. Virulent and avirulent strains of equine arteritis virus induce different quantities of TNF-alpha and other proinflammatory cytokines in alveolar and blood-derived equine macrophages. Virology 2003;314:662–70.

52. Go YY, Cook RF, Fulgencio JQ, et al. Assessment of correlation between in vitro CD3+ T cell susceptibility to EAV infection and clinical outcome following experimental infection. Vet Microbiol 2012;157:220–5.

53. Go YY, Bailey E, Cook DG, et al. Genome-wide association study among four horse breeds identifies a common haplotype associated with in vitro CD3+ T cell susceptibility/resistance to equine arteritis virus infection. J Virol 2011;85: 13174–84.

54. Go YY, Bailey E, Timoney PJ, et al. Evidence that in vitro susceptibility of CD3+ T lymphocytes to equine arteritis virus infection reflects genetic predisposition of naturally infected stallions to become carriers of the virus. J Virol 2012;86: 12407–10.

55. McCollum WH. Vaccination for equine viral arteritis. In: Bryans JT, Gerber H, editors. Proceedings of the 2nd International Conference on Equine Infectious Diseases. Basel (Switzerland): S. Karger; 1970. p. 143–51.

56. Fukunaga Y, McCollum WH. Complement-fixation reactions in equine viral arteritis. Am J Vet Res 1977;38:2043–6.

57. Balasuriya UB, Snijder EJ, van Dinten LC, et al. Equine arteritis virus derived from an infectious cDNA clone is attenuated and genetically stable in infected stallions. Virology 1999;260:201–8.

58. MacLachlan NJ, Balasuriya UB, Hedges JF, et al. Serologic response of horses to the structural proteins of equine arteritis virus. J Vet Diagn Invest 1998;10: 229–36.

59. Go YY, Snijder EJ, Timoney PJ, et al. Characterization of equine humoral antibody response to the nonstructural proteins of equine arteritis virus. Clin Vaccine Immunol 2011;18:268–79.

60. McCollum WH. Development of a modified virus strain and vaccine for equine viral arteritis. J Am Vet Med Assoc 1969;155:318–22.

61. McCollum WH. Studies of passive immunity in foals to equine viral arteritis. Vet Microbiol 1976;1:45–54.

62. Hullinger PJ, Wilson WD, Rossitto PV, et al. Passive transfer, rate of decay, and protein specificity of antibodies against equine arteritis virus in horses from a Standardbred herd with high seroprevalence. J Am Vet Med Assoc 1998;213: 839–42.

63. Castillo-Olivares J, Tearle JP, Montesso F, et al. Detection of equine arteritis virus (EAV)-specific cytotoxic CD8[+] T lymphocyte precursors from EAV-infected ponies. J Gen Virol 2003;84:2745–53.

64. World Organization for Animal Health (OIE) 2013. Equine Viral Arteritis. OIE Manual of Diagnostic Tests and Vaccines for Terrestrial Animals, 8th edition, vol. 2. Office International des Epizooties, Paris, France. Chapter 2.5.10, p.1–16.

65. Balasuriya UB, Leutenegger CM, Topol JB, et al. Detection of equine arteritis virus by real-time TaqMan reverse transcription-PCR assay. J Virol Methods 2002;101:21–8.

66. Lu Z, Branscum AJ, Shuck KM, et al. Comparison of two real-time reverse transcription polymerase chain reaction assays for the detection of *Equine*

arteritis virus nucleic acid in equine semen and tissue culture fluid. J Vet Diagn Invest 2008;20:147–55.

67. Miszczak F, Shuck KM, Lu Z, et al. Evaluation of two magnetic-bead-based viral nucleic acid purification kits and three real-time reverse transcription-PCR reagent systems in two TaqMan assays for equine arteritis virus detection in semen. J Clin Microbiol 2011;49:3694–6.

68. Chung C, Wilson C, Timoney P, et al. Validation of an improved competitive enzyme-linked immunosorbent assay to detect Equine arteritis virus antibody. J Vet Diagn Invest 2013;25:727–35.

69. Lopez JW, Del Piero F, Glaser A, et al. Immunoperoxidase histochemistry as a diagnostic tool for detection of equine arteritis virus antigen in formalin fixed tissues. Equine Vet J 1996;28:77–9.

70. Del Piero F. Diagnosis of equine arteritis virus infection in two horses by using monoclonal antibody immunoperoxidase histochemistry on skin biopsies. Vet Pathol 2000;37:486–7.

71. Little TV, Holyoak GR, McCollum WH, et al. Output of equine arteritis virus from persistently infected stallions is testosterone dependent. In: Plowright W, Rossdale PD, Wade JF, editors. Proceedings of the 6th International Conference on Equine Infectious Diseases. Buckinghamshire (UK): R & W Publications (Newmarket) Ltd; 1991. p. 225–9.

72. Holyoak GR, Little TV, Vernon M, et al. Correlation between ultrasonographic findings and serum testosterone concentration in prepubertal and peripubertal colts. Am J Vet Res 1994;55:450–7.

73. Fortier G, Vidament M, DeCraene F, et al. The effect of GnRH antagonist on testosterone secretion, spermatogenesis and viral excretion in EVA-virus excreting stallions. Theriogenology 2002;58:425–7.

74. Zhang J, Stein DA, Timoney PJ, et al. Curing of HeLa cells persistently infected with equine arteritis virus by a peptide-conjugated morpholino oligomer. Virus Res 2010;150:138–42.

75. Harry TO, McCollum WH. Stability of viability and immunizing potency of lyophilized, modified equine arteritis live-virus vaccine. Am J Vet Res 1981;42:1501–5.

76. Annonymous. EVA vaccine granted animal test certificate. Vet Rec 1993;133: 26–7.

77. McKinnon AO, Colbern GT, Collins JK, et al. Vaccination of stallions with a modified live equine arteritis virus vaccine. J Equine Vet Sci 1986;6:66–9.

78. Timoney PJ, Umphenour NW, McCollum WH. Safety evaluation of a commercial modified live equine arteritis virus vaccine for use in stallions. In: Powell David G, editor. Proceedings of the 5th International Conference of Equine Infectious Diseases. Lexington (KY): The University Press of Kentucky; 1988. p. 19–27.

79. Summers-Lawyer KA, Go YY, Lu Z, et al. Response of stallions to primary immunization with a modified live equine viral arteritis vaccine. J Equine Vet Sci 2011; 31:10.

80. Timoney PJ, Fallon L, Shuck K, et al. The outcome of vaccinating five pregnant mares with a commercial equine viral arteritis vaccine. Equine Vet Educ 2007; 19:6.

81. Broaddus CC, Balasuriya UB, White JL, et al. Evaluation of the safety of vaccinating mares against equine viral arteritis during mid or late gestation or during the immediate postpartum period. J Am Vet Med Assoc 2011;238:741–50.

82. Moore BD, Balasuriya UB, Nurton JP, et al. Differentiation of strains of equine arteritis virus of differing virulence to horses by growth in equine endothelial cells. Am J Vet Res 2003;64:779–84.

83. McCollum WH, Timoney PJ, Roberts AW, et al. Response of vaccinated and non-vaccinated mares to artificial insemination with semen from stallions persistently infected with equine arteritis virus. In: Powell David G, editor. Proceedings of 5th International Conference on Equine Infectious Diseases. Lexington (KY): The University Press of Kentucky; 1987. p. 13–8.

84. Castillo-Olivares J, Wieringa R, Bakonyi T, et al. Generation of a candidate live marker vaccine for equine arteritis virus by deletion of the major virus neutralization domain. J Virol 2003;77:8470–80.

85. Anonymous. Equine viral arteritis uniform methods and rules, effective April 19, 2004. USDA-APHIS, Washington DC, USA; 2004. p. 1–19.

86. Timoney PJ, McCollum WH, Roberts AW, et al. Status of equine viral arteritis in Kentucky for 1986. Vet Rec 1987;120:282.

87. Timoney PJ. Factors influencing the international spread of equine diseases. Vet Clin North Am Equine Pract 2000;16:537–51, x.

88. Timoney PJ. The increasing significance of international trade in equids and its influence on the spread of infectious diseases. Ann N Y Acad Sci 2000;916: 55–60.

89. Balasuriya UB, Maclachlan NJ. The immune response to equine arteritis virus: potential lessons for other arteriviruses. Vet Immunol Immunopathol 2004;102: 107–29.

90. Zhang J, Go YY, Huang CM, et al. Development and characterization of an infectious cDNA clone of the modified live virus vaccine strain of equine arteritis virus. Clin Vaccine Immunol 2012;19:1312–21.

Equine Infectious Anemia in 2014: Live with It or Eradicate It?

Charles J. Issel, DVM, PhDa,*, R. Frank Cook, PhDa, Robert H. Mealey, DVM, PhDb,
David W. Horohov, MS, PhDa

KEYWORDS

- Equine infectious anemia • Serology • Host immune response
- Agar gel immunodiffusion test • Transmission by insects and man

KEY POINTS

- Equine infectious anemia (EIA) control programs in the United States have been effective, although they are now at a crossroads in that the mobile and tested population is mostly segregated and, therefore, at low risk from untested equids that constitute the remaining reservoir for EIA virus (EIAV).
- Consequently, the goals of testing should be reexamined, "smarter" testing conducted by increasing the intervals between tests for frequently tested equid populations, and strategies developed to increase testing of the untested reservoir population.
- In many areas, required testing at change of ownership has proved invaluable in the identification of new cases.
- In areas of the world where working equids are still important agricultural animals and EIA is endemic, strategies other than destruction without compensation must be developed if control of EIA in more than localized situations is the goal.
- Additional research is required to improve direct detection techniques such as polymerase chain reaction–based methods for amplification of EIAV genetic material.
- The most important recommendation is to assume that all equid contacts are infected with EIAV.

INTRODUCTION

Clinical signs of swamp fever or equine infectious anemia were first described in 1843, with research published in 1904 proving it was caused by a filterable agent or virus (EIAV) that persisted in its equid hosts and was transmitted in blood.[1] Mechanical transmission by large hematophagus insect vectors (horse flies and deer flies) was demonstrated by the 1940s.[2] Despite these early advances, there were no practical control measures for EIAV until 1972 when Leroy Coggins and coworkers

a Department of Veterinary Science, Maxwell H. Gluck Equine Research Center, University of Kentucky, Lexington, KY 40546, USA; b Department of Veterinary Microbiology and Pathology, College of Veterinary Medicine, Washington State University, PO Box 647040, Pullman, WA 99164–7040, USA
* Corresponding author.
E-mail address: cissel@uky.edu

Vet Clin Equine 30 (2014) 561–577
http://dx.doi.org/10.1016/j.cveq.2014.08.002   vetequine.theclinics.com

demonstrated that antibodies to the virus were detectable in an agar gel immunodiffusion test (AGIDT) using antigen extracted from spleens of acutely infected horses.[3] Furthermore, these antibodies were correlated with the presence of EIAV by horse inoculation tests.[4] This test received rapid international acceptance, and is known as the Coggins test by the veterinary community and horse owners alike.

What have we learned since the early 1970s when testing was adopted on a wide scale? During the first 10 years of widespread official AGIDT use, more than 57,000 positive results were reported to the US Department of Agriculture (USDA) with most of the infected equids being removed from the population by nonmandatory slaughter. However, from 2007 to 2012 more than 8 million samples were tested in the United States, with 485 identified as positive for EIAV, meaning that it costs about $650,000 to find each positive animal. Are we using the investment the horse industry makes for this passive EIA surveillance wisely?

In the absence of an effective vaccine, the success of the test and removal approach for the control of EIA cannot be overstated, at least in those areas where testing has been traditionally routine. This article addresses 4 main questions:

1. What have we learned about EIAV, host control of its replication, and inapparent carriers?
2. Where do we stand internationally in the control of EIA?
3. Are we doing our best at diagnosing the infection when samples are submitted to the laboratory?
4. How can veterinarians reduce the chance that they are spreading blood-borne infections?

This article attempts to put these issues into practical contemporary perspectives for the equine practitioner. The reader is referred to recent reviews for more detailed information on EIA and EIAV.[5,6]

ETIOLOGY
Taxonomy

EIAV is classified within the *Lentivirus* genus of the subfamily Orthoretrovirinae in the family Retroviridae, and as such has been designated the "country cousin" of human immunodeficiency virus (HIV).[6]

Morphology

Each circular or oval 115-nm EIAV particle contains 2 copies of a single-stranded positive-sense genomic RNA enclosed within a conical-shaped core (**Fig. 1**A). The shape of the core is one of the defining features of lentiviruses, and provided some of the first evidence that HIV or "lymphadenopathy-associated virus," as it was originally labeled, is a member of the lentiviral genus.[7,8] Surrounding the core component is a proteinaceous matrix that in turn is bounded by a host-cell–derived lipid membrane containing numerous 6- to 8-nm projections.[9,10]

Equine Infectious Anemia Virus and Its Relationship with Other Lentiviruses

At approximately 8.2 kbp, EIAV (see **Fig. 1**B) has the smallest genome[11–13] of all known living lentiviruses, yet is a highly successful pathogen despite possessing just 84% of the coding capacity of HIV. The proviral DNA of all retroviruses consists of 3 major structural genes, *gag, pol* and *env*, bounded at each end by long terminal repeats. Lentiviruses are known as complex retroviruses because they possess several open reading frames (ORFs) in addition to the 3 major structural genes. These ORFs encode molecules termed accessory proteins; they perform regulatory

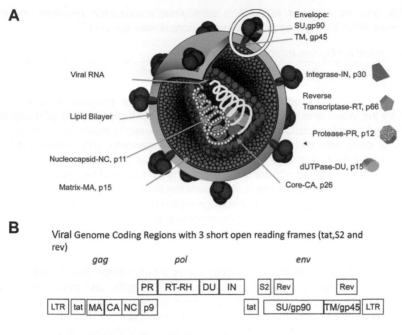

A

Envelope:
SU,gp90
TM, gp45

Viral RNA

Integrase-IN, p30

Reverse
Transcriptase-RT, p66

Lipid Bilayer

Protease-PR, p12

Nucleocapsid-NC, p11

dUTPase-DU, p15

Matrix-MA, p15

Core-CA, p26

B

Viral Genome Coding Regions with 3 short open reading frames (tat,S2 and rev)

gag   pol   env

| PR | RT-RH | DU | IN | | S2 | Rev | | Rev |

| LTR | tat | MA | CA | NC | p9 | | tat | SU/gp90 | TM/gp45 | LTR |

C   Major viral proteins for diagnosis

MW	Nomenclature	Tests using this antigen
p26	Core Antigen	AGID, ELISA, Immunoblot
gp45	Transmembrane	ELISA, Immunoblot
gp90	Surface Unit	Immunoblot

Fig. 1. (*A*) The equine infectious anemia virion structure showing location and identity of structural proteins. (*B*) The 8 kbp equine infectious anemia virus (EIAV) provirus is shown, with long terminal repeats (LTR) and protein-coding regions (*gag, pol, env, tat,* S2, and *rev*), with protein names added. (*C*) Major protein antigens of EIAV used in current commercial test kits (all p26 based; one commercial ELISA kit includes p26 and a determinant of gp45, but no discrimination is made). The immunoblot test is mainly a research test today, but can detect immune responses against all 3 major proteins of EIAV. AGID, agar gel immunodiffusion; ELISA, enzyme-linked immunosorbent assay.

functions, counter host defenses, and/or enhance pathogenicity. EIAV is again unusual in that it contains the least number of ORFs (3 compared with, eg, 4 in bovine immunodeficiency virus and 6 in HIV), giving it the simplest genome organization of any extant lentivirus (see **Fig. 1**B). Although 2 of the accessory proteins (Tat, Rev) are common to all lentiviruses, the third (S2) is unique to EIAV.[11–13] Furthermore, the equine lentivirus is the only surviving member of the genus that does not possess an additional ORF encoding a Vif orthologue. This protein is directed against important host retroviral defense proteins of the apolipoprotein β editing complex 3 family

(APOβEC3), and its absence in EIAV is somewhat unexpected because horses possess more APOβEC3 genes than any other nonprimate species.[14]

Proteins Encoded by Equine Infectious Anemia Virus

Gag/Pol

Gag and Pol proteins are produced from a genomic full-length viral mRNA. Gag proteins (see **Fig. 1**B) are produced following cleavage of a polyprotein precursor (PR55^{gag}) by the virally encoded proteinase (Pr) to yield p15 matrix (MA), p26 capsid antigen (CA), p11 nucleocapsid (NC), and the p9 "late domain" protein. These proteins form the viral core, with p11 binding to the viral RNA genome, p26 comprising the conical core structure, and p15 forming the matrix that surrounds the core (see **Fig. 1**A). In addition, p15 and p26 are essential for the formation of viral particles while p9 is critical for the release of progeny virus particles from the host cell. The Pol proteins are also produced by proteolytic cleavage (again by the viral Pr) of a polyprotein precursor (PR180$^{gag/pol}$), and consist of Pr, reverse transcriptase (RT), Integrase (IN), and other enzymes important in viral replication.

Env

The EIAV *env* gene products are also produced as a polyprotein that is cleaved by cellular endoproteinases to yield the surface unit (SU) or gp90 and transmembrane (TM) or gp45 envelope glycoproteins. These proteins are involved in binding to the cellular receptor (recently identified as equine lentivirus receptor-1 [ELR-1], a member of the tumor necrosis factor receptor family[15]) and subsequent infection of host cells.

Accessory proteins

Tat recruits host cell proteins that are essential for the elongation of nascent viral RNA transcripts by RNA Pol II while Rev promotes the nuclear export of full-length genomic and singly spliced viral RNAs. Although the mode of action of S2 is not completely understood, deletion of this accessory protein results in attenuation of EIAV, with peak viral replication rates in vivo reduced by several orders of magnitude. It is possible that S2 may enhance inflammatory cytokine production.[16–21]

Host Cells

In common with all other members of the genus, EIAV infects cells of the monocyte/macrophage lineage, although viral protein expression and progeny virus production only occur in mature tissue macrophages or dendritic cells. However, in contrast to HIV, EIAV cannot infect CD4$^+$ T-helper lymphocytes and so does not cause long-term immunodeficiency in equids. In addition, some strains may infect endothelial cells,[22] and a recent report has demonstrated EIAV antigen expression in lung epithelial cells from infected horses in Romania.[23] The significance of this finding in terms of the potential for aerosol transmission remains to be determined, although field strains of EIAV can be adapted under laboratory conditions to replicate this process in equine or canine fibroblastic cells, resulting in attenuation in vivo.

Mechanisms of Persistence

EIAV can resist immunologic and other forms of host defense, including retroviral restriction factors (RRF), to persist for life. Several strategies have evolved to achieve this goal:

- Integration of proviral DNA into host cell chromatin.
- EIAV infects monocytes but is not transcriptionally active, which permits a period of latency whereby it can be transported around the body without being subjected to immunologic surveillance.

- Innate resistance to RRFs. A recent report suggests that EIAV Env proteins are resistant to the equine orthologue of tetherin, an RRF that anchors progeny viral particles to the host cell membrane, thereby preventing them from continuing the infection.[24] It has also been suggested EIAV is resistant to equine APOβEC3 proteins.[14] However, another study has questioned this finding, instead presenting evidence that the most effective members of the APOβEC3 family against EIAV are simply not expressed in horse macrophages.[25]
- Structural resistance to neutralizing antibodies. EIAV SU is the only protein known to contain epitopes recognized by neutralizing antibodies. The fact that SU is innately resistant to this class of antibody is suggested by the finding that neutralization titers of postinfection serum samples are increased 1000- to 10,000-fold by introduction of specific amino acid substitutions within this glycoprotein.[26]
- Genetic and antigenic variation. The RT of retroviruses is error prone, and as the enzyme has no proofreading ability it is unable to correct mistakes. In the case of EIAV the error rate is such that 1 nucleotide substitution is likely to occur during each replication cycle. As mutations are also introduced by frequent recombination events between the 2 copies of genomic RNA within each virus particle, the viral population rapidly becomes a "swarm" or quasispecies consisting of many different but related genotypes. This process enables EIAV to respond quickly to selection pressure such as that from the immune system.

EPIDEMIOLOGY

EIAV has a worldwide distribution. The virus appears to infect all equids, but clinical responses depend on viral, individual host, and host species factors. For example, donkeys infected with horse-adapted EIAV strains have lower viral loads, mild or no clinical responses, and mount slower, lower antibody responses than horses infected under identical conditions.[27] Viral factors are suggested by the fact that virulence can be increased by sequential passages in vivo.[4,28]

EIAV Is a blood-borne virus that is naturally transmitted mechanically (no insect viral replication step) by blood-feeding insects (**Box 1**), especially members of the Tabanidae (horse flies and deer flies). For transmission to occur feeding must be interrupted, with the fly seeking and finding a second host to feed to repletion. Whether a fly returns to the original host or seeks a new host is determined by proximity. Experimentally it has been determined that 99% of horse flies will return to the original host if an alternative is more than 50 m away.[29] Factors controlling insect-mediated EIAV transmission include the volume of blood retained on insect mouthparts, and the time taken to reach a second host and blood-associated viral loads (see **Box 1**), with optimal conditions for transfer being high virus titers, high vector populations, and a high density of susceptible hosts. Infectious microorganisms that employ mosquitoes as vectors generally have the ability to replicate in Culicidae cells and migrate though the gut to reach the salivary gland so that they can be injected into a new host when the insect feeds. Lentiviruses do not possess these abilities, so when mosquitoes feed on EIAV-infected equids, virus particles that are ingested will be destroyed by contact with digestive enzymes. Furthermore, the volume of blood retained by mosquitoes is significantly lower than the small volumes (10 ± 5 nL) of bloodmeal residue that have been measured on the mouthparts of horse flies such as *Tabanus fuscicostatus*,[30] thereby making it unlikely the *Culicidae* are major contributors to the mechanical transmission of EIAV. However, another extremely important mode of transmission is that mediated through the actions of humans. For comparison of risks from insects and humans, see **Box 1**.

Box 1
Major factors comparing vector potential for transmitting EIAV

Vector Parameter

Vector mouthparts

- Painful bites induce defensive behavior and interrupt feeding: this favors tabanids because of mouthpart design

Individual vector

- Blood on mouthparts: Up to 0.00001 mL; probably less than 10% efficiency in transfer
- Virus content: Up to 10 50% horse infectious doses (HID_{50}) on mouthparts after partial feeding on acute case

Space and time

- Distance to second host important
- Likelihood of transmission decreases exponentially with increased distance from source after interrupted feeding
- Transit time: Virus can remain viable on mouthparts for at least 30 minutes

Human Involvement

Multiuse needles, syringes, veterinary equipment, plasma transfusions

Volume potential up to 10^7 greater than 1 horse fly feeding

Virus survival longer on needles than vector mouthparts

Summary

	Insect Vector Group			
	Tabanids	Stable Flies	Mosquitoes	Man
Overall importance	High	High	Low to None	Highest
Rate of Interrupted feeding	Highest	High	Low	No data
Blood volume transferred	High	Lower	Lower	Highest
Unassisted flight distance	Longer	Shorter	Shorter	Longest

Molecular Epidemiology

Intraisolate variation in equine infectious anemia virus

In infected equids, *gag* and *pol* are relatively conserved over time while extensive genetic variation occurs in *env* and the ORF encoding Rev.[31–34] It has been demonstrated that EIAV undergoes antigenic drift,[35,36] in that each febrile episode in an infected animal is associated with a different antigenic variant or "immunologic escape mutant." This conclusion is supported by nucleotide sequence analysis of SU isolated during sequential clinical episodes from individual horses or ponies,[34,37] and shows that most amino acid substitutions are within 8 hypervariable domains.

Interisolate variation in equine infectious anemia virus

To date only 4 complete genomic sequences from EIAV field isolates have been published (EIAV$_{LIA}$ [China], EIAV$_{IRE}$ [Ireland], EIAV$_{MIY}$ [Japan], EIAV$_{WY}$ [United States]). These sequences share 80% or more nucleotide sequence identity, with each comprising a separate clade, suggesting they all evolved independently since diverging from a common ancestor.[11–13] However, phylogenetic analysis based on more numerous available *gag* sequences (13 clades from just 23 samples) suggest the molecular epidemiology of EIAV is likely to be far more complex, posing considerable difficulties for future vaccine development programs.

Variation between EIAV isolates is not distributed evenly throughout the genome, with Gag p26 and *pol* gene products being relatively conserved (80%–89% amino acid identity), whereas amino acid identity between Gag p9 and S2 is less than 50%. Conservation of p26 is somewhat fortuitous because this antigen forms the basis for almost all commercially available serologic tests for the detection of EIAV-infected equids. Although there is significant genetic variation between isolates, most of the previously identified structural/functional motifs within viral proteins are either maintained or contain highly conservative amino acid substitutions.[11,12,38] For example, despite significant variation, the late domain in Gag p9 (tyrosine [Y], proline [P], aspartic acid [D], leucine [L]) that is implicated in the release of progeny virions from the host cell[11,12,38,39] is present in all strains analyzed to date.[11,12,38] Analysis of the immunologically important SU glycoprotein demonstrates that amino acid substitutions between strains are distributed throughout the molecule with the exception of the amino terminus. The only other conserved feature is the presence of cysteine residues, suggesting that disulfide bridges are essential to the structural and functional integrity of SU.[12]

PATHOGENESIS

Clinical disease is initially caused by proinflammatory cytokines that include tumor necrosis factor α (TNFα), interleukin-1α and -β (IL-1α, IL-1β), interleukin 6 (IL-6), and transforming growth factor β (TGFβ). These cytokines are released when viral loads reach a critical threshold level that equates experimentally with plasma-associated EIAV RNA burdens (**Fig. 2**) of 5×10^7 to 1×10^8 copies/mL[40] (or viremia exceeding 10^5 median horse infective doses per milliliter of plasma). IL-6 and TNFα induce febrile responses by activating the arachidonic pathway to increase production of prostaglandin E$_2$, while TNFα/TGFβ contribute to thrombocytopenia by suppressing

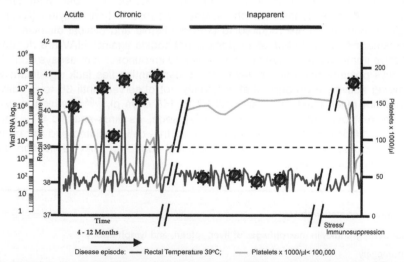

Fig. 2. Kinetics of events following intravenous inoculation of a horse with 10^3 median horse infective doses of a horse-pathogenic laboratory strain of EIAV. Virus load (plasma viremia in copies of viral RNA/mL) is designated by cartoons of virus particles. The first positive test for antibody against EIAV is shown as a + on the timeline shortly after the first febrile episode.

equine megakaryocyte growth and TNFα promotes anemia by downregulating erythropoiesis.[41–44] Furthermore, in some species TNFα induces severe thrombocytopenia by stimulating release of platelet agonists including thrombin, plasmin, and serotonin.[45] During later stages of the disease adaptive immune responses may also contribute to pathogenesis (**Box 2**) by immune-mediated destruction of antibody-coated platelets and phagocytosis of complement C3–coated erythrocytes, resulting in the presence of hemosiderin granules in macrophages and thickened glomerular tufts within the kidney caused by excess levels of C3.[46–48] Induction of oxidative stress produced by changes in glutathione peroxidase and uric acid levels may also play a role in the pathogenesis of EIAV infections by escalating inflammatory responses while simultaneously decreasing immune cell proliferation.[49]

CLINICAL SIGNS

That EIA can have 3 distinct clinical phases designated acute (first disease episode), chronic (multiple sequential disease episodes), and inapparent (see **Fig. 2**; **Table 1**) was first described in 1904.[1] Depending on the virulence and inoculum size of the infecting EIAV strain, acute disease can occur following a 1- to 4-week incubation period. However, signs of disease may be completely absent, or limited to mild febrile episodes that go undetected. When they do occur (see **Fig. 2**), the most common acute clinical signs include fever, thrombocytopenia, lethargy, and inappetance. In severe cases, petechiation, hemolytic anemia, and epistaxis can occur. Classical chronic disease signs include anemia, thrombocytopenia, weight loss, dependent edema, and occasionally neurologic signs (ataxia and/or encephalitis) (see earlier discussion for pathologic lesions that may be associated with EIA).

HOST IMMUNE RESPONSES

Studies in horses with severe combined immunodeficiency (SCID), which have intact innate immunity but lack functional B and T lymphocytes, have demonstrated that adaptive immune responses (which include cytotoxic T lymphocytes [CTL] and neutralizing antibodies) are required to control viremia and clinical disease.[50–53] In experimental infections in horses or ponies, antibodies against EIAV are detectable in sensitive immunoblot assays or enzyme-linked immunosorbent assays (ELISA) 14 to 28 days postinfection (pi). However, these early antibodies lack significant viral-neutralizing activity, a property that is usually not observed until 38 to 87 days pi and may not reach maximal levels until 90 to 148 days pi,[35,54,55] which is usually long after resolution of the acute disease episode. As virus-specific CTL can be detected at 14 days pi,[56] it is currently believed that cell-mediated and not humoral immune responses are responsible for the initial control of EIAV replication, along with alleviating clinical signs.

Box 2
Pathology associated with EIA
Hemosiderin granules in macrophages of liver, spleen, and lymph nodes
Splenomegaly
Hepatomegaly (nonsupportive hepatitis with periportal lymphocytic/monocytic infiltration)
Glomerulonephritis (immune complex deposition)
Interstitial lung lesions

Table 1
Three clinical phases of EIA

Phase	Viral Loads	Predominant Clinical Signs
Acute (transient)	High ($\geq 5 \times 10^7$ viral RNA copies or $\geq 10^5$ HID_{50}/mL blood)	Fever ($\geq 102.5°F$, $39°C$) Thrombocytopenia
Chronic (≥ 12 mo) ($\geq 102.5°F$, $39°C$)	High ($\geq 5 \times 10^7$ viral RNA copies or $\geq 10^5$ HID_{50}/mL blood)	Multiple sequential fever episodes Thrombocytopenia Anemia Edema Neurologic depression Cachexia Petechial hemorrhages
Inapparent (months to years)	Low ($\leq 10^2$ viral RNA copies/mL blood)	No overt signs

Initial mammalian immune responses are limited by the phenomenon of immunodominance to just a few of the many potential epitopes that are present within microbial organisms.[57–59] Although such restricted host immune responses seem to be sufficient against most infectious agents, they may constitute a weakness that is exploited by highly mutable pathogens such as EIAV, because only a relatively few genetic substitutions are required in the viral genome for escape from immunologic surveillance. As mentioned earlier, viruses associated with each new febrile episode are not neutralized by antibodies generated against previous virus isolates from the same infected equid. Furthermore, not all immune responses are created equal, in that control of viral loads and clinical disease is often associated with CTL that bind to their respective epitopes with high avidity, whereas those that have weaker binding are significantly less effective. It has been observed that epitopes recognized by high-avidity CTL are subject to rapid mutational changes in EIAV-infected individuals, whereas those bound by their less avid counterparts may persist for years.[56,60]

The ability of EIAV to evade initial immunodominant-restricted responses forces the equid host into a cycle of "catch-up" whereby its immune system must respond to the emergence of each new antigenic viral variant. However, this cycle can be broken by maturation and broadening of the immune response. There is increased recognition in terms of the number of epitopes associated with cell-mediated immune responses while humoral immune responses evolve from low-avidity interactions with linear epitopes, to high-avidity binding, to more conformational epitopes.[54] Furthermore, transition from the chronic to the inapparent clinical phase of EIA is associated with a switch from strain-specific to cross-reactive neutralizing antibodies.[35,61] If present at high enough titer before infection, these cross reactive or broadly neutralizing antibodies have the potential to protect against genetically diverse EIAV strains.[50,53] Overall, the fact active immune responses are required for maintenance of the inapparent carrier state is demonstrated by the fact immunosuppression with corticosteroids results in a significant increase in plasma-associated viral loads and, very often, recrudescence of clinical disease.[62–64]

DIAGNOSIS

As no pathognomonic signs or lesions exist for EIA, reliance on laboratory tests is imperative. Traditional virus isolation techniques using equine monocyte–derived macrophage cultures are not practical because of viability coupled with sensitivity issues, and no laboratories offer this service. Several systems based on the polymerase chain reaction (PCR) technique have been developed to detect EIAV genetic material (directly in the case of proviral DNA or coupled with an RT step with viral RNA), and some have been used successfully with field isolates.[38,65–68] However, before these techniques can be adopted routinely it must be shown: (1) that the primers (and probes) used in these assays are located in highly conserved regions of the viral genome, as variation in these sequences can either prevent or significantly reduce the sensitivity of detection; and (2) that PCR-based techniques are sensitive enough to detect the extremely low levels of EIAV-specific nucleic acids present in some inapparent carrier animals. Unfortunately there is no conclusive evidence demonstrating that any of the PCR-based assays described to date meets these criteria. Therefore, current diagnostic techniques for EIA are reliant on serologic detection (see **Fig. 1**C). Although this is an indirect approach and is unable to detect recent infections before the development of antibodies, it is the only viable option at present.

In many countries the only officially recognized test for diagnosis of EIAV infections is the AGIDT. However, in some countries such as the United States, several commercial ELISA-based tests are also approved for use. Furthermore, the United States permits the immunoblot (or Western blot) assay to be used as a supplemental test at specific reference laboratories (National Veterinary Services Laboratories and University of Kentucky) to reach consensus when other diagnostic tests have yielded contradictory results. The immunoblot test has proved to be highly sensitive and capable of detecting antibodies directed against 3 major EIAV antigens (p26, gp90, gp45; see **Fig. 1**C).

Although the AGIDT is highly specific, it is relatively insensitive. Recent studies conducted in Italy demonstrated that the number of EIA positive cases identified increased by 17% when serum samples were screened by ELISA instead of AGIDT.[69,70] Results from these studies have prompted the development of a 3-tiered testing scheme for EIA. In this scheme, all samples are screened by ELISA tests with those found positive for EIA are confirmed by AGIDT. In the few cases where these results do not agree, additional immunoblot tests are performed. Thus, the sensitivity of ELISA tests is combined with the specificity of the AGIDT and the power of the immunoblot test for the accurate diagnosis of EIA.

THERAPEUTIC STRATEGIES

Supportive therapy may be administered to aid in recovery from febrile episodes and associated signs. Treatment with corticosteroids is contraindicated because of the resultant increase in viral load and clinical disease. Because supportive therapy has no effect on the virus itself and the virus persists for life, most bodies including the American Association of Equine Practitioners (AAEP) recommend the humane destruction of EIAV test–positive equids.

CONTROL STRATEGIES

There are currently no vaccines against EIAV in clinical use. Major impediments to developing a uniformly effective EIAV vaccine include tremendous strain diversity worldwide, antigenic variation, neutralization resistance, periodic viral latency, and proviral integration into the host genome. Although experimental inactivated, subunit, and recombinant vaccines have had variable or disappointing results, an experimental live attenuated vaccine has shown efficacy against challenge.[71–73] A live attenuated vaccine was developed in China in the 1970s by serial passage of a virulent virus strain through donkey leukocyte cultures.[74] This vaccine was used in millions of Chinese horses between 1975 and 1990 and was credited with controlling EIA in China, after which the vaccine program was discontinued.[74–77] The protective immunity elicited by these live vaccines most likely involves broadly active CTL, helper T-cell, and neutralizing antibody responses. Although attenuated EIAV vaccines can protect against viremia and clinical disease, they do not guarantee sterile protection in every vaccinate, and vaccine strains can persist in vivo. Because of the interference with diagnostic testing, in addition to the potential for modified live viruses to revert to virulence (a concern for lentiviruses given their ability to mutate and recombine), vaccination is not a component of current EIA control strategies. It is possible that continued research will lead to a future vaccine, perhaps a novel viral vectored vaccine that overcomes the aforementioned obstacles. This vaccine might play a role in future EIA control programs, especially in endemic countries.

In the absence of effective immune-prophylactic approaches, breaking the cycle of transmission depends on detection and removal (euthanasia or lifelong segregation) of infected equids. Segregation generally entails application of a permanent form of visible identification coupled with keeping the infected animal 200 m from all other equids, as at this distance it is generally accepted that blood-feeding insect vectors will invariably return to the original and will not seek an alternative host should feeding be interrupted. As these required constraints cannot usually be met, most owners opt for humane destruction as recommended by the AAEP and other regulatory bodies. In some jurisdictions, mandatory destruction is required.

Insect-mediated mechanical transmission of EIAV is not efficient, as blood contamination of insect mouthparts is generally below one hundred thousandth of a milliliter of blood. This figure is especially relevant in the case of inapparent carriers where viremia levels may be less than one 50% horse-infective dose per milliliter (HID_{50}/mL). In limited studies under field conditions whereby human involvement was strictly controlled, transmission between adult reproductively active inapparent carriers and sentinels was minimal and progeny were raised free of the infection at a high rate, even in areas of high vector pressures. However, intervention by man can radically alter this situation, especially in areas of the world where education about transmission of infectious diseases is lacking. That being said, even the best education can be ignored, as most cases in well-publicized outbreaks in 2006 appeared to be mediated by man, including veterinarians.

If control of EIA in highly mobile populations (where testing is required in most areas) is the goal, the test and segregate/remove strategy has been proved to be very successful (witness the statistics in the United States available in the USDA video[78]). If eradication of EIA is the goal, different approaches must be taken. This statement is made because in many countries of the world where EIA is endemic, working equid inapparent carriers may be required as agricultural animals, and their testing and removal without compensation may not be possible or practical. In these circumstances, other strategies must be used.

SUMMARY

Four questions are posed in the introduction of this review. It is hoped that it will be apparent from the foregoing discussion that almost all new cases of EIA are inapparent carriers and are associated with host-mediated, long-term control of viral replication. Although the mechanisms associated with this control are not fully understood, they depend on active immune responses, as shown by higher viral loads and frequent recrudescence of disease following corticosteroid induced immunosuppression.

EIA control programs in the United States have been effective, although they are now at a crossroads in that the mobile and tested population is mostly segregated and, therefore, at a low risk from untested equids that constitute the remaining reservoir for EIAV. Consequently, the goals of testing should be reexamined; "smarter" testing should be conducted by increasing the intervals between tests for frequently tested equid populations and the development of strategies for increased testing of the untested reservoir population. In many areas, required testing at change of ownership has proved invaluable in the identification of new cases. In areas of the world where working equids are still important agricultural animals and EIA is endemic, strategies other than destruction without compensation must be developed if control of EIA in more than localized situations is the goal.

Recent evidence, particularly from the Italian National Surveillance Program, demonstrates that EIA diagnostic approaches based on AGIDT alone can generate up to 17% false-negative results. In this situation veterinarians are clearly not doing their best to detect EIA when samples are submitted to the laboratory. Although our armamentarium of laboratory tools for EIA diagnostics is currently limited to serologic tests, accuracy can be dramatically improved by adoption of a 3-tier system in which samples are initially screened by EIA-ELISA, with test-positives confirmed by AGIDT and those producing discordant results analyzed using the immunoblot test. However, even the best serologic diagnostic tests cannot detect very recent infections before humoral responses have developed. Therefore, additional research is required to improve direct detection techniques such as PCR-based methods for amplification of EIAV genetic material.

Finally, what can veterinarians do in their practices and hospitals to reduce the chance that they are contributing to the spread of blood-borne infections? The most important recommendation is to assume that all equid contacts are infected with EIAV. Although this seems to be out of proportion to the risk, it is the authors' belief that making this assumption is the only way to effectively adopt and faithfully follow methods designed to minimize and eliminate the risk. This point was brought into sharp focus during the outbreak of EIA in Ireland in 2006. Unfortunately the virus was not on the radar, as there had not been a serologic test–positive case in the country since the 1970s. As a result, several horses became infected through iatrogenic means. The equine community would be wise to develop and adopt standard or universal precautions similar to those adopted after the advent of AIDS, especially in reference to transmission of EIA, piroplasmosis, Theiler disease, and other blood-borne conditions.

REFERENCES

1. Vallee H, Carre H. Sur la natur infectieuse de l'anenie du cheval. CR Acad Sci 1904;139:331–3.
2. Stein CD, Lotze JC, Mott LO. Transmission of equine infectious anemia by the stablefly, Stomoxys calcitrans, the horsefly, Tabanus sulcifrons (Macquart), and by injection of minute amounts of virus. Am J Vet Res 1942;3:183–93.
3. Coggins L, Norcross NL, Nusbaum SR. Diagnosis of equine infectious anemia by immunodiffusion test. Am J Vet Res 1972;33(1):11–8.
4. Kemeny LJ, Mott LO, Pearson JE. Titration of equine infectious anemia virus. Effect of dosage on incubation time and clinical signs. Cornell Vet 1971;61(4):687–95.
5. Cook RF, Leroux C, Issel CJ. Equine infectious anemia and equine infectious anemia virus in 2013: a review. Vet Microbiol 2013;167(1–2):181–204.
6. Leroux C, Cadore JL, Montelaro RC. Equine infectious anemia virus (EIAV): what has HIV's country cousin got to tell us? Vet Res 2004;35(4):485–512.

7. Montagnier L, Dauguet C, Axler C, et al. A new type of retrovirus isolated from patients presenting with lymphadenopathy and acquired immune deficiency syndrome: structural and antigenic relatedness with equine infectious anemia virus. Annales de Virologie Paris 1984;135(1):119–34.

8. Gelmann EP, Popovic M, Blayney D, et al. Proviral DNA of a retrovirus, human T-cell leukemia virus, in two patients with AIDS. Science 1983;220(4599):862–5.

9. Matheka HD, Coggins L, Shively JN, et al. Purification and characterization of equine infectious anemia virus. Arch Virol 1976;51(1–2):107–14.

10. Weiland F, Matheka HD, Coggins L, et al. Electron microscopic studies on equine infectious anemia virus (EIAV). Arch Virol 1977;55(4):335–40 Ref.

11. Dong JB, Zhu W, Cook FR, et al. Identification of a novel equine infectious anemia virus field strain isolated from feral horses in southern Japan. J Gen Virol 2013;94(Pt 2):360–5.

12. Quinlivan M, Cook F, Kenna R, et al. Genetic characterization by composite sequence analysis of a new pathogenic field strain of equine infectious anemia virus from the 2006 outbreak in Ireland. J Gen Virol 2013;94(Pt 3):612–22.

13. Liang H, He X, Shen RX, et al. Combined amino acid mutations occurring in the envelope closely correlate with pathogenicity of EIAV. Arch Virol 2006;151(7): 1387–403.

14. Bogerd HP, Tallmadge RL, Oaks JL, et al. Equine infectious anemia virus resists the antiretroviral activity of equine APOBEC3 proteins through a packaging-independent mechanism. J Virol 2008;82(23):11889–901.

15. Zhang B, Jin S, Jin J, et al. A tumor necrosis factor receptor family protein serves as a cellular receptor for the macrophage-tropic equine lentivirus. Proceedings of the National Academy of Sciences of the United States of America 2005;102(28):9918–23.

16. Dorn P, DaSilva L, Martarano L, et al. Equine infectious anemia virus tat: insights into the structure, function, and evolution of lentivirus trans-activator proteins. J Virol 1990;64(4):1616–24.

17. Belshan M, Harris ME, Shoemaker AE, et al. Biological characterization of Rev variation in equine infectious anemia virus. J Virol 1998;72(5):4421–6.

18. Belshan M, Park GS, Bilodeau P, et al. Binding of equine infectious anemia virus rev to an exon splicing enhancer mediates alternative splicing and nuclear export of viral mRNAs. Mol Cell Biol 2000;20(10):3550–7.

19. Li F, Puffer BA, Montelaro RC, et al. The S2 gene of equine infectious anemia virus is dispensable for viral replication in vitro. J Virol 1998;72(10):8344–8, 8330 ref.

20. Li F, Leroux C, Craigo JK, et al. The S2 gene of equine infectious anemia virus is a highly conserved determinant of viral replication and virulence properties in experimentally infected ponies. J Virol 2000;74(1):573–9.

21. Covaleda L, Fuller FJ, Payne SL. EIAV S2 enhances pro-inflammatory cytokine and chemokine response in infected macrophages. Virology 2010;397(1): 217–23.

22. Maury W, Thompson RJ, Jones Q, et al. Evolution of the equine infectious anemia virus long terminal repeat during the alteration of cell tropism. J Virol 2005; 79(9):5653–64.

23. Bolfa P, Nolf M, Cadore JL, et al. Interstitial lung disease associated with Equine Infectious Anemia Virus infection in horses. Vet Res 2013;44:113.

24. Yin X, Hu Z, Gu Q, et al. Equine tetherin blocks retrovirus release and its activity is antagonized by equine infectious anemia virus envelope protein. J Virol 2014; 88(2):1259–70.

25. Zielonka J, Bravo IG, Marino D, et al. Restriction of equine infectious anemia virus by equine APOBEC3 cytidine deaminases. J Virol 2009;83(15):7547–59.
26. Cook RF, Berger SL, Rushlow KE, et al. Enhanced sensitivity to neutralizing antibodies in a variant of equine infectious anemia virus is linked to amino acid substitutions in the surface unit envelope glycoprotein. J Virol 1995;69(3):1493–9.
27. Cook SJ, Cook RF, Montelaro RC, et al. Differential responses of *Equus caballus* and *Equus asinus* to infection with two pathogenic strains of equine infectious anemia virus. Vet Microbiol 2001;79(2):93–109.
28. Rwambo PM, Issel CJ, Hussain KA, et al. In vitro isolation of a neutralization escape mutant of equine infectious anemia virus (EIAV). Arch Virol 1990; 111(3–4):275–80.
29. Issel CJ, Foil LD. Studies on equine infectious anemia virus transmission by insects. J Am Vet Med Assoc 1984;184(3):293–7.
30. Foil LD, Adams WV, McManus JM, et al. Bloodmeal residues on mouthparts of *Tabanus fuscicostatus* (Diptera: Tabanidae) and the potential for mechanical transmission of pathogens. J Med Entomol 1987;24(6):613–6.
31. Belshan M, Baccam P, Oaks JL, et al. Genetic and biological variation in equine infectious anemia virus Rev correlates with variable stages of clinical disease in an experimentally infected pony. Virology 2001;279(1):185–200.
32. Salinovich O, Payne SL, Montelaro RC, et al. Rapid emergence of novel antigenic and genetic variants of equine infectious anemia virus during persistent infection. J Virol 1986;57(1):71–80.
33. Leroux C, Hammond SA, Singh M, et al. Recurring nature of equine infectious anemia (EIA) is associated with dynamic evolution in the principal neutralizing domain (PND) of the EIAV surface glycoprotein. Proceedings of the 8th International Conference on Equine Infectious Diseases. Newmarket, United Kingdom: R&W Publications (Newmarket) Ltd; 1999. p. 404–5.
34. Zheng YH, Sentsui H, Nakaya T, et al. In vivo dynamics of equine infectious anemia viruses emerging during febrile episodes: insertions/duplications at the principal neutralizing domain. J Virol 1997;71(7):5031–9.
35. Rwambo PM, Issel CJ, Adams WV, et al. Equine infectious anemia virus (EIAV) humoral responses of recipient ponies and antigenic variation during persistent infection. Arch Virol 1990;111(3–4):199–212.
36. Kono Y. Antigenic variation of equine infectious anemia virus as detected by virus neutralization. Brief report. Arch Virol 1988;98(1–2):91–7.
37. Leroux C, Issel CJ, Montelaro RC. Novel and dynamic evolution of equine infectious anemia virus genomic quasispecies associated with sequential disease cycles in an experimentally infected pony. J Virol 1997;71(12):9627–39.
38. Capomaccio S, Willand ZA, Cook SJ, et al. Detection, molecular characterization and phylogenetic analysis of full-length equine infectious anemia (EIAV) gag genes isolated from Shackleford Banks wild horses. Vet Microbiol 2012; 157(3–4):320–32.
39. Puffer BA, Parent LJ, Wills JW, et al. Equine infectious anemia virus utilizes a YXXL motif within the late assembly domain of the GAP p9 protein. J Virol 1997;71(9):6541–6.
40. Cook RF, Cook SJ, Berger SL, et al. Enhancement of equine infectious anemia virus virulence by identification and removal of suboptimal nucleotides. Virology 2003;313(2):588–603.
41. Tornquist SJ, Oaks JL, Crawford TB. Elevation of cytokines associated with the thrombocytopenia of equine infectious anaemia. J Gen Virol 1997;78(Pt 10): 2541–8.

42. Sellon DC, Russell KE, Monroe VL, et al. Increased interleukin-6 activity in the serum of ponies acutely infected with equine infectious anaemia virus. Res Vet Sci 1999;66(1):77–80.

43. Costa LR, Santos IK, Issel CJ, et al. Tumor necrosis factor-alpha production and disease severity after immunization with enriched major core protein (p26) and/or infection with equine infectious anemia virus. Vet Immunol Immunopathol 1997;57(1–2):33–47.

44. Tornquist SJ, Crawford TB. Suppression of megakaryocyte colony growth by plasma from foals infected with equine infectious anemia virus. Blood 1997; 90(6):2357–63.

45. Tacchini-Cottier F, Vesin C, Redard M, et al. Role of TNFR1 and TNFR2 in TNF-induced platelet consumption in mice. J Immunol 1998;160(12):6182–6.

46. Sentsui H, Kono Y. Phagocytosis of horse erythrocytes treated with equine infectious anemia virus by cultivated horse leukocytes. Arch Virol 1987;95(1–2):67–78.

47. Perryman LE, McGuire TC, Banks KL, et al. Decreased C3 levels in a chronic virus infection: equine infectious anemia. J Immunol 1971;106(4):1074–8.

48. Henson JB, McGuire TC. Immunopathology of equine infectious anemia. Am J Clin Pathol 1971;56(3):306–13.

49. Bolfa PF, Leroux C, Pintea A, et al. Oxidant-antioxidant imbalance in horses infected with equine infectious anaemia virus. Vet J 2012;192(3):449–54.

50. Taylor SD, Leib SR, Wu W, et al. Protective effects of broadly neutralizing immunoglobulin against homologous and heterologous equine infectious anemia virus infection in horses with severe combined immunodeficiency. J Virol 2011; 85(13):6814–8.

51. Perryman LE, O'Rourke KI, McGuire TC. Immune responses are required to terminate viremia in equine infectious anemia lentivirus infection. J Virol 1988; 62(8):3073–6.

52. Mealey R, Fraser D, Oaks J, et al. Immune reconstitution prevents continuous equine infectious anemia virus replication in an Arabian foal with severe combined immunodeficiency: Lessons for control of lentiviruses. Clin Immunol 2001;101(2):237–47.

53. Taylor SD, Leib SR, Carpenter S, et al. Selection of a rare neutralization-resistant variant following passive transfer of convalescent immune plasma in equine infectious anemia virus-challenged SCID horses. J Virol 2010;84(13):6536–48.

54. Hammond SA, Cook SJ, Lichtenstein DL, et al. Maturation of the cellular and humoral immune responses to persistent infection in horses by equine infectious anemia virus is a complex and lengthy process. J Virol 1997;71(5):3840–52.

55. Ball JM, Rushlow KE, Issel CJ, et al. Detailed mapping of the antigenicity of the surface unit glycoprotein of equine infectious anemia virus by using synthetic peptide strategies. J Virol 1992;66(2):732–42.

56. Mealey RH, Sharif A, Ellis SA, et al. Early detection of dominant Env-specific and subdominant Gag-specific CD8+ lymphocytes in equine infectious anemia virus-infected horses using major histocompatibility complex class I/peptide tetrameric complexes. Virology 2005;339(1):110–26.

57. Busch DH, Pamer EG. MHC class I/peptide stability: implications for immunodominance, in vitro proliferation, and diversity of responding CTL. J Immunol 1998; 160(9):4441–8.

58. Borysiewicz LK, Hickling JK, Graham S, et al. Human cytomegalovirus-specific cytotoxic T cells. Relative frequency of stage-specific CTL recognizing the 72-kD immediate early protein and glycoprotein B expressed by recombinant vaccinia viruses. J Exp Med 1988;168(3):919–31.

59. Kedl RM, Kappler JW, Marrack P. Epitope dominance, competition and T cell affinity maturation. Curr Opin Immunol 2003;15(1):120–7.

60. Mealey RH, Zhang B, Leib SR, et al. Epitope specificity is critical for high and moderate avidity cytotoxic T lymphocytes associated with control of viral load and clinical disease in horses with equine infectious anemia virus. Virology 2003;313(2):537–52.

61. Sponseller BA, Sparks WO, Wannemuehler Y, et al. Immune selection of equine infectious anemia virus env variants during the long-term inapparent stage of disease. Virology 2007;363(1):156–65.

62. Tumas DB, Hines MT, Perryman LE, et al. Corticosteroid immunosuppression and monoclonal antibody-mediated CD5+ T lymphocyte depletion in normal and equine infectious anaemia virus-carrier horses. J Gen Virol 1994;75(Pt 5): 959–68.

63. Kono Y, Hirasawa K, Fukunaga Y, et al. Recrudescence of equine infectious anemia by treatment with immunosuppressive drugs. Natl Inst Anim Health Q (Tokyo) 1976;16(1):8–15.

64. Craigo JK, Durkin S, Sturgeon TJ, et al. Immune suppression of challenged vaccinates as a rigorous assessment of sterile protection by lentiviral vaccines. Vaccine 2007;25(5):834–45.

65. Cappelli K, Capomaccio S, Cook FR, et al. Molecular detection, epidemiology, and genetic characterization of novel European field isolates of equine infectious anemia virus. J Clin Microbiol 2011;49(1):27–33.

66. Dong JB, Zhu W, Cook FR, et al. Development of a nested PCR assay to detect equine infectious anemia proviral DNA from peripheral blood of naturally infected horses. Arch Virol 2012;157(11):2105–11.

67. Nagarajan MM, Simard C. Detection of horses infected naturally with equine infectious anemia virus by nested polymerase chain reaction. J Virol Methods 2001;94(1–2):97–109.

68. Quinlivan M, Cook RF, Cullinane A. Real-time quantitative RT-PCR and PCR assays for a novel European field isolate of equine infectious anaemia virus based on sequence determination of the gag gene. Vet Rec 2007;160(18): 611–8.

69. Scicluna MT, Issel CJ, Cook FR, et al. Is a diagnostic system based exclusively on agar gel immunodiffusion adequate for controlling the spread of equine infectious anaemia? Vet Microbiol 2013;165(1–2):123–34.

70. Issel CJ, Scicluna MT, Cook SJ, et al. Challenges and proposed solutions for more accurate serological diagnosis of equine infectious anaemia. Vet Rec 2013;172(8):210.

71. Craigo JK, Li F, Steckbeck JD, et al. Discerning an effective balance between equine infectious anemia virus attenuation and vaccine efficacy. J Virol 2005; 79(5):2666–77.

72. Li F, Craigo JK, Howe L, et al. A live attenuated equine infectious anemia virus proviral vaccine with a modified S2 gene provides protection from detectable infection by intravenous virulent virus challenge of experimentally inoculated horses. J Virol 2003;77(13):7244–53.

73. Craigo JK, Zhang B, Barnes S, et al. Envelope variation as a primary determinant of lentiviral vaccine efficacy. Proceedings of the National Academy of Sciences of the United States of America 2007;104(38):15105–10.

74. Shen DT. Equine infectious anemia vaccine. In: Salzman LA, editor. Animal models of retrovirus infection and their relationship to AIDS. Orlando (FL): Academic Press; 1986. p. 387–92.

75. Zhang X, Wang Y, Liang H, et al. Correlation between the induction of Th1 cytokines by an attenuated equine infectious anemia virus vaccine and protection against disease progression. J Gen Virol 2007;88(Pt 3):998–1004.
76. Lin YZ, Shen RX, Zhu ZY, et al. An attenuated EIAV vaccine strain induces significantly different immune responses from its pathogenic parental strain although with similar in vivo replication pattern. Antiviral Res 2011;92(2):292–304.
77. Shen T, Liang H, Tong X, et al. Amino acid mutations of the infectious clone from Chinese EIAV attenuated vaccine resulted in reversion of virulence. Vaccine 2006;24(6):738–49.
78. Available at: http://mfile3.akamai.com/88068/wmv/ocbmtcmedia.download.akamai.com/88068/aphis/EIA_final_HDCAP.asx. Accessed September 26, 2014.

Hendra Virus

Deborah Middleton, BVSc, MVSc, PhD

KEYWORDS

- Hendra • Horse • Pathogenesis • Vaccine • Emerging • Zoonotic • Infectious
- Disease

KEY POINTS

- Hendra virus infection is a serious emerging zoonosis, and human infection is acquired through contact with acutely infected horses.
- The natural reservoirs of Hendra virus are Australian mainland flying foxes, and horses are infected following exposure to flying fox secretions.
- The increasing number of equine outbreaks and associated human risk exposures exacerbate community concerns and heighten pressure to cull flying fox populations.
- Use of an inactivated Hendra virus subunit vaccine in horses reduces the potential for virus replication and thus the risk of transmission of infection to people.
- Improved infection control procedures and a heightened awareness of the possibility of Hendra virus infection need to be maintained for dealing with sick horses, particularly those whose vaccination status is uncertain.

EMERGENCE

Hendra virus (HeV) is a zoonotic paramyxovirus that emerged in 1994 in the Brisbane suburb of Hendra, Queensland, Australia.[1] It was the first member to be characterized within a new viral genus Henipavirus in the order Mononegavirales and family Paramyxoviridae, wherein it forms a distinct clade with Nipah virus and Cedar virus.[2,3] HeV was initially isolated from equine lung tissue during investigation of an outbreak of severe febrile respiratory disease in horses that led to the natural death or euthanasia of 14 out of 21 affected animals. Two people (a horse trainer and a stablehand) who had close contact with the infected horses developed an influenza-like illness (ILI), and one of these patients died with severe interstitial pneumonia. HeV was also isolated from the kidney of the fatal human case. On inoculation into experimental horses, HeV induced a similar disease to that observed in the field; the virus was able

Funding Sources: National Health and Medical Research Council grants 1022516, National Institutes of Health grants U01-A107795, Commonwealth of Australia, Queensland State Government, Intergovernmental Hendra Virus Taskforce.
Conflict of Interest: Nil.
Australian Animal Health Laboratory, CSIRO, PB 24, Geelong, Victoria 3220, Australia
E-mail address: Deborah.middleton@csiro.au

to be reisolated from their tissues including lung, kidney, and lymph nodes thereby confirming that HeV was the etiologic agent of the field event.

There were further sporadic HeV outbreaks in horses between 1994 and 2010, with 14 events identified overall each involving up to five horses; all occurred in coastal Queensland or the northeastern corner of New South Wales (NSW) (**Fig. 1**A). Then, during 2011 and 2012, there were 26 HeV incidents in horses including the first case west of the Great Dividing Range (**Fig. 1**B). Together with discovery of the first field infection in a dog on a property undergoing a HeV disease investigation[4] these events substantially raised the community profile of HeV infection as an unmanaged emerging zoonotic disease. The following year saw eight HeV incidents overall and, for the first time, equal numbers of equine cases were seen in NSW as Queensland. A second canine case was also found on an outbreak property.[5]

ZOONOTIC INFECTION

There have been five HeV outbreaks in horses that have been associated with transmission of infection to people, and there is a strong epidemiologic connection between infection of people and direct contact with horses. Six of the seven affected humans have been exposed to the blood or secretions of terminally ill horses or have been contaminated with body fluids during postmortem examination of infected horses; three were veterinarians. In the seventh patient, a veterinary nurse, the high-risk exposure was assessed to have occurred while performing daily nasal cavity lavage (for management of another condition) on a horse during the last 3 days of its HeV incubation period.[6] The HeV attack rate for people exposed to potentially

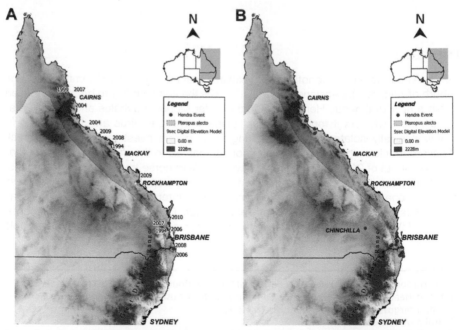

Fig. 1. (A) Locations of HeV events between 1994 and 2010 highlighting the distribution of *Pteropus alecto* and the low-lying coastal regions on the nine-section digital elevation model. (B) Locations of HeV events between 2011 and 2013 highlighting the distribution of *P alecto*; the low-lying coastal regions on the nine-sec digital elevation model; and Chinchilla, the first case west of the Great Dividing Range.

infected equine body fluids has been estimated at 10%.[6] HeV infection in people has an estimated incubation period of 9 to 16 days and is associated with ILI that can progress to encephalitis, which may be fatal. The current human case fatality rate is 57%, with death of one patient attributed to multiorgan failure (with interstitial pneumonia) and the remainder to encephalitis. In one of these individuals, the episode of encephalitis that proved fatal had been preceded 13 months earlier by an ILI with meningitis from which he seemed to have made a full recovery.[7] Serum obtained during both illnesses was positive for neutralizing antibodies to HeV and for viral genome, and HeV antigen was identified in brain at necropsy. Relapsing encephalitis may also occur in people infected with the closely related Nipah virus,[8] the second of only three viruses isolated within the Henipavirus genus. At present it is unclear whether recrudescence of central nervous system disease, presumably as a complication of virus persistence in the central nervous system, is a feature of Henipavirus infection in species other than humans. Currently there is no evidence for long-term viral shedding in survivors of HeV infection.[9]

THE VIRAL RESERVOIR

A serologic study conducted soon after the discovery of HeV did not show evidence of neutralizing antibody in the Queensland horse population suggesting that the virus was not being maintained within this species, and so the possibility of another source for the virus was investigated.[10] In an initial survey, sera from 46 species including 34 species of fauna were sampled and none were positive for antibody against HeV, but extension of the work to fruit bats (flying foxes) revealed a seroprevalence of more than 25% in these animals.[11] There are four species of mainland Australian flying fox, namely the grey-headed flying fox (*Pteropus poliocephalus*), black flying fox (*P alecto*), little red flying fox (*P scapulatus*), and the spectacled flying fox (*P conspicillatus*) and there is serologic evidence that each harbors HeV. Interestingly, all spillover events to horses have occurred within the natural range of the black flying fox, and transmission from any other flying fox species cannot account for each and every recognized equine infection (see **Fig. 1**).[12]

In free-living bats, HeV was first isolated from a fetus (*P alecto*) and a fetus and uterine fluid (*P poliocephalus*)[13] and subsequently also from urine collected beneath flying fox roosts.[14] Although these findings are consistent with systemic infection of flying foxes by HeV, no associated clinically significant disease has been recognized in them. These observations have been reinforced by experimental studies in *P poliocephalus* and *P alecto*,[15–17] wherein no clinical abnormalities were recorded, although sporadic virally induced vasculitis was identified in some animals, including in the placenta of a pregnant *P poliocephalus*. Although in these studies HeV was also reisolated from a fetus and sporadically from pregnant animals, the data overall did not support pregnancy as a significant factor in increasing shedding or transmission opportunity.

Similarly, a longitudinal field study of the occurrence HeV RNA in pooled bat urine from under roosts found that shedding varied from year to year, occurred periodically and at any time of the year, and that HeV was not present in all flying fox colonies all the time.[18] These authors also observed that positive findings for HeV in bat urine did not associate in time with spillover events to horses, consistent with a requirement for other factors to precipitate such transmission. The identity of these factors is currently unknown.

HENDRA VIRUS INFECTION IN HORSES

HeV infection of horses is believed to be acquired following direct exposure to the virus in flying fox secretions; however, the precise way in which this occurs is not known.

The infection is sporadic, commonly involving only a single horse within a group. Occasional multihorse outbreaks where there is evidence of horse-to-horse transmission (most likely via contamination of surfaces or equipment by infectious fluids) have permitted an estimation of the field incubation period between 4 and 16 days.[1,19,20] There is an acute onset of disease, with fever, depression, inappetance, tachycardia, tachypnea, dyspnea, facial edema, aimless pacing, muscle fasciculation, and ataxia; death follows within 48 to 72 hours in approximately 75% of cases. In animals that are terminally ill a copious frothy nasal discharge may also be seen as a reflection of severe pulmonary edema. Some affected horses may be found dead. In horses that survive the acute infection clinical recovery may seem to be complete but, because the current national policy is to euthanize convalescent horses, no long-term follow-up has been carried out on such cases, especially with respect to the potential for recrudescence of virus replication in the central nervous system.

Both neurologic and respiratory signs have been a feature of HeV infection in horses since the original outbreak in 1994 where, although the dominant clinical presentation was respiratory disease, two convalescent seropositive horses exhibited myoclonic twitches.[21] However, in later years the appearance of field cases of acute HeV infection were even more strongly associated with signs that localized to the respiratory system. Combined with the nonspecific nature of many other clinical signs, differential diagnosis (especially from more common disorders, such as pneumonia, pleuropneumonia, and colic) was and remains challenging and complex. In contrast to a respiratory syndrome presentation, a multihorse outbreak developed in an equine referral practice in 2008 where the predominant clinical signs were attributable to involvement of the central nervous system.[22] These included ataxia, disorientation, hypersensitivity, head tilt, facial nerve paralysis, stranguria, head pressing, and circling. This outbreak event reinforced the need to also consider HeV in the differential diagnosis of neurologic disease in horses.

Experimental exposure of horses to an HeV isolate (Hendra virus/Australia/Horse/2008/Redlands) recovered from the spleen of a horse exhibiting such neurologic disease was carried out under Biosafety Level (BSL) 4 conditions at the CSIRO Australian Animal Health Laboratory, Geelong, Victoria, Australia.[23] Clinical signs and pathologic findings were generally consistent with those recorded for earlier spillover events, and for similar experimental studies conducted using the original HeV isolate (Hendra virus/Australia/Horse/1994/Hendra), suggesting that there had been no significant evolution in virus pathogenicity for horses in intervening years. These authors also commented that three of the five horses presenting with neurologic manifestations of acute HeV infection had pre-existing lesions of the head (corneal lesion, nasal granuloma, and mandibular fracture), and so there was potential for HeV exposure in a manner that may have bypassed mucosal protective mechanisms thereby influencing the course of infection.

Moreover, in special consideration of the dominant neurologic manifestations associated with field infection involving Hendra virus/Australia/Horse/2008/Redlands, phylogenetic analysis was conducted on HeV isolates from horses obtained between 1994 and 2008.[24] Sequence analysis revealed a high level of conservation at genome and amino acid levels with, in particular, a lower level of nucleotide changes than observed in other RNA viruses and also no correlation between relatedness of isolates and time. Results of assessment of the complete genetic sequence of HeV recovered from the natural bat host since 2008 are consistent with several virus variants circulating within them at, on occasion, multiple locations over the same time period.[14] Overall, however, the viral genome seemed to be stable in its reservoir. Interestingly, HeV isolates recovered from disease outbreaks in horses were genetically aligned to diverse flying fox virus variants, suggesting that such spillover events are not attributable to the genetic sequence characteristics of a single HeV variant.

Pathogenesis and Pathology

In the preclinical stage of infection, viral genetic material can be recovered on nasal swabs from experimental horses after as little as 2 days postexposure to HeV by oral and nasal routes.[23] Gene copy numbers in nasal secretions steadily increase through the incubation period and into the clinical phase of infection, consistent with local replication in the upper respiratory tract or nasopharynx. Viremia ensues, followed rapidly by the onset of fever, and soon afterward viral genome can also be recovered from oral secretions and urine. Signs of systemic illness develop shortly after that as HeV replication becomes more widely established in tissues and organs.

There is comparatively little pathologic data available from field postmortems and most information has been recorded from experimental studies. In peracute cases there may be few gross abnormalities at postmortem examination. Where described, postmortem lesions in acutely affected animals have included pulmonary edema, congestion, and consolidation, with blood-tinged foam in the airways,[1,19,21] dilation of subpleural lymphatics,[25] subpleural hemorrhage,[23] congestion of intra-abdominal lymph nodes,[15] and enlarged, edematous submandibular, sternal, and bronchial lymph nodes.[23] The dominant light microscopic lesion in natural and experimental HeV infection of horses is vasculitis that affects predominantly smaller blood vessels in a wide range of tissues including lung, brain (and meninges), lymphoid tissues, kidney (glomeruli), and female reproductive tract but also nasal mucosa, adrenal gland, liver, heart, and gastrointestinal tract. Necrotizing lymphadenitis is common, as is extensive lung involvement including widespread necrotizing alveolitis with marked fibrinous alveolar exudates. Syncytial cells are regularly identified within renal glomeruli, lymphoid tissues, vascular endothelium, lymphatic endothelium, and in alveolar walls. HeV antigen is readily visualized in affected tissues using appropriate immunohistochemical techniques (**Fig. 2**). Virus may also be recovered from the fresh carcass, especially from lung, kidney, and lymphoid tissues but also brain and spinal

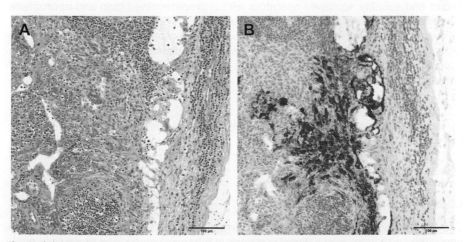

Fig. 2. (A) Histologic section of lymph node from horse with acute HeV infection showing lymphadenitis with syncytial cell formation (hematoxylin and eosin, original magnification × 20). (B) HeV antigen in section adjacent to Fig. 2A (anti-Nipah N antibody, original magnification × 20).

cord, cerebrospinal fluid, meninges, upper respiratory tract, heart, and adrenal gland. As would be expected, delays in postmortem examination may adversely impact on the success of virus isolation attempts.

A few field cases of HeV that have clinically recovered from acute disease (associated with the development of virus neutralizing antibodies) have been euthanized in line with current national policy. Each had shown neurologic signs during the clinical phase of infection and, at the time of postmortem examination, had mild to moderately severe, focal, nonsuppurative meningoencephalitis with gliosis and perivascular cuffing; low levels of HeV genome were also recovered from the brain. The significance of these findings with respect to the possibility of virus persistence in the equine brain is not yet understood. However, in the context of potential transmission risk it is relevant to note that infectious virus has not been recovered from human patients with relapsing HeV[7] or Nipah virus encephalitis.[8]

Laboratory Diagnosis

Because the clinical signs associated with HeV infection are not pathognomonic, laboratory confirmation of the diagnosis is essential. Consideration of the zoonotic potential of the virus should guide the process of collection of samples for submission to diagnostic laboratories, and should only be undertaken if the associated risks can be effectively managed. This is especially important because the often peracute nature of the disease is such that results of laboratory testing may not be available until the after the horse has died, meaning that any significant human exposure is likely to have already occurred. In the live horse, samples should include blood in EDTA and nasal, oral, and rectal swabs for polymerase chain reaction testing and, if indicated from the polymerase chain reaction result, virus isolation attempts in a BSL4 laboratory. Whole blood should also be collected for serologic testing by enzyme-linked immunosorbent assay or by neutralization test in a BSL4 laboratory.[26] Postmortem examination of the recently dead horse is a particularly hazardous activity because the HeV viral load is highest at this time, but it may be indicated when atypical disease is observed or when confirmation of the diagnosis is essential, for example when a human exposure risk has been identified. Necropsy can be safely conducted by experienced and suitably equipped operators with a predetermined plan and appropriate infrastructure for preventing exposure of personnel, for carcass removal, and for environmental decontamination. However, if those criteria cannot be met then suitable risk reduction measures might include limiting specimen collection to such tissues as the superficial mandibular lymph nodes and a jugular vein blood sample, and swabs of nasal, oral, and rectal orifices.

Therapy

No specific therapy exists for horses with HeV infection, and if diagnostic confirmation precedes death, euthanasia is carried out. Appropriate considerations around infection control should guide any welfare interventions in ill horses suspected of being infected by HeV.

COMMUNITY IMPACT

The 18 equine HeV incidents of 2011 and the first reported field infection of a dog were associated with increased national coverage in the mass media, and those communications to the public sent the message that burgeoning infection risk to the community was attributable to expansion of flying fox populations into urban areas[27] rather than to direct contact with infected horses. As a result, there was increasing pressure to instigate measures for the control or extermination of flying fox populations, despite their key environmental role in pollination of native forests and any attendant practical and ethical considerations. Mendez and colleagues[28] also reported increasing numbers of veterinarians and other equine health care staff to be departing equine practice because they believed that they were unable to adequately manage HeV-associated risks and liability within their workplace. Follow-on effects included increased occupational risk for some equine veterinarians, especially practice principals who elected to undertake all the equine work themselves and those veterinarians who elected to work in a less than ideal environment to meet animal welfare needs. A growing level of resentment was also described that was attributed to some practices that would only deliver preventative medicine services to healthy horses.

A HENDRA VIRUS VACCINE FOR HORSES

There is no straightforward means of preventing exposure of horses to HeV that is shed by flying foxes. Factors influencing interspecies transmission are likely complex, are poorly understood, and the interface between bats and horses cannot be eliminated within periurban and rural communities. Thus, a more direct approach has been introduced to protect the health of horses and to reduce the risk of human infection, namely vaccination of horses. The aim of suppression of HeV virus replication in animals exposed to field virus is to remove the acutely ill horse from the chain of onward transmission to people.

HeV G attachment glycoprotein is one of the two major envelope glycoproteins that are required for infection of the host cell, and in 2005, Bossart and coauthors[29] reported development of a recombinant soluble HeV G (sG) that elicited virus-neutralizing antibodies in rabbits. A candidate vaccine based on the antigen HeVsG was first efficacy tested in cats against Nipah virus[30,31] and subsequently in ferrets against HeV,[32] and the success of the outcomes to virus exposure in these species encouraged translation of the work into the horse.[33] For use in the horse, sG was specifically reformulated with a proprietary adjuvant approved for use in that species and delivered as an inactivated subunit vaccine. Data gathered after using a prime-boost immunization regime confirmed development of neutralizing antibody in vaccinated horses, and all immunized horses were protected from disease following exposure to an otherwise lethal HeV challenge under BSL4 conditions. In addition, there was no evidence of virus replication in vaccinated animals apart from transient low HeV N gene copy number detected in the nasal swabs of one horse exposed to virus 6 months after booster vaccination. However, viral genome was not recovered from the tissues of any horse. More recent serologic studies using different vaccination regimes suggest that antibody titer persists at high level 12 months after a priming series that comprises three immunizations (Day 0, Day 21, 6 months); horses exposed to HeV 12 months after receiving a third vaccine showed no evidence of HeV replication in swabs, blood, or tissues (Deborah Middleton, unpublished observations, 2014).

The equine HeV vaccine (Equivac HeV; Zoetis, Parkville, Vic, Australia) was released for administration by veterinarians late in 2012. As expected vaccine uptake has been greatest in the regions of highest perceived risk, notably coastal Queensland and northeastern NSW but, because HeV events are sporadic, it may be some time before the impact of vaccination on the incidence of acute HeV infection of horses can be assessed. Complete HeV vaccine coverage of the Australian horse herd will not be achieved for several reasons, including the cost of its administration and varying perceptions around which horse populations are at risk of disease. Accordingly, improved infection control procedures and a heightened awareness of the possibility of HeV infection need to be maintained for dealing with sick horses, particularly when HeV vaccination status is uncertain.

POSTEXPOSURE THERAPEUTICS FOR PEOPLE

Exposure of humans to infectious doses of HeV from acutely affected horses may occur in the future. Not all horses will be vaccinated against HeV and outbreaks occur in temperate to tropical climates where continual compliance with certain items of personal protective equipment may be difficult to achieve. The emotional attachment of humans to their horses leads to regular close contact where use of personal protective equipment is usually impractical, and the occupational exposure limits by contact and/ or inhalation are, and will remain, unknown.

In 2008, Zhu and coauthors[34] screened a large nonimmune human antibody library and described the identification and characterization of a human monoclonal antibody, m102.4, which neutralized HeV and Nipah virus in vitro. When given postexposure to laboratory animals, m102.4 has been shown to prevent acute Nipah- and Hendra-associated morbidity and mortality in ferrets[35] (Deborah Middleton, unpublished observations, 2012) and in African Green monkeys,[36] although infection is not prevented. In addition, amelioration of disease signs in both species is optimal when m102.4 is administered within 24 hours of exposure to virus, before the detection of Hendra viral RNA in blood or its recovery from oropharyngeal secretions, and before the onset of fever or other clinical signs[36] (Deborah Middleton, unpublished observations, 2012).

These studies encouraged the initiation of preclinical safety testing of m102.4 and a phase 1 human clinical trial that will commence in 2014. However, the value of m102.4 in management of human infection after the onset of clinical illness, especially the complication of encephalitis, is yet to be assessed.

OTHER SUSCEPTIBLE ANIMAL HOSTS

Diverse species have proved susceptible to HeV infection under experimental conditions including cats, ferrets, hamsters, pigs, and guinea pigs. Each exhibits disease generally similar to that observed in horses, with ferrets and hamsters in particular used in efficacy assessment of antihenipavirus vaccines and therapeutics.[37–40] More recently, Dups and colleagues[41] reported encephalitis in wild-type laboratory mice in the absence of significant systemic infection; this model holds great promise as a tool for investigation of the neurologic complications of HeV infection that are a particular feature of the human disease. Field infections have not yet been recorded in pigs, cats, or guinea pigs (ferrets are not permitted as pets in Queensland), but during 2011 a dog sampled on an outbreak property was found to have antibody to HeV without having shown signs of disease. A similar canine case was identified in NSW in 2013 during investigation of the HeV-associated death of a horse.

To better assess the impact of HeV infection in dogs and their potential for transmission risk, dogs were exposed to HeV under BSL4 containment conditions (Deborah Middleton, unpublished observations, 2013). Dogs proved to be reliably susceptible to infection under the conditions of exposure, and showed only subtle or no clinical signs of illness; development of neutralizing antibody was associated with virus clearance. Virus replication in the pharynx led to shedding of infectious virus that, for a short period of time, was sufficient to transmit infection to naive ferrets. As yet, all human cases of HeV infection have had a strong epidemiologic connection to close contact with an infected horse. The level of risk posed by field exposure to HeV-infected dogs has not yet been ascertained.

SUMMARY

The incidence of emerging zoonotic diseases has been increasing for several decades[42] and significant predictors of emergence, such as increasing human population growth and density, will persist in the foreseeable future. Thus, it is to be expected that further new and highly pathogenic infections will enter the human population, that companion or agricultural animals may be the immediate source, and that a wildlife species will prove to be the pathogen's reservoir host. As for HeV, mitigating the impact of such events on the community will require ongoing acknowledgment of the interconnectedness of human, animal, and environmental health that is harnessed to interdisciplinary approaches to management of disease outbreaks, definition of knowledge gaps, and prioritization of research needs.

REFERENCES

1. Murray K, Selleck P, Hooper P, et al. A morbillivirus that caused fatal disease in horses and humans. Science 1995;268:94–7.
2. Chua KB, Goh KJ, Wong KT. Fatal encephalitis due to Nipah virus among pig-farmers in Malaysia. Lancet 1999;354:1256–9.
3. Marsh GA, de Jong C, Barr JA, et al. Cedar virus: a novel henipavirus isolated from Australian bats. PLoS Pathog 2012;8:e1002836.
4. Symons R. Re: Canine case of Hendra virus and Hendra virus vaccine. Aust Vet J 2011;89(10):N24.
5. Hendra virus, equine – Australia (18): (Queensland) canine. Available at: http://www.promedmail.org. ProMed Arch No: 20130721.1837123. Accessed March 14, 2014.
6. Playford EG, McCall B, Smith G, et al. Human Hendra virus encephalitis associated with equine outbreak, Australia, 2008. Emerg Infect Dis 2010;16(2):219–23.
7. O'Sullivan JD, Allworth AM, Paterson DL, et al. Fatal encephalitis due to novel paramyxovirus transmitted from horses. Lancet 1997;349:93–5.
8. Tan CT, Goh KJ, Wong KT, et al. Relapsed and late-onset Nipah encephalitis. Ann Neurol 2002;51:703–8.
9. Taylor C, Playford EG, McBride WJ, et al. No evidence of prolonged Hendra virus shedding by 2 patients, Australia. Emerg Infect Dis 2012;18:2025–7.
10. Young PL, Halpin K, Selleck PW, et al. Serologic evidence for the presence in Pteropus bats of a paramyxovirus related to equine morbillivirus. Emerg Infect Dis 1996;2:239–40.
11. Field H, Young P, Yob JM, et al. The natural history of Hendra and Nipah viruses. Microbes Infect 2001;3:307–14.
12. Hutson T, Suyanto A, Helgen K, et al. Pteropus alecto. In: IUCN 2013. IUCN red list of threatened species. Version 2013.2. 2008. Available at: www.iucnredlist.org. Accessed February 07, 2013.
13. Halpin K, Young PL, Field HE, et al. Isolation of Hendra virus from pteropid bats: a natural reservoir of Hendra virus. J Gen Virol 2000;81:1927–32.
14. Smith I, Broos A, de Jong C, et al. Identifying Hendra virus diversity in pteropid bats. PLoS One 2011;6:e25275.
15. Williamson MM, Hooper PT, Selleck PW, et al. Transmission studies of Hendra virus (equine morbillivirus) in fruit bats, horses and cats. Aust Vet J 1998;76:813–8.
16. Williamson MM, Hooper PT, Selleck PW, et al. Experimental Hendra virus infection in pregnant guinea-pigs and fruit bats (Pteropus poliocephalus). J Comp Pathol 1999;122:201–7.

17. Halpin K, Hyatt AD, Fogarty R, et al. Pteropid bats are confirmed as the reservoir hosts of henipaviruses: a comprehensive experimental study of virus transmission. Am J Trop Med Hyg 2011;85:946–51.
18. Field H, de Jong C, Melville D, et al. Hendra virus infection dynamics in Australian fruit bats. PLoS One 2011;6:e28678.
19. Selvey LA, Wells RM, McCormack JG, et al. Infection of humans and horses by a newly described morbillivirus. Med J Aust 1995;162:642–5.
20. Baldock FC, Douglas IC, Halpin K, et al. Epidemiological investigations into the 1994 equine morbillivirus outbreaks in Queensland, Australia. Singapore Vet J 1996;20:57–61.
21. Rogers RJ, Douglas IC, Baldock FC, et al. Investigation of a second focus of equine Morbillivirus infection in coastal Queensland. Aust Vet J 1996;74:243–4.
22. Field H, Schaaf K, Kung N, et al. Hendra virus outbreak with novel clinical features, Australia. Emerg Infect Dis 2010;16(2):338–40.
23. Marsh GA, Haining J, Hancock TJ, et al. Experimental infection of horses with Hendra virus/Australia/Horse/2008/Redland. Emerg Infect Dis 2011;17: 2232–8.
24. Marsh GA, Todd S, Foord A, et al. Genome sequence conservation of Hendra virus isolates during spillover to horses, Australia. Emerg Infect Dis 2010;11: 1767–9.
25. Hooper PT, Ketterer PJ, Hyatt AD, et al. Lesions of experimental equine morbillivirus pneumonia in horses. Vet Pathol 1997;34:312–22.
26. Guidelines for veterinarians handling potential Hendra virus infection in horses Version 5.0. 2013. Available at: http://www.daff.qld.gov.au/__data/assets/pdf_file/0009/97713/2355-guidelines-for-veterinarians-sept-2013.pdf. Accessed March 14, 2014.
27. Degeling C, Kerridge I. Hendra in the news: public policy meets public morality in times of zoonotic uncertainty. Soc Sci Med 2013;82:156–63.
28. Mendez DH, Judd J, Speare R. Unexpected result of Hendra virus outbreaks for veterinarians, Queensland, Australia. Emerg Infect Dis 2012;18:83–5.
29. Bossart KN, Crameri G, Dimitrov AS, et al. Receptor binding, fusion inhibition and induction of cross-reactive neutralizing antibodies by a soluble G glycoprotein of Hendra virus. J Virol 2005;79(11):6690–702.
30. Mungall BA, Middleton D, Crameri G, et al. Feline model of acute Nipah virus infection and protection with a soluble glycoprotein-based subunit vaccine. J Virol 2006;80:12293–302.
31. McEachern JA, Bingham J, Crameri G, et al. A recombinant subunit vaccine formulation protects against lethal Nipah virus challenge in cats. Vaccine 2008; 26:3842–52.
32. Pallister J, Middleton D, Wang LF, et al. A recombinant Hendra virus G glycoprotein-based subunit vaccine protects ferrets from lethal Hendra virus challenge. Vaccine 2011;29:5623–30.
33. Middleton D, Pallister J, Klein R, et al. Hendra virus vaccine, a one-health approach to protecting horse, human, and environmental health. Emerg Infect Dis 2014;20:372–9.
34. Zhu Z, Bossart KN, Bishop KA, et al. Exceptionally potent cross-reactive neutralisation of Nipah and Hendra viruses by a human monoclonal antibody. J Infect Dis 2008;197:846–53.
35. Bossart KN, Zhu Z, Middleton D, et al. A neutralizing monoclonal antibody protects against lethal disease in a new ferret model of acute Nipah virus infection. PLoS Pathog 2009;10:e1000642.

36. Bossart KN, Geisbert TW, Feldmann H, et al. A neutralizing human monoclonal antibody protects African green monkeys from Hendra virus challenge. Sci Transl Med 2011;3:1–17.
37. Hooper PT, Westbury HA, Russell GM. The lesions of experimental equine morbillivirus disease in cats and guinea pigs. Vet Pathol 1997;34:323–9.
38. Westbury HA, Hooper PT, Brouwer SL, et al. Susceptibility of cats to equine morbillivirus. Aust Vet J 1996;74:132–4.
39. Guillaume V, Wong KY, Looi RY, et al. Acute Hendra virus infection: analysis of the pathogenesis and passive antibody protection in the hamster model. Virology 2009;387:459–65.
40. Li M, Embury-Hyatt C, Weingartl HM. Experimental inoculation study indicates swine as a potential host for Hendra virus. Vet Res 2010;41:33.
41. Dups J, Middleton D, Yamada M, et al. A new model for Hendra virus encephalitis in the mouse. PLoS One 2012;7:e40308.
42. Jones KE, Patel NG, Levy MA, et al. Global trends in emerging infectious diseases. Nature 2008;451:990–3.

New Perspectives for the Diagnosis, Control, Treatment, and Prevention of Strangles in Horses

Andrew S. Waller, BSc, PhD

KEYWORDS

- Strangles • *Streptococcus equi* • ELISA • qPCR • Vaccine

KEY POINTS

- The ability of *Streptococcus equi* to establish persistent infection, usually within the guttural pouches, is critical to interepizootic transmission, the recurrence of strangles, and the high incidence of this disease around the world.
- The lack of clinical signs shown by persistently infected carriers emphasizes the need to implement effective quarantine and testing procedures for their identification and treatment before they come into contact with an existing herd.
- A blood sample taken on arrival can be tested to identify horses that may have been recently exposed to, or are persistently infected with, *S equi*, and that require further investigation.
- Quantitative polymerase chain reaction tests for *S equi* are now regarded as the gold standard for the detection of *S equi*.
- The development of effective vaccines against strangles that permit the differentiation of infected from vaccinated animals remains a significant unmet objective.

INTRODUCTION

Strangles was first reported in 1251 by Jordanus Ruffus,[1] an officer in the imperial court of Emperor Frederick II, although the disease almost certainly has older origins. Despite improvements in the health and management of horse populations, strangles remains the most frequently diagnosed infectious disease of horses worldwide. Only

Disclosure: The author has received support from the Animal Health Trust, the Horse Trust (ref: G1606), the Horserace Betting Levy Board (ref: vet/prj/730, 734, 751 and 758), the British Horse Society, the Wellcome Trust (ref: 86970), the European Breeders Fund, the Anne Duchess of Westminster's Charitable Trust, the Margaret Giffen Charitable Trust, and the PetPlan Charitable Trust.
Centre for Preventive Medicine, Animal Health Trust, Lanwades Park, Kentford, Newmarket, Suffolk CB8 7UU, UK
E-mail address: andrew.waller@aht.org.uk

Vet Clin Equine 30 (2014) 591–607
http://dx.doi.org/10.1016/j.cveq.2014.08.007   **vetequine.theclinics.com**

the geographically isolated Icelandic horse population remains free of strangles, a situation that has been maintained through a virtual absence of horse imports for more than 1000 years. In excess of 600 outbreaks of strangles are estimated to occur in the United Kingdom alone each year.[2] Outbreaks can involve all of the horses on a yard, require movement restrictions that often remain in force for more than 2 months, and incur an economic cost to some premises that may exceed £250,000 ($425,000).

THE CAUSAL AGENT

Strangles is caused by infection with *Streptococcus equi* subspecies *equi* (*S equi*), which, despite the inference from its name, is a subgroup of the diverse population of *S equi* subspecies *zooepidemicus* (*Streptococcus zooepidemicus*), with which it shares more than 97% DNA identity.[3] Nonequine infections with *S zooepidemicus* can be severe, including cases of acute fatal hemorrhagic pneumonia in dogs,[4–6] and septicemia, meningitis, and toxic shock syndrome in humans.[7–10] However, despite its ability to cause severe clinical signs and its close relationship with *S equi*, *S zooepidemicus* is often regarded as a commensal organism of the equine upper respiratory tract. *S zooepidemicus* is associated with a variety of diseases in horses, including uterine infections of mares[11,12] and ulcerative keratitis.[13] Investigations of outbreaks of respiratory disease caused by *S zooepidemicus* have been confounded by the diversity of this group of bacteria and the ability of outbreak strains to persistently infect the tonsils of recovered horses.[14] Emerging evidence supports epidemiologic studies that suggested a causal role for *S zooepidemicus* in cases of respiratory disease,[15] and modern typing methods[16] have directly linked specific strains to individual outbreaks.[17,18] Such data indicate that the population of *S zooepidemicus* that is resident in the tonsils of horses includes pathogenic strains and provides a snapshot of the history of infection within an individual animal.[19] The differentiation of *S equi* from the resident population of *S zooepidemicus* and the immune responses to these closely related pathogens is a particular challenge for modern diagnostic techniques and is described in more detail later.

CLINICAL SIGNS OF STRANGLES

Strangles is characterized by pyrexia, followed by abscessation of lymph nodes in the head and neck.[20] The name strangles was coined from the signs of dysphagia that some horses experience. Some of these horses are suffocated by the enlarged lymph nodes, which can obstruct the airway. Affected animals develop pharyngitis, which may lead to them being reluctant to eat, particularly dried food, resulting in anorexia. Some affected horses stand with their necks extended and depression is common.

Following entry of *S equi* via the nose or mouth, the organism attaches to and invades the tonsillar crypts of the oropharynx and nasopharynx and can be detected in the lymph nodes of the head and neck within 3 hours after infection.[21] The transient attachment of *S equi* to the oropharynx and nasopharynx before invasion into adjacent lymphoid tissue is highlighted by an inability to detect *S equi* using nasopharyngeal swabs or washes taken 24 hours after infection. Clusters of *S equi* are apparent in the lamina propria after 48 hours.[21] Superantigens,[22,23] phospholipase A_2 toxins,[3] streptolysin S,[24] and several other surface and secreted proteins[25–29] produced by *S equi* modulate the proliferation and activity of neutrophils, leading to a failure of innate immune defences.[21] For example, the SeM surface protein is known to bind fibrinogen and immunoglobulin, providing an increased resistance to phagocytosis.[25,30–34]

Lymph node abscesses increase in size and develop a thick fibrous capsule that walls off the infection. Growth of the bacterium in these abscesses may be increased through the production of a secreted molecule, equibactin, which enhances the capacity of S equi to import iron.[35] Bacterial proliferation and an ineffective immune response induce an increase in body temperature. The onset of pyrexia can vary from a few days to several weeks after infection, depending on the infectious dose received, and from one individual animal to another, but can usually be detected before bacteria begin to shed from infected lymph nodes. Therefore, once a strangles outbreak is confirmed, presumptively infected pyretic horses may be identified and isolated before the organism is passed to in-contact animals. Fever normally persists and increases, exceeding 42°C (107.6°F) in some cases, as abscesses mature in infected lymph nodes.

Abscesses formed in the retropharyngeal or submandibular lymph nodes typically rupture between 7 days and 4 weeks after infection. Retropharyngeal lymph node abscesses usually rupture into the guttural pouches, which drain via the eustachian tube into the nasopharynx, resulting in the profuse mucopurulent nasal discharge typically associated with strangles. Abscesses may also form in the cervical and tracheal/bronchial lymph nodes, rupturing externally through the skin over a process of several weeks. S equi is particularly resistant to phagocytosis and killing by the equine immune system[25,26,28,36,37] and the process of abscess rupture that permits drainage of purulent material is important for the resolution of the infection. Older horses often have a milder, atypical form of the disease, possibly as a result of cross-protection/partial protection caused by prior infection with different strains of S zooepidemicus or S equi[38] or through differences in the infecting strain.[39,40]

CONVALESCENCE AND THE CARRIER STATE

Despite the severity of clinical signs during the acute phase of disease, most horses (~98%) recover from strangles over a period of weeks. An adaptive immune response can be detected 2-weeks after infection,[41] assisting mucosal clearance of S equi.[42] An estimated 75% of recovered horses develop protective immunity to S equi.[43,44] However, despite the development of antibody responses, approximately 10% of convalescent horses fail to clear all abscess material from their guttural pouches or sinus tracts. Residual pus dries and hardens to form chondroids that can remain in the horse for several years, and potentially for the remaining lifetime of that animal.[45,46] Live S equi persists in chondroids, or possibly as a biofilm on mucosal surfaces, and can intermittently shed from carrier animals into the environment.

S equi does not survive for long in the environment, particularly on surfaces exposed to direct sunlight.[47] However, S equi shed from an acutely or persistently infected individual may gain access to naive horses via the nose or mouth, or through contaminated drinking water (in which it can persist for up to 1 month), tack, and other fomites. The ability of S equi to establish persistent infection is critical to interepizootic transmission, the recurrence of strangles, and the high incidence of this disease around the world.

THERAPEUTIC TREATMENT OF HORSES WITH STRANGLES

Although S equi is sensitive to all antibiotics, with the exception of aminoglycosides, veterinary opinion remains divided as to whether antibiotic treatment is useful. On identification of an index case, the isolation of healthy in-contact animals and the immediate administration of antibiotics to them for 3 to 5 days may prevent these animals from developing clinical signs of disease. However, treated animals are unlikely to develop immunity to S equi infection and remain susceptible,[38] and the use of antibiotics in horses with subclinical infection in which abscesses have already formed only delays the onset of clinical signs and extends the time taken to resolve the outbreak.

The use of antibiotic therapy may provide temporary clinical improvement in fever and lethargy, which may assist the management of severe cases, particularly if the animal presents with dyspnea as a result of partial upper airway obstruction. Penicillin is considered the drug of choice and antibiotic resistance has not yet been reported in S equi. However, antibiotic resistance has begun to emerge in some strains of S zooepidemicus[5] and appropriate consideration should be given before sanctioning their use.

THERAPEUTIC TREATMENT OF PERSISTENTLY INFECTED CARRIERS

Elimination of S equi from the guttural pouches of persistently infected horses can be accomplished by endoscopic guttural pouch lavage. Sedation aids in implementation of endoscopy and facilitates drainage of flush material from the guttural pouches by lowering the horse's head. Chondroids present in the guttural pouch can be removed using a memory-helical polyp retrieval basket through the biopsy channel of the endoscope (**Fig. 1**).[46] Surgical hyovertebrotomy and ventral drainage through the Viborg triangle carry inherent risks of general anesthesia and surgical dissection around major blood vessels and nerves and S equi contamination of the hospital environment, but is practical if large numbers of chondroids are identified within the guttural pouch. Empyema of the guttural pouch can be resolved by repeated lavages with isotonic saline or polyionic fluid using rigid or indwelling catheters or through the use of a suction pump attached to the endoscope. Topical installation of 20% (weight/volume) acetylcysteine solution may assist the treatment of empyema. Topical benzylpenicillin (see **Box 1**) is instilled into the guttural pouches via an endoscope guided into the pouch opening. The administration of systemic antibiotics may further improve treatment success. The guttural pouches are resampled 2 weeks later to confirm lack of infection following analysis by quantitative polymerase chain reaction (qPCR).

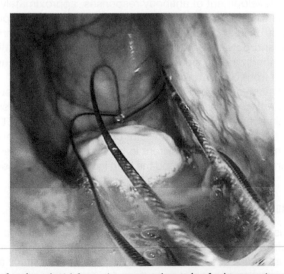

Fig. 1. Recovery of a chondroid from the guttural pouch of a horse using a memory-helical polyp retrieval basket through the biopsy channel of the endoscope.

Box 1
Preparation of a gelatin/penicillin solution for topical treatment of persistent infection of the guttural pouch

Weigh out 2 g of gelatin and add 40 mL of sterile water.

Heat or microwave to dissolve the gelatin.

Cool gelatin to 45 to 50°C.

Add 10 mL of sterile water to 10,000,000 units (10 Mega units) of sodium benzylpenicillin G.

Mix penicillin solution with the cooled gelatin to make a total volume of 50 mL.

Dispense into syringes and leave overnight at 4°C to set.

COMPLICATIONS

Bastard strangles occurs when the infection spreads to lymph nodes or tissues distant from the lymph nodes of the head and neck, and can be difficult to diagnose. A history of exposure to S equi and laboratory results consistent with chronic infection, anemia, fever responsive to penicillin, hyperfibrinogenemia, and hyperglobulinemia support the diagnosis of metastatic abscessation. Treatment requires long-term antimicrobial therapy, and appropriate local treatment or drainage of abscesses if possible. However, metastatic infection often results in the death of the affected animal, particularly when abscesses form in the lungs, liver, spleen, kidneys, or brain.

Purpura hemorrhagica is an aseptic necrotizing vasculitis resulting in edema of the head, ventral abdomen, and limbs, and petechial hemorrhages of the mucous membranes. Although often associated with S equi infection, purpura hemorrhagica is thought to be caused by the deposition of immune complexes in blood vessels and can occur in response to several different antigens,[48] including an excessive anti-SeM antibody response.[49] Treatment usually consists of dexamethasone and supportive care, including the administration of intravenous fluids, hydrotherapy, and bandaging. Mortalities of between 8% and 25% have been documented, but most horses can recover from purpura given good veterinary care.[48–50]

PREVENTING INFECTION

Recent research has cataloged the genetic differences between S equi and S zooepidemicus strains.[3] Although much of this work lies outside the scope of this article, knowledge of the S equi genome is shedding new light on how this organism causes disease[51,52] and has enabled the identification of novel targets leading to the development of fast, sensitive, and specific diagnostic tests[41,53,54] and new preventative vaccines.[55]

CULTURE TEST FOR STREPTOCOCCUS EQUI

The diagnosis of S equi infection has traditionally relied on the inoculation of blood agar containing colistin and nalidixic acid with clinical material recovered from swabs, washes, or abscesses and overnight incubation at 37°C in a 5% CO_2 atmosphere. Beta-hemolytic colonies of S equi are picked and used to inoculate Todd-Hewitt nutrient broth, which is incubated overnight at 37°C in a 5% CO_2 atmosphere. In addition, the turbid cultures are used to inoculate purple broth cultures containing trehalose, lactose, or sorbitol. S equi fails to ferment these sugars, whereas S zooepidemicus usually ferments lactose and sorbitol, and Streptococcus dysgalactiae subspecies *Streptococcus equisimilis* (*S equisimilis*), another common beta-hemolytic *Streptococcus*, ferments trehalose.[56] The isolation and identification of *S equi* using this method is therefore time consuming and requires a minimum of 48 hours from receipt of clinical samples. This reporting delay often has consequences for the isolation of infected horses, providing *S equi* with greater opportunity to transmit through naive populations. The isolation of *S equi* is confounded by the presence of other beta-hemolytic bacteria, most notably *S zooepidemicus* and *S equisimilis*. Advances in polymerase chain reaction (PCR) technology have highlighted deficiencies in the culture test, showing that it is no longer the gold-standard method for the detection of *S equi* or diagnosis of strangles.

POLYMERASE CHAIN REACTION ASSAYS

The first PCR-based tests developed for *S equi* targeted the 5′ region of the SeM gene and were estimated to be around 3 times more sensitive than the traditional culture assay.[57,58] However, this region is highly variable[39,40] and some strains of *S equi* isolated from persistently infected carriers lack the target region.[40,59] Advances in PCR technology have led to the development of qPCR assays. These assays can be completed in less than 2 hours from sample receipt and benefit from even greater levels of sensitivity. The superantigen-encoding genes have been exploited as diagnostic targets for the detection of *S equi* by qPCR.[53] However, there is a certain level of functional redundancy in *S equi*[3,23] that permitted the loss of at least 1 of these target genes in an outbreak of strangles identified in the United States (R. Holland, personal communication, 2012).

A triplex qPCR assay has recently been developed[54] that targets 2 *S equi*–specific genes: *eqbE*, encoding part of the equibactin biosynthesis system,[3,35] and SEQ2190, encoding a unique surface protein.[3] An internal control strain of *S zooepidemicus* is added to the clinical sample before DNA extraction to serve as a within-assay control to eliminate the risk of false-negative reporting through failures in DNA extraction or the presence of PCR inhibitors. The triplex assay has an overall sensitivity of 93.9% and specificity of 96.6% and detects 10-fold fewer quantities of *S equi* than the limit of the culture assay, regardless of the presence of contaminating bacteria.[54]

The culture assay failed to identify 39.7% of qPCR-positive samples. In the past, the poor sensitivity of the culture assay and its failure to correctly identify qPCR-positive samples was excused by the claim that PCR detects so-called dead DNA.[38] Although technically this is correct and qPCR can detect killed *S equi* following insufficient cleaning and sterilization of endoscopy equipment, DNA does not persist on mucosal surfaces in vivo and any culture-positive or qPCR-positive result should be taken seriously (**Box 2**). The presence of contaminating beta-hemolytic streptococci explained 56% of triplex-positive/culture-negative results, and poor assay sensitivity explained the remaining 44% of false-negative culture results reported by Webb and colleagues[54] in 2013. Therefore, the triplex qPCR sets a new benchmark for quality control and sensitivity and is now regarded as the new gold-standard test for the detection of *S equi*.

SEROLOGY TESTS FOR EXPOSURE TO *STREPTOCOCCUS EQUI*

Persistence of *S equi* in the guttural pouches of horses is associated with follicular hyperplasia,[60] suggesting that it may be possible to identify persistently infected carriers in the absence of bacterial shedding through the quantification of a specific antibody response.

> **Box 2**
> **Example case report 1**
>
> A convalescent mare was sampled at weekly intervals by nasopharyngeal swab and the samples analyzed by both culture and qPCR. The third sample taken on the 4th August 2010 tested positive by both qPCR and culture (**Fig. 2**) but, despite advice to the attending veterinarian to examine the mare by guttural pouch endoscopy, the horse was resampled at weekly intervals until the 29th September 2010 when 3 consecutive negative nasopharyngeal swab samples had been obtained. The horse was pronounced infection free and permitted to move to a new yard where a new outbreak of strangles began on the 25th October 2010. In this example, the qPCR and culture assays agreed and highlight the intermittent nature of shedding S equi from the guttural pouch. This case also emphasizes the need to examine positive horses by guttural pouch endoscopy to ensure that persistently infected horses are not inadvertently missed.

Vaccination with SeM-containing vaccines has been linked with complications such as purpura hemorrhagica[48] and this perceived risk led to the development of a SeM-based indirect enzyme-linked immunosorbent assay (iELISA) for the identification of horses with high anti-SeM antibody levels before vaccination with SeM-containing vaccines.[38] The SeM iELISA has subsequently been exploited for the identification of horses infected with S equi, with high antibody titers being suggested to indicate disseminated disease.[38] However, the SeM protein has a homologue in S zooepidemicus, SzM,[40] which raises the possibility that antibodies directed against SzM could cross-react with the SeM iELISA leading to the identification of false-positive horses. Preincubating sera with heat-killed S zooepidemicus removes cross-reactive antibodies to SzM before the detection of SeM-specific antibody responses.[61] However, this process, although successful in reducing assay background, has not been adopted in assays based on full-length SeM.

To overcome the problem of cross-reactivity with S zooepidemicus, an iELISA assay using the N-terminal portion of SeM, which is unique to S equi, has been developed.[41] The new assay is performed alongside a second iELISA to quantify the levels of antibodies against the S equi–specific portion of SEQ2190 and a positive result is issued if either or both of the iELISAs exceed the positive cutoff.[41] Comparison of the dual-antigen iELISA with a commercial iELISA marketed by IDvet (which is based on the full SeM protein) showed that, although the IDvet iELISA had comparable sensitivity (89.9% vs 93.3%), it incorrectly identified 23% of negative sera as being positive when they originated from the Icelandic horse biobank at Keldur, which had no possibility of containing S equi–specific antibodies. In contrast, the dual iELISA yielded a specificity of 99.3%, highlighting its application to identify potentially infected animals before they can transmit the infection.[41]

A prototype of the dual iELISA test, based on antigen A (SEQ2190) and antigen B, has previously been used to determine the prevalence of exposure to S equi in

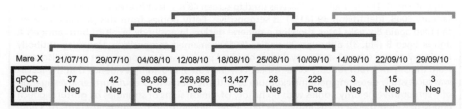

Mare X	21/07/10	29/07/10	04/08/10	12/08/10	18/08/10	25/08/10	10/09/10	14/09/10	22/09/10	29/09/10
qPCR	37	42	98,969	259,856	13,427	28	229	3	15	3
Culture	Neg	Neg	Pos	Pos	Pos	Neg	Pos	Neg	Neg	Neg

Fig. 2. Culture and qPCR results following sampling of a convalescent mare over time. Neg, negative; Pos, positive.

different horse populations. A study of 109 horses in Lesotho identified 11 seropositive horses (10.1%).[62] Another study identified 133 seropositive animals among 319 healthy horses (42%) at 31 unregulated events and yards in Ireland.[63] Some yards had no seropositive horses, whereas the prevalence at others was as high as 90%, highlighting premises with endemic infection (**Box 3**). The iELISA also identified all 10 horses that had recently had clinical signs of strangles in a UK study.[64]

USING THE DIAGNOSTIC TESTS TO MINIMIZE THE IMPACT OF *STREPTOCOCCUS EQUI* INFECTION

Horses that are persistently infected seem clinically normal and may remain unaffected during outbreaks of disease. Following resolution of clinical signs in affected animals, the screening of unaffected animals is often regarded as an unnecessary expense. However, if left untreated, these animals remain a source of future infection.

The lack of clinical signs shown by persistently infected carriers emphasizes the need to implement effective quarantine and testing procedures for their identification and treatment before they come into contact with an existing herd. The quarantine area should be separated from the rest of the premises and clearly marked equipment (brushes, water buckets, and so forth) should be used to maintain biosecurity. Regular disinfection of equipment and water can minimize the opportunity for *S equi* to persist in the environment. Horses in quarantine should ideally be attended only by dedicated staff who do not deal with other horses, or, failing that, be seen only by staff after they have dealt with other horses in order to minimize transmission of any infectious agent from potentially infectious quarantined animals. Body temperatures should be obtained twice daily to identify signs of pyrexia at the earliest opportunity, which can then be investigated further. A blood sample taken on arrival can be used to identify recently exposed or persistently infected horses (**Box 4**). If negative, a second blood sample taken 2 weeks later should be tested to identify horses that have seroconverted and may have been incubating the infection. If this is also negative and the horse remains free from clinical disease, then it should be safe to enter the herd. Horses testing positive via the blood test should be investigated further. The guttural pouches should ideally be visually examined by endoscopy to identify obvious signs of persistent infection and a saline wash should be taken for analysis by qPCR. If qPCR tests on these samples are negative, then it should be safe for the horse to enter the herd. If any of the samples test qPCR positive or chondroids are visible on endoscopy, then these should be treated as described earlier before entry onto the premises.

Box 3
Example case report 2

A yard of 52 polo ponies had recurrent problems with strangles including cases in August 2007, 8th and 13th December 2007, and 5th and 16th January 2008. However, the clinical signs were generally mild. The strangles iELISA was used to screen 48 resident horses sampled on the 17th January 2008, identifying 39 (81%) as seropositive. Forty ponies from this population were sampled again 8 weeks later, showing a general decline in antibody levels to both antigen A and antigen B (**Fig. 3**), although 20 ponies (50%) remained seropositive. However, antibody levels in 2 ponies (pony 1 and pony 2) that had had pyrexia and mucopurulent nasal discharge from the 5th and 16th January 2008 respectively increased, providing evidence that the iELISA was successfully detecting genuine exposure to and infection with *S equi*. Further investigation of 6 seropositive healthy ponies with no history of clinical signs of strangles by guttural pouch endoscopy identified a persistently infected carrier, highlighting the endemic status of *S equi* infection on this yard.

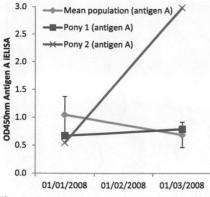 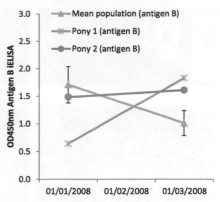

Fig. 3. Seroconversion of 2 clinically affected polo ponies while resident on a yard with endemic *S equi* infection. Error bars indicate the 95% confidence interval. A positive antigen A result is greater than or equal to 0.5 OD_{450nm} and a positive result for the antigen B iELISA is greater than or equal to 1.0 OD_{450nm}. OD, optical density.

The first clinical signs of strangles (pyrexia, nasal discharge, and enlarged submandibular lymph nodes) can be highly variable in appearance from one horse to another and are not restricted to *S equi* infection. However, if *S equi* infection is suspected, the horse should be isolated immediately to minimize the risk of transmission to in-contact animals. A needle aspirate from an enlarged or abscessed lymph node is the optimal sample for confirmation of *S equi* infection. *S equi* rapidly invades the lymph nodes of infected horses and is often not isolated from nasal swabs or washes taken during the early stages of disease,[38] so a negative nasal swab/wash result by culture or even qPCR does not necessarily mean that the animal is not infected with *S equi*, particularly if clinical signs suggest otherwise. Create 3 color-coded groups, even if limited space dictates that horses must remain in the same paddock only separated by 2 layers of electric fence to avoid nose-to-nose contact. The red group includes horses that have shown 1 or more clinical signs consistent with strangles. Amber group horses are those that have had direct or indirect contact with an infected horse in the red group and may be incubating the infection. The remaining green group horses have had no known direct or indirect contact with affected animals. The body temperatures of all horses in the green and amber groups should be obtained twice daily and any febrile horse should be moved to the red group. Color code buckets and other equipment to ensure that mixing between groups does not occur and wherever possible use dedicated staff for each color-coded group. If separate staff are not an option, staff should always move from the lowest risk to highest risk groups (ie, green to amber to red groups in that order and not back again). No horses should be allowed into, or out of, the yard at this time.

Screening procedures to identify those horses persistently infected with *S equi* should commence no sooner than 3 weeks after the resolution of the last clinical

---

Box 4
Example case report 3

Seven of 56 newly acquired horses arriving at a rescue center were found to be seropositive and later confirmed to be persistently infected by guttural pouch endoscopy and lavage (**Fig. 4**). All carriers were treated and no clinical cases of strangles occurred on mixing with resident horses.

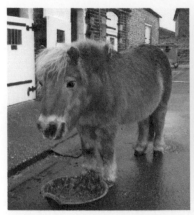 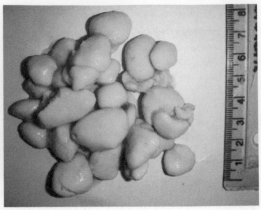

Fig. 4. Twenty-eight chondroids recovered from a healthy Shetland pony with serology assay OD_{450nm} of 2.5 for antigen A and 3.9 for antigen C.

case. Screening of horses in the amber and green groups using the dual iELISA test identifies other horses that were exposed before or during the outbreak that could be subclinical carriers and that, if left untreated, could trigger subsequent outbreaks (**Box 5**). Animals testing positive by iELISA and those in the red group should be investigated by guttural pouch endoscopy or, if this is not possible, nasopharyngeal swabbing/washing to establish whether they are persistently infected with *S equi*. Samples should be tested by qPCR to maximize sensitivity and carriers treated as described earlier.

VACCINATION AGAINST STRANGLES

Horses are among the most widely traveled animals on the planet and vaccination could play an important role in protecting horses from the inadvertent exposure to *S equi* while attending equine events or sales. Therefore, the ideal strangles vaccine would confer adequate levels of protection against the currently circulating strains of *S equi* with a long duration of immunity. Most equine vaccinations are administered via intramuscular injection and so, ideally, a strangles vaccine should be safe to administer via this route. It should have the capability to differentiate infected from vaccinated animals (DIVA) in order for the vaccine to be used alongside existing management strategies that incorporate qPCR and iELISA diagnostic tests. DIVA not only enables the normal movement of vaccinated horses but also permits the identification of vaccinated horses that were exposed to and successfully protected from *S equi*. Such data would build confidence in a vaccine, facilitating its wider use and leading to increased herd immunity.

Box 5
Example case report 4

An outbreak of strangles in livery yard in Scotland of unknown source resolved and all horses and ponies were screened using the dual iELISA to identify unaffected horses for further investigation, alongside those affected in the outbreak. Guttural pouch endoscopy confirmed that a healthy Shetland pony was persistently infected with *S equi*. The pony was treated and the infection eradicated.

KILLED AND CELL EXTRACT STRANGLES VACCINES

The first documented vaccine against strangles was developed by Bazeley[65-69] working with the Australian military in the 1940s. His vaccine was based on a culture of S equi that was heat killed at 55°C for 12 minutes and administered subcutaneously. Severe injection site reactions and pyrexia were frequently observed in vaccinated animals. However, 29 of approximately 2500 vaccinated horses developed strangles compared with 101 of approximately 1900 unvaccinated animals ($P<.0001$).[67] Analysis of formalin-killed or S equi extracts failed to show protection in this study.[67]

Cell-free versions of this early vaccine are available in some parts of the world and include Equivac S (Zoetis New Zealand), Strepguard (MSD Animal Health), and Strepvax II (Boehringer Ingelheim), which are administered by the intramuscular route. However, few data on the efficacy of these vaccines are publically available. One study found that 17 of 59 (29%) foals vaccinated with an SeM-based vaccine and 39 of 55 (71%) controls had clinical signs of strangles when observed 2 weeks after the third vaccination ($P<.0001$). However, 32 of 60 (53%) foals vaccinated with the same vaccine and 29 of 60 (48%) controls had clinical signs of strangles ($P = .72$) when observed 6 weeks after the third vaccination. These data suggest that any protection conferred by this vaccine was short lived. Furthermore, 44% and 29% of vaccinates, respectively, developed adverse reactions at the injection site in this study.[70] None of these vaccines have DIVA capability.

LIVE-ATTENUATED VACCINES

The only strangles vaccine available in Europe is Equilis StrepE (MSD Animal Health). Equilis StrepE is a live-attenuated aroA deletion mutant, which is based on a 1990 isolate from Holland.[40,71] In 2 separate studies in which all nonvaccinated control animals developed strangles, 2 doses of 10^9 colony-forming units of Equilis StrepE administered via submucosal (SM) injection into the upper lip protected 5 of 5 and 2 of 4 horses from developing lymph node abscesses following intranasal challenge 2 weeks after the second SM vaccination ($P = .0476$ and $P = .4286$, respectively).[71] Intramuscular administration of this vaccine seemed to be efficacious, protecting all 3 vaccinated animals.[71] However, injection site reactions, from which the vaccine strain was recovered, precluded administration via this more conventional and convenient route.[40,71,72] Adverse reactions following SM vaccination with Equilis StrepE have been reported.[72] The vaccine contains the same genetic material as virulent strains of S equi (excluding aroA), and so interferes with culture and qPCR tests while the vaccine strain persists, and iELISA tests by triggering positive test results that cannot readily be differentiated from those arising from natural infection. The lack of DIVA capability confounds the identification of vaccinated horses that are infected with virulent strains of S equi. Therefore, all vaccinated animals triggering a positive iELISA result are required to be examined further to eliminate the possibility that they may be persistently infected (**Box 6**).

A second live-attenuated vaccine, Pinnacle IN (Zoetis), for intranasal administration, is available in the United States and some other territories. The vaccine is based on the CF32 strain that was isolated from a horse in New York during 1981 and attenuated via treatment with nitrosoguanidine. As with Equilis StrepE, Pinnacle causes adverse effects if injected intramuscularly and does not have DIVA capability. The vaccine strain has been linked to lymph node abscesses and can be shed up to 46 days after vaccination of young (<1 year old) ponies.[73] Furthermore, S equi resembling the Pinnacle IN vaccine strain was isolated from recently vaccinated horses in New Zealand that had subsequently developed strangles, suggesting that some horses may have increased

> **Box 6**
> **Example case report 5**
>
> A pregnant mare in good health tested positive using the dual iELISA described earlier, despite the owner having no knowledge of a prior history of strangles or exposure to *S equi*. The horse had been vaccinated 5 years previously with Equilis StrepE. However, it was decided that it was unlikely that the observed antibody response was caused by vaccination. The mare was examined further by guttural pouch endoscopy and lavage. Washes recovered from the guttural pouches tested qPCR positive, indicating persistent infection. On further discussion with the owner it became clear that the horse had been stationed at the Defence Animal Centre at Melton Mowbray, United Kingdom, at the time of a strangles outbreak. The mare was treated to eliminate the persistent infection in the guttural pouch, which was confirmed by qPCR analysis of guttural pouch lavages 2 weeks later.

sensitivity to the vaccine, or that the strain can revert to virulence.[74] No data on efficacy have been published, but at the Getting to Grips with Strangles meeting in Stockholm in 2010, Zoetis stated that, following experimental challenge, 9 of 15 controls developed strangles compared with 3 of 22 high-dose vaccinates ($P = .0049$) and 2 of 22 low-dose ($P = .0023$) vaccinates 3 weeks after the second vaccination. Therefore, the commercial live-attenuated vaccines for strangles can confer significant levels of protection. However, they lack DIVA capability and have been linked to adverse reactions in some animals.

Early research data suggested that all *S equi* strains were identical because sera from a convalescent horse cross-reacted with other isolates and there was no variation in *Hind* III restriction pattern between different *S equi* isolates on Southern blot analysis using an SeM gene probe.[34] However, sequence analysis of the SeM gene identified differences between strains of *S equi*,[2,39,40,74,75] with 128 different alleles currently identifiable in the online database at http://pubmlst.org/cgi-bin/mlstdbnet/agdbnet.pl?file=sz_seM.xml (last accessed 10th April 2014). Evidence suggests that the population of *S equi* is changing over time as the organism continues to evolve, with domination of SeM-9 strains of *S equi* within the United Kingdom.[2,75] Equilis StrepE and Pinnacle were derived from strains that cluster into groups of *S equi* distantly related to the dominant SeM-9 strains. Although an antibody response is likely to cross-react between different strains of *S equi*,[34] the level of protection conferred by these vaccines against currently circulating strains of *S equi* remains unknown.

SUBUNIT VACCINES

Subunit vaccines are based on recombinant *S equi* proteins produced in and purified from *Escherichia coli* strains. These vaccines generally have excellent safety profiles because only the desired target proteins are used in the vaccine. Subunit vaccines do not contain *S equi* DNA and can be designed to avoid the particular antigens used in diagnostic tests, conferring the ability to DIVA. However, the identification of protective antigens represents a significant challenge for vaccine design. The vaccination of mice with recombinant SeM conferred protection against challenge with *S equi*,[76] but these promising results were not repeated following the vaccination and challenge of horses.[77] Two subunit vaccines consisting of 6 *S equi*–specific proteins or 5 *S equi* adhesin proteins also failed to confer protection in ponies, despite the generation of promising serum antibody responses.[78] However, a combination of 7 *S equi* surface and secreted proteins, Septavac, which were identified through analysis of the *S equi* genome[3] and mouse studies,[79] protected 6 of 7 vaccinated Welsh mountain ponies 2 weeks after their third vaccinations ($P = .0047$).[55] The inclusion of the immunoglobulin-cleaving proteins IdeE and IdeE2 in the vaccine were found to be important to efficacy and a 5-component vaccine, Pentavac, lacking these components protected only 1 of 7 ponies 2 weeks after the fourth vaccination.[55] The combination of proteins used did not include SeM or SEQ2190 and so this vaccine is likely to have DIVA capability.[41] The Septavac vaccine (now known as Strangvac) is based on a SeM-9 strain of *S equi* recovered from a horse in Sweden in 2000,[55] which is more closely related to the dominant strains circulating the UK horse population.

SUMMARY AND FUTURE PERSPECTIVES

S equi has evolved to exploit the anatomy of the horse producing abscesses in the lymph nodes, which enable the organism to persistently infect a proportion of convalescent animals. Shedding of *S equi* from carrier animals enables the onward transmission of this pathogen and further outbreaks of disease. Therefore, the identification and treatment of persistently infected carriers is critical if the cycle of infection is to be broken and *S equi* eradicated. The improvements to the available diagnostic tests greatly assist the identification of persistently infected animals and are preventing new outbreaks of disease. However, further work is required to permit their use alongside effective vaccines, which can increase herd immunity and reduce the number of strangles outbreaks occurring in horse populations around the world.

REFERENCES

1. Rufus J. De medicina equorum, 1251.
2. Parkinson NJ, Robin C, Newton JR, et al. Molecular epidemiology of strangles outbreaks in the UK during 2010. Vet Rec 2011;168:666.
3. Holden MT, Heather Z, Paillot R, et al. Genomic evidence for the evolution of *Streptococcus equi*: host restriction, increased virulence, and genetic exchange with human pathogens. PLoS Pathog 2009;5:e1000346.
4. Chalker VJ, Brooks HW, Brownlie J. The association of *Streptococcus equi* subsp. *zooepidemicus* with canine infectious respiratory disease. Vet Microbiol 2003;95:149–56.
5. Chalker VJ, Waller A, Webb K, et al. Genetic diversity of *Streptococcus equi* subsp. *zooepidemicus* and doxycycline resistance in kennelled dogs. J Clin Microbiol 2012;50:2134–6.
6. Pesavento PA, Hurley KF, Bannasch MJ, et al. A clonal outbreak of acute fatal hemorrhagic pneumonia in intensively housed (shelter) dogs caused by *Streptococcus equi* subsp. *zooepidemicus*. Vet Pathol 2008;45:51–3.
7. Abbott Y, Acke E, Khan S, et al. Zoonotic transmission of *Streptococcus equi* subsp. *zooepidemicus* from a dog to a handler. J Med Microbiol 2010;59:120–3.
8. Bradley SF, Gordon JJ, Baumgartner DD, et al. Group C streptococcal bacteremia: analysis of 88 cases. Rev Infect Dis 1991;13:270–80.
9. Downar J, Willey BM, Sutherland JW, et al. Streptococcal meningitis resulting from contact with an infected horse. J Clin Microbiol 2001;39:2358–9.
10. Hashikawa S, Iinuma Y, Furushita M, et al. Characterization of group C and G streptococcal strains that cause streptococcal toxic shock syndrome. J Clin Microbiol 2004;42:186–92.
11. Hong CB, Donahue JM, Giles RC Jr, et al. Equine abortion and stillbirth in central Kentucky during 1988 and 1989 foaling seasons. J Vet Diagn Invest 1993;5:560–6.
12. Smith KC, Blunden AS, Whitwell KE, et al. A survey of equine abortion, stillbirth and neonatal death in the UK from 1988 to 1997. Equine Vet J 2003;35:496–501.

13. Brooks DE, Andrew SE, Biros DJ, et al. Ulcerative keratitis caused by beta-hemolytic *Streptococcus equi* in 11 horses. Vet Ophthalmol 2000;3:121–5.

14. Anzai T, Walker JA, Blair MB, et al. Comparison of the phenotypes of *Streptococcus zooepidemicus* isolated from tonsils of healthy horses and specimens obtained from foals and donkeys with pneumonia. Am J Vet Res 2000;61:162–6.

15. Wood JL, Newton JR, Chanter N, et al. Association between respiratory disease and bacterial and viral infections in British racehorses. J Clin Microbiol 2005;43: 120–6.

16. Webb K, Jolley KA, Mitchell Z, et al. Development of an unambiguous and discriminatory multilocus sequence typing scheme for the *Streptococcus zooepidemicus* group. Microbiology 2008;154:3016–24.

17. Lindahl SB, Aspan A, Baverud V, et al. Outbreak of upper respiratory disease in horses caused by *Streptococcus equi* subsp. *zooepidemicus* ST-24. Vet Microbiol 2013;166:281–5.

18. Velineni S, Desoutter D, Perchec AM, et al. Characterization of a mucoid clone of *Streptococcus zooepidemicus* from an epizootic of equine respiratory disease in New Caledonia. Vet J 2014;200:82–7.

19. Waller AS. Equine respiratory disease: a causal role of *Streptococcus zooepidemicus*. Vet J 2014;201:3–4.

20. Timoney JF. Strangles. Vet Clin North Am Equine Pract 1993;9:365–74.

21. Timoney JF, Kumar P. Early pathogenesis of equine *Streptococcus equi* infection (strangles). Equine Vet J 2008;40:637–42.

22. Artiushin SC, Timoney JF, Sheoran AS, et al. Characterization and immunogenicity of pyrogenic mitogens SePE-H and SePE-I of *Streptococcus equi*. Microb Pathog 2002;32:71–85.

23. Paillot R, Robinson C, Steward K, et al. Contribution of each of four superantigens to *Streptococcus equi*-induced mitogenicity, gamma interferon synthesis, and immunity. Infect Immun 2010;78:1728–39.

24. Flanagan J, Collin N, Timoney J, et al. Characterization of the haemolytic activity of *Streptococcus equi*. Microb Pathog 1998;24:211–21.

25. Galan JE, Timoney JF. Molecular analysis of the M protein of *Streptococcus equi* and cloning and expression of the M protein gene in *Escherichia coli*. Infect Immun 1987;55:3181–7.

26. Lannergard J, Guss B. IdeE, an IgG-endopeptidase of *Streptococcus equi* ssp. *equi*. FEMS Microbiol Lett 2006;262:230–5.

27. Timoney JF, Yang J, Liu J, et al. IdeE reduces the bactericidal activity of equine neutrophils for *Streptococcus equi*. Vet Immunol Immunopathol 2008;122:76–82.

28. Tiwari R, Qin A, Artiushin S, et al. Se18.9, an anti-phagocytic factor H binding protein of *Streptococcus equi*. Vet Microbiol 2007;121:105–15.

29. Turner CE, Kurupati P, Jones MD, et al. Emerging role of the interleukin-8 cleaving enzyme SpyCEP in clinical *Streptococcus pyogenes* infection. J Infect Dis 2009; 200:555–63.

30. Lewis MJ, Meehan M, Owen P, et al. A common theme in interaction of bacterial immunoglobulin-binding proteins with immunoglobulins illustrated in the equine system. J Biol Chem 2008;283:17615–23.

31. Meehan M, Lewis MJ, Byrne C, et al. Localization of the equine IgG-binding domain in the fibrinogen-binding protein (FgBP) of *Streptococcus equi* subsp. *equi*. Microbiology 2009;155:2583–92.

32. Meehan M, Lynagh Y, Woods C, et al. The fibrinogen-binding protein (FgBP) of *Streptococcus equi* subsp. *equi* additionally binds IgG and contributes to virulence in a mouse model. Microbiology 2001;147:3311–22.

33. Boschwitz JS, Timoney JF. Inhibition of C3 deposition on *Streptococcus equi* subsp. *equi* by M protein: a mechanism for survival in equine blood. Infect Immun 1994;62:3515–20.

34. Galan JE, Timoney JF. Immunologic and genetic comparison of *Streptococcus equi* isolates from the United States and Europe. J Clin Microbiol 1988;26: 1142–6.

35. Heather Z, Holden MT, Steward KF, et al. A novel streptococcal integrative conjugative element involved in iron acquisition. Mol Microbiol 2008;70:1274–92.

36. Boschwitz JS, Timoney JF. Characterization of the antiphagocytic activity of equine fibrinogen for *Streptococcus equi* subsp. *equi*. Microb Pathog 1994; 17:121–9.

37. Walker JA, Timoney JF. Construction of a stable non-mucoid deletion mutant of the *Streptococcus equi* Pinnacle vaccine strain. Vet Microbiol 2002;89:311–21.

38. Sweeney CR, Timoney JF, Newton JR, et al. *Streptococcus equi* infections in horses: guidelines for treatment, control, and prevention of strangles. J Vet Intern Med 2005;19:123–34.

39. Anzai T, Kuwamoto Y, Wada R, et al. Variation in the N-terminal region of an M-like protein of *Streptococcus equi* and evaluation of its potential as a tool in epidemiologic studies. Am J Vet Res 2005;66:2167–71.

40. Kelly C, Bugg M, Robinson C, et al. Sequence variation of the SeM gene of *Streptococcus equi* allows discrimination of the source of strangles outbreaks. J Clin Microbiol 2006;44:480–6.

41. Robinson C, Steward KF, Potts N, et al. Combining two serological assays optimises sensitivity and specificity for the identification of *Streptococcus equi* subsp. *equi* exposure. Vet J 2013;197:188–91.

42. Galan JE, Timoney JF. Mucosal nasopharyngeal immune responses of horses to protein antigens of *Streptococcus equi*. Infect Immun 1985;47:623–8.

43. Hamlen HJ, Timoney JF, Bell RJ. Epidemiologic and immunologic characteristics of *Streptococcus equi* infection in foals. J Am Vet Med Assoc 1994;204: 768–75.

44. Todd AG. Strangles. J Comp Pathol Ther 1910;23:212–29.

45. Newton JR, Wood JL, Dunn KA, et al. Naturally occurring persistent and asymptomatic infection of the guttural pouches of horses with *Streptococcus equi*. Vet Rec 1997;140:84–90.

46. Verheyen K, Newton JR, Talbot NC, et al. Elimination of guttural pouch infection and inflammation in asymptomatic carriers of *Streptococcus equi*. Equine Vet J 2000;32:527–32.

47. Weese JS, Jarlot C, Morley PS. Survival of *Streptococcus equi* on surfaces in an outdoor environment. Can Vet J 2009;50:968–70.

48. Pusterla N, Watson JL, Affolter VK, et al. Purpura haemorrhagica in 53 horses. Vet Rec 2003;153:118–21.

49. Sweeney CR, Whitlock RH, Meirs DA, et al. Complications associated with *Streptococcus equi* infection on a horse farm. J Am Vet Med Assoc 1987;191: 1446–8.

50. Heath SE, Geor RJ, Tabel H, et al. Unusual patterns of serum antibodies to *Streptococcus equi* in two horses with purpura hemorrhagica. J Vet Intern Med 1991;5:263–7.

51. Waller AS. Strangles: taking steps towards eradication. Vet Microbiol 2013;167: 50–60.

52. Waller AS, Paillot R, Timoney JF. *Streptococcus equi*: a pathogen restricted to one host. J Med Microbiol 2011;60:1231–40.

53. Baverud V, Johansson SK, Aspan A. Real-time PCR for detection and differentiation of *Streptococcus equi* subsp. *equi* and *Streptococcus equi* subsp. *zooepidemicus*. Vet Microbiol 2007;124:219–29.
54. Webb K, Barker C, Harrison T, et al. Detection of *Streptococcus equi* subspecies *equi* using a triplex qPCR assay. Vet J 2013;195:300–4.
55. Guss B, Flock M, Frykberg L, et al. Getting to grips with strangles: an effective multi-component recombinant vaccine for the protection of horses from *Streptococcus equi* infection. PLoS Pathog 2009;5:e1000584.
56. Bannister MF, Benson CE, Sweeney CR. Rapid species identification of group C streptococci isolated from horses. J Clin Microbiol 1985;21:524–6.
57. Newton JR, Verheyen K, Talbot NC, et al. Control of strangles outbreaks by isolation of guttural pouch carriers identified using PCR and culture of *Streptococcus equi*. Equine Vet J 2000;32:515–26.
58. Timoney JF, Artiushin SC. Detection of *Streptococcus equi* in equine nasal swabs and washes by DNA amplification. Vet Rec 1997;141:446–7.
59. Chanter N, Talbot NC, Newton JR, et al. *Streptococcus equi* with truncated M-proteins isolated from outwardly healthy horses. Microbiology 2000;146(Pt 6):1361–9.
60. Waller AS, Jolley KA. Getting a grip on strangles: recent progress towards improved diagnostics and vaccines. Vet J 2007;173:492–501.
61. Davidson A, Traub-Dargatz JL, Magnuson R, et al. Lack of correlation between antibody titers to fibrinogen-binding protein of *Streptococcus equi* and persistent carriers of strangles. J Vet Diagn Invest 2008;20:457–62.
62. Ling AS, Upjohn MM, Webb K, et al. Seroprevalence of *Streptococcus equi* in working horses in Lesotho. Vet Rec 2011;169:72.
63. Walshe N, Johnston J, MacCarthy E, et al. "Strangles" in less regulated sectors of the Irish horse industry. J Equine Vet Sci 2012;32:S3–95.
64. Knowles EJ, Mair TS, Butcher N, et al. Use of a novel serological test for exposure to *Streptococcus equi* subspecies equi in hospitalised horses. Vet Rec 2010;166: 294–7.
65. Bazeley PL. Studies with equine streptococci 1. Aust Vet J 1940;16:140–6.
66. Bazeley PL. Studies with equine streptococci 2. Aust Vet J 1940;16:243–59.
67. Bazeley PL. Studies with equine streptococci 3. Aust Vet J 1942;18:141–55.
68. Bazeley PL. Studies with equine streptococci 4. Aust Vet J 1942;18:189–94.
69. Bazeley PL. Studies with equine streptococci 5. Aust Vet J 1943;19:62–85.
70. Hoffman AM, Staempfli HR, Prescott JF, et al. Field evaluation of a commercial M-protein vaccine against *Streptococcus equi* infection in foals. Am J Vet Res 1991;52:589–92.
71. Jacobs AA, Goovaerts D, Nuijten PJ, et al. Investigations towards an efficacious and safe strangles vaccine: submucosal vaccination with a live attenuated *Streptococcus equi*. Vet Rec 2000;147:563–7.
72. Kemp-Symonds J, Kemble T, Waller A. Modified live *Streptococcus equi* ('strangles') vaccination followed by clinically adverse reactions associated with bacterial replication. Equine Vet J 2007;39:284–6.
73. Borst LB, Patterson SK, Lanka S, et al. Evaluation of a commercially available modified-live *Streptococcus equi* subsp *equi* vaccine in ponies. Am J Vet Res 2011;72:1130–8.
74. Patty O, Cursons R. The molecular identification of *Streptococcus equi* subsp. *equi* strains isolated within New Zealand. N Z Vet J 2014;62:63–7.
75. Ivens PA, Matthews D, Webb K, et al. Molecular characterisation of 'strangles' outbreaks in the UK: the use of M-protein typing of *Streptococcus equi* ssp. *equi*. Equine Vet J 2011;43:359–64.

76. Meehan M, Nowlan P, Owen P. Affinity purification and characterization of a fibrinogen-binding protein complex which protects mice against lethal challenge with *Streptococcus equi* subsp. *equi*. Microbiology 1998;144:993–1003.
77. Sheoran AS, Artiushin S, Timoney JF. Nasal mucosal immunogenicity for the horse of a SeM peptide of *Streptococcus equi* genetically coupled to cholera toxin. Vaccine 2002;20:1653–9.
78. Timoney JF, Qin A, Muthupalani S, et al. Vaccine potential of novel surface exposed and secreted proteins of *Streptococcus equi*. Vaccine 2007;25: 5583–90.
79. Flock M, Karlstrom A, Lannergard J, et al. Protective effect of vaccination with recombinant proteins from *Streptococcus equi* subspecies equi in a strangles model in the mouse. Vaccine 2006;24:4144–51.

Rhodococcus equi Foal Pneumonia

Noah D. Cohen, VMD, MPH, PhD

KEYWORDS

- Foal • Pneumonia • Rhodococcus equi • Antimicrobial therapy
- Extrapulmonary disorders • Thoracic ultrasound

KEY POINTS

- Environmental factors such as density of mares and foals and airborne concentrations of virulent Rhodococcus equi increase the odds of foals developing R equi pneumonia.
- Extrapulmonary disorders can be common.
- Diagnosis is established in foals with clinical signs of pneumonia by microbiologic culture of R equi from fluid obtained by tracheobronchial aspiration (TBA).
- Emergence of resistance to macrolides and absence of effective alternatives represent important challenges in the treatment of R equi pneumonia.
- Highly effective methods for preventing R equi pneumonia in foals are lacking.

INTRODUCTION

Infection of the respiratory tract and other extrapulmonary sites by the bacterium *Rhodococcus equi* continues to be an important cause of disease and death for foals. The objective of this article was to review information regarding the epidemiology, clinical signs, diagnostic testing, and control and prevention of R equi infections of foals.

ETIOLOGY

R equi is a gram-positive, facultative intracellular pathogen that preferentially infects macrophages.[1]

EPIDEMIOLOGY

R equi pneumonia has been described as occurring recurrently at some farms, whereas other farms experience either only sporadic occurrence of the disease or are spared from having affected foals.[1] At farms that experience the disease on a recurrent basis (hereafter termed *endemic farms*), there is considerable variation in

Department of Large Animal Clinical Sciences, College of Veterinary Medicine & Biomedical Sciences, Texas A&M University, College Station, TX 77843-4475, USA
E-mail address: ncohen@cvm.tamu.edu

Vet Clin Equine 30 (2014) 609–622
http://dx.doi.org/10.1016/j.cveq.2014.08.010
0749-0739/14/$ – see front matter © 2014 Elsevier Inc. All rights reserved.

vetequine.theclinics.com

the cumulative incidence of disease among farms[2-4] and between years.[5] Moreover, diagnosis at farms with recurrent cases of R equi pneumonia is often presumptive because veterinarians or farm managers eschew the use of tracheobronchial aspiration (TBA) and laboratory testing in some or all foals because of health risks for foals, time and physical effort for the procedure, or costs for TBA and associated cytologic and microbiological testing. Consequently, case definitions generally do not meet the standard recommendations for diagnosis of R equi[6] at many farms. Thus, it is difficult to accurately characterize the burden of disease in foals caused by R equi infections at the population level. In general, cumulative incidences tend to be around 10% to 20% from birth through weaning, although higher cumulative incidences are reported.[2-5]

Use of ultrasonographic screening is increasingly common at endemic farms to identify foals with pulmonary consolidation or abscess formation attributed to R equi infection. When foals are treated for R equi pneumonia based on the results of ultrasonographic screening, an increased apparent cumulative incidence of disease occurs because foals that will not develop clinical signs of pneumonia are included with those that will subsequently develop pneumonia. For example, it was recently reported that among 270 foals at a large breeding farm in Texas, 80% (216/270) developed ultrasonographic evidence of pulmonary consolidations or abscesses greater than 10 mm in diameter; of these 216 foals, only 46 (21%) ultimately developed clinical signs of pneumonia.[7]

The epidemiology of infectious diseases is often characterized in terms of factors relating to the infectious agent, the environment, and the host.[8] Isolates that are virulent in foals bear a plasmid that encodes a virulence-associated surface-expressed protein (VapA) that is necessary but not sufficient to cause disease.[9,10] It seems that a wide array of genotypically distinct virulent (and avirulent) isolates of R equi may be found in the air, equine feces, soil, and water at horse breeding farms.[11-13] Moreover, within a given foal it is possible to identify genotypically distinct isolates from the same organ or different organs.[14,15] Thus, it seems likely that all isolates with the plasmid encoding VapA are capable of causing disease in foals. Recent evidence indicates that macrolide-resistant isolates of R equi are associated with a worse prognosis in foals.[16] Although it is biologically plausible that macrolide-resistant isolates are more difficult to treat and thus are more likely to cause severe disease, it is also possible and plausible that these isolates are more likely to be recovered from foals that are treated for longer periods of time or are more likely to be recovered from foals that have been treated long term. It is also conceivable that macrolide-resistant isolates might also be more virulent for mechanisms other than susceptibility to macrolides.

From the standpoint of the environment, evidence exists that the disease occurs primarily at large breeding farms that use management practices desirable for control and prevention of contagious diseases.[2-4] Thus, the occurrence of R equi does not seem to be explained simply by poor hygiene or suboptimal management. The density of mares and foals has been positively associated with increased odds of R equi pneumonia.[2-4,17] The concentration of virulent R equi in the feces of mares during the perinatal period was not directly correlated with development of disease in their foals.[18] Nevertheless, mares represent an important source of R equi for their foals because most if not all mares shed R equi in their feces.[18,19] Although soil concentrations of virulent R equi are not associated with the cumulative incidence of R equi pneumonia, there is evidence that airborne concentrations of virulent R equi are positively associated with disease.[20] In general, airborne concentrations of R equi tend to be higher in stalls and barns than paddocks or pastures.[21,22] Airborne concentrations of virulent R *equi* are higher in the stalls of foals that subsequently develop *R equi* pneumonia than in the stalls of foals that do not develop the disease.[23,24] Early exposure to higher concentrations of virulent *R equi* in foaling stalls may be a risk factor for subsequent disease development, and may explain reports indicating that foals that are born and maintained in pastures are at lower risk of *R equi* pneumonia.[4,25] Use of more refined methods for quantifying airborne exposures could improve our understanding of the association of risk of *R equi* pneumonia with airborne concentrations of virulent *R equi* (and other particulates) in foaling stalls and paddocks.

The findings that virulent *R equi* are widely distributed in the environment at horse breeding farms yet only some foals develop disease indicate that host factors are important for this disease. Pneumonia caused by *R equi* seems to be restricted to foals: Horses older than 1 year are rarely affected, and when mature horses are affected, there is usually an accompanying immunodeficiency. These observations suggest that young foals may be predisposed because their immune system is either naïve or deficient. Evidence of deficiencies in innate and adaptive immunity has been described for neonates of other species.[26,27] Evidence regarding immune function of newborn foals is conflicting. Foals express markedly less interferon-γ than older foals or adult horses,[28,29] and gene expression of leukocytes to *R equi* changes with age.[30] Neonatal foals do not respond as strongly as older foals to vaccination with either inactivated viral vaccines or live, intracellularly replicating bacteria.[31,32] On the other hand, evidence exists that stimulated interferon-γ responses of 10-day-old foals are similar to those of older foals and adults.[33] Thus, conclusive evidence of an immunodeficiency (rather than mere naivety) remains to be demonstrated. Moreover, the correlates of protective immunity against *R equi* in foals also remain to be determined.

Anecdotally, some stallions and mares seem to be more likely to produce affected foals than other mares and stallions from the same farms. These data suggest a genetic basis for susceptibility to *R equi* infection. Using a candidate gene approach, polymorphisms in the *SLC11A1* gene (formerly known as *NRAMP1*) and the transferrin gene have been associated with *R equi* pneumonia in Arabian and Thoroughbred foals, respectively.[34,35] An association with the interleukin-7 receptor gene was significantly associated with heavier burden of virulent *R equi* recovered from TBA fluid (>5000 CFU/mL) relative to foals that did not have *R equi* recovered from their TBA fluid.[36] Microsatellite markers also have been identified that were significantly associated with higher *R equi* concentrations in TBA fluid,[37] including some that were associated with immune response genes.[38] None of these reported associations is particularly large (ie, the magnitude of the resultant odds ratios are all quite modest). This is not surprising, because it is unlikely that the genetic basis of susceptibility to *R equi* is a simple Mendelian trait. Rather, it is likely a complex trait with modest contributions from multiple genes involving a number of biological pathways and processes. Nevertheless, collectively these results suggest that immune-related and iron-mediated processes play a role in the pathogenesis of *R equi*.

Much remains to be understood regarding the epidemiology of *R equi* pneumonia. Of particular interest from the standpoint of the agent is the extent of emergence and dissemination of macrolide resistance and the impact on foal health of these macrolide-resistant isolates.[12,16] Further evaluation of the role in *R equi* pneumonia of environmental factors such as density of mares and foals, foaling and maintaining foals at pasture, and airborne concentrations are much needed, including intervention trials. Finally, host factors, including neonatal immunity, genetics, and their intersection, are also needed to unravel the complex epidemiology of foal pneumonia caused by *R equi*.

CLINICAL SIGNS

The most common clinical signs in foals with *R equi* pneumonia reflect lower respiratory tract infection and include coughing, fever, increased respiratory rate and effort (including flared nostrils and an abdominal component to their breathing), increased heart rate, and abnormal airway sounds in the trachea (often referred to as tracheal rattling) and in the lungs (crackles, wheezes, or both may be heard).[1,39] Nasal discharge is not a common finding in infected foals. Affected foals are most commonly between 1 and 3 months of age when clinical signs become apparent. Progression of pneumonia is insidious and pulmonary lesions may be quite extensive before the onset of clinical signs. On rare occasions, a subacute form of the disease may be recognized in which previously healthy foals present with sudden onset of respiratory distress that progresses rapidly to death in less than 48 hours; some of these foals may be found dead with little or no prodromal findings.[39]

Foals also may manifest extrapulmonary signs of infection with *R equi*. A wide array of extrapulmonary disorders (EPDs) associated with *R equi* infection have been reported (**Box 1**).[40] These EPDs are often found concurrently with pneumonia, but also may be found independent of pneumonia. Foals may have more than 1 EPD concurrently.[40] The most common EPDs are (1) diarrhea, (2) ulcerative enterotyphlocolitis, (3) presumed immune-mediated synovitis, (4) intra-abdominal lymphadenitis or abscessation, and (5) uveitis.[40] Establishing whether *R equi* is the cause of diarrhea can be confusing because many foals shed *R equi* in feces, and the level of shedding has not been convincingly associated with presence of enteritis, typhlitis, or colitis or with diarrheal disease. Moreover, the antimicrobials used to treat *R equi* pneumonia can cause diarrhea.[41] Interestingly, it has been reported that more than half of foals with ulcerative enterotyphlocolitis caused by *R equi* have diarrhea.[40]

Polysynovitis can occur in 40% or more of affected foals.[40] The most commonly affected sites include the tarsocrural joints, carpal joints, and fetlock joints; other synovial structures can be involved (**Fig. 1**). These swellings generally result in no more than mild pain and decreased range of motion, whereas foals with septic polyarthritis are generally quite lame. Generally, synovitis resolves concurrent with the clinical signs of pneumonia.[40] Intra-articular treatment is seldom if ever warranted; however, topical, enteral, or parenteral nonsteroidal anti-inflammatory drugs may help to reduce swelling and improve the comfort of severely affected foals.

The frequency with which intra-abdominal lymphadenitis and lymph node abscessation develop among foals at breeding farms is unknown. Nevertheless, it may be prudent to consider abdominal ultrasonography of *R equi*-affected foals because the prognosis for foals with intra-abdominal abscess development is generally grave.[40] Uveitis also has been associated with a poor prognosis,[40] possibly reflecting a manifestation of more severe systemic disease among affected foals.

DIAGNOSIS

The so-called gold standard for diagnosis is the microbiologic culture of *R equi* from fluid obtained by TBA.[6] Whenever possible, these findings should be supported by cytologic evidence of septic inflammation and pleomorphic, gram-positive rods found intracellularly in TBA fluid, and results of thoracic imaging that reveal pulmonary abscesses or consolidations.[6] The purpose of obtaining these supportive cytologic and imaging results is to reduce the likelihood of false-positive results that can occur because of the ubiquity of *R equi* in the environment of foals. Use of polymerase chain reaction (PCR) testing of TBA fluid for *R equi* offers advantages: Results are rapidly available (within hours of receipt, whereas microbiologic culture requires days);

Box 1
Extrapulmonary disorders identified in foals infected with *Rhodococcus equi*

More common

Diarrhea

Intra-abdominal abscesses

Intra-abdominal lymphadenitis

Polysynovitis

Pyogranulomatous hepatitis

Ulcerative enterotyphlocolitis

Uveitis

Less common

Bacteremia

Cellulitis/lymphangitis

Granulomatous meningitis

Immune-mediated hemolytic anemia and/or thrombocytopenia

Intracranial abscess(es)

Mediastinal lymphadenitis

Osteomyelitis (including vertebral osteomyelitis)

Pericarditis

Peripheral lymphadenitis

Peritonitis

Pleuritis

Pyogranulomatous nephritis

Septic arthritis

Septic synovitis

Subcutaneous abscesses (including paravertebral abscesses and submandibular lymph node abscesses)

---

virulent strains can be specifically identified by amplifying the *vapA* gene of *R equi*; and PCR can be more sensitive than microbiologic culture.[42] Disadvantages of PCR testing for *R equi* include that one cannot identify other bacterial species that may be present, and that one does not retain live *R* equi, which can be tested for antimicrobial susceptibility or for genotyping or phenotyping of strains for clinical or epidemiologic purposes.

Because of the expense, labor, and risks to foals, many veterinarians eschew performing TBAs to confirm a diagnosis. To date, suitable noninvasive alternatives have not been identified. Serologic testing is not accurate for diagnosis.[43,44] Although sensitivity of fecal PCR was relatively high in a small group of affected foals, a large-scale, systematic evaluation of fecal PCR testing has not been reported (to the author's knowledge). Testing nasal swabs either by culture or PCR for *R equi* is not useful for diagnosis.[45] Because alternatives to TBA are lacking, many if not most veterinarians make a diagnosis of *R equi* presumptively in the field based on signalment, clinical signs, and results of thoracic ultrasonography revealing peripheral pulmonary

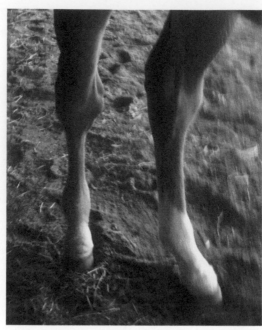

Fig. 1. Effusion of tarsocrural joints in a foal with *Rhodococcus equi* pneumonia. This foal also had effusion of its carpal joints and fetlock joints (all 4 limbs).

abscesses or consolidations. Although prone to misclassification, it is likely that the positive predictive value of this approach is high at farms, with recurrent confirmed cases of *R equi* pneumonia and where the cumulative incidence of disease is high.

THERAPEUTIC STRATEGIES

Administration of a macrolide in combination with rifampin has been the standard of care for about 30 years. For the first 10 to 15 years, erythromycin was the macrolide of choice (15–37.5 mg/kg orally every 6–12 hours).[6] In recent years, azithromycin (10 mg/kg orally every 24 hours for 5–7 days, followed by the same dosage every 48 hours) and clarithromycin (7.5 mg/kg orally every 12 hours) have been used more commonly based on considerations of both pharmacokinetics and drug distribution, ease of administration (ie, longer interval between doses), and retrospective comparison of efficacy.[6,46] Recently, intramuscular administration of gamithromycin has been demonstrated to provide concentrations above the minimum inhibitory concentration required to inhibit the growth of 90% of organisms of *R equi* in bronchoalveolar lavage fluid cells and neutrophils for about 9 days, indicating that weekly administration of gamithromycin might be feasible.[47] Anecdotally, some practitioners are using this antimicrobial to treat pneumonia in foals because of the convenience of weekly administration. Use of other macrolides such as tulathromycin or tilmicosin does not seem warranted.[48,49]

Controversy exists regarding the value of including rifampin with macrolides. The combination was first proposed for clinical use in the mid 1980s based on synergy between erythromycin and rifampin observed in vitro,[50] which was bolstered by expert opinion,[51] a case series,[52] and a study using historical controls treated with the combination of penicillin and gentamicin.[53] Subsequently, it was demonstrated that the combination was superior to either drug alone in reducing tissue concentrations of

R equi in experimentally infected immunodeficient mice.[54] More recently, it was demonstrated that the combination of a macrolide plus rifampin had a lower mutant prevention concentration than any of the macrolides alone.[55]

Despite the aforementioned evidence supporting the combination, there is also evidence to question the value of the combination. Coadministration of rifampin to foals lowers concentrations of macrolides in plasma and bronchoalveolar lavage fluids, in large part by inhibiting intestinal absorption of macrolides.[56,57] Clinical studies of foals with mild clinical signs and varying sizes of pulmonary abscesses or consolidations at a large breeding farm in Germany have failed to demonstrate a benefit of combining macrolides with rifampin versus macrolides alone.[58–60] Interestingly, only 1 of these 3 studies[60] documented that macrolide treatment (with or without rifampin) was superior to placebo, indicating that many foals with mild or no clinical signs but with ultrasonographic lesions may recover without treatment. This finding is consistent with observations from a large breeding farm in Texas.[7]

A well-designed, large-scale clinical trial is needed to answer the question regarding the benefit (or detriment) of combining a macrolide with rifampin for treating foals with *R equi* pneumonia. Such a study is unlikely to be performed because of the logistical and financial requirements for its conduct. In the absence of strong clinical evidence of reduced efficacy associated with using the combination, and in light of the specter of emerging resistance to macrolides, it is recommended that macrolides be combined with rifampin based on historical experience and evidence that the combination lowers the mutant prevention concentration of macrolides against *R equi*.

CONTROL STRATEGIES

Although the case for curative medicine is often perceived as being more compelling than that for prevention, prophylaxis is likely to be the most effective approach for controlling *R equi* pneumonia at horse breeding farms. Unfortunately, to date, highly effective prevention of *R equi* pneumonia is lacking. Although there are anecdotal reports of decreased incidence after reducing the density of mares and foals at farms, controlled, well-designed intervention trials of management practices for reducing *R equi* pneumonia have not been reported. Although successful chemoprophylaxis with macrolides has been reported,[61] conflicting evidence exists.[62] The reasons for these discrepant results are unknown, but the point is likely moot because prophylactic use of macrolides cannot be recommended in light of the apparent emergence of resistance to macrolides by *R equi* associated with their widespread use in a control and prevention program implemented at a breeding farm.[12] As noted, macrolide-resistant isolates seem to be associated with a poorer prognosis in foals.[16] Nevertheless, the results of successful chemoprophylaxis indicate that intervention during early life can decrease the cumulative incidence of *R equi* pneumonia.

Transfusion with hyperimmune plasma has been documented in experimental and observational studies to reduce the cumulative incidence of *R equi* pneumonia; however, success is not complete, and at least 1 study failed to identify evidence of relative risk reduction.[63–67] Transfusion of hyperimmune plasma carries some risks for foals, including transfusion reactions, transfusion-associated hepatitits,[68] and harm to foals resulting from being handled. The procedure also is expensive and labor intensive. Despite these limitations, transfusion of hyperimmune plasma continues to be a mainstay for the control and prevention of *R equi* at breeding farms because of the absence of other more effective strategies.

To date, there are no licensed vaccines available in North America to prevent *R equi* pneumonia, despite several decades of effort using a variety of strategies including inactivated vaccines, subunit vaccines, DNA vaccines, and genetically engineered modified live bacteria.[69-78] The only method repeatedly (twice) documented to protect foals against experimental intrabronchial R equi infection has been intragastric administration of live, virulent R equi.[79,80] Although this approach will not be acceptable for commercial application because of concerns for environmental dissemination and contamination and potential to cause disease in foals, it indicates that intragastric vaccination may lead to protection of foals. Recently, a reduced-virulence mutant of R equi was demonstrated to protect 2 of 4 foals against subsequent intrabronchial challenge with virulent R equi.[81] An effective vaccine would be a boon to the equine breeding industry and foal health.

Based on the postulate that innate immune responses of foals are deficient, and that innate immune responses promote adaptive responses, it has been proposed that nonspecific immunomodulation of foals might promote immunity to R equi. Products evaluated for their ability to stimulate innate immune responses of foals include mycobacterial cell wall extracts, cytosine–phosphate–guanine oligodeoxynucleotides, and inactivated Parapox ovis virus.[82-85] To date, only the killed P ovis product has been systematically evaluated, and it failed to protect foals against R equi pneumonia when administered 3 times to foals during the first 10 days after birth.[86]

In the absence of highly effective prevention, many veterinarians have turned to early detection by applying screening tests to evaluate foals against R equi pneumonia. A variety of methods for screening have been proposed, including physical inspection or examination, evaluation of results of hematology, serology or serum biochemical testing, and thoracic imaging.[6] To the author's knowledge, the sensitivity and specificity of physical inspection or examinations (including recording rectal temperatures and thoracic auscultation) have not been systematically evaluated in well-designed epidemiologic studies. Results of white blood cell concentration have been inconsistent. A study at 1 Thoroughbred farm in Florida indicated that white blood cell concentration provided reasonably good sensitivity (approximately 90%) and acceptable specificity (approximately 80%) using a cutpoint of 15,000 cells/μL[87]; however, a study at a large Quarter Horse farm in Texas revealed relatively modest sensitivity and specificity when using a white blood cell concentration of 13,000 cells/μL.[88] Both these studies indicated that fibrinogen concentration did not have any clinically adequate combinations of sensitivity and specificity at any cutpoint.[65,66] Evaluation of 5 serologic tests indicated that none provided clinically acceptable combinations of sensitivity and specificity for screening purposes.[43] An immunoassay for serum amyloid A failed to demonstrate adequate sensitivity or specificity as a screening test for R equi in a study from Texas[44]; controlled, independent evaluation of the commercially available patient/stall-side semiquantitative serum amyloid A assay as a screening test for R equi pneumonia in foals has not been reported, to the author's knowledge.

Ultrasonographic screening to detect pulmonary consolidation or abscess formation has been advocated as a method for reducing mortality associated with R equi and as a means for reducing the duration of treatment. Although there are some anecdotal data that support the former purported advantage,[89] there is no convincing evidence that the latter is true. More important, treatment of foals with macrolides (with or without rifampin) based on positive results of ultrasonographic screening seems to be fairly common at farms that employ screening (**Fig. 2**). Such treatment results in larger numbers (and proportions) of foals being treated with antimicrobials, many of which would not require treatment. For example, in a recent study conducted at a large Quarter Horse farm where thoracic ultrasonographic screening was performed but where no treatment was implemented in foals based on positive screening test results, the proportion of foals with ultrasonographic evidence of

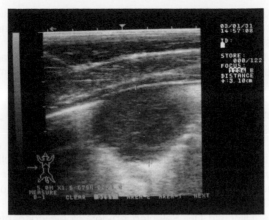

Fig. 2. Ultrasonographic lesion in a foal that was known to be infected with *Rhodococcus equi* but did not develop clinical signs of pneumonia; this foal had other lesions with the same appearance. Similar lesions may be observed in foals that do not develop clinical signs.

lesions was high (80%; 216/270), but only 46 (21%) of these 216 ultrasonographically-positive foals required treatment. If this farm had elected to treat ultrasound-positive foals, approximately 3 or 4 foals would have been needlessly treated for every foal that developed clinical signs for which treatment was indicated.[7] Thus, the low specificity of ultrasonographic screening contributes to more extensive use of antimicrobials, and this practice has been linked to development of macrolide resistance.[12] Thus, the authors do not recommend the practice of ultrasonographic screening and treating foals until an approach incorporating ultrasonography that provides both high sensitivity and specificity for detecting foals that will develop clinical signs of pneumonia is developed.

Highly effective prevention for *R equi* foal pneumonia remains elusive. In the absence of effective prevention, screening for earlier detection and intervention of foals that will develop clinical pneumonia should be pursued; however, currently available approaches lack adequate combinations of sensitivity and specificity to be either effective or adequately safe.

SUMMARY

Pneumonia caused by *R equi* remains an important cause of disease and death in foals. Important challenges for treatment, control, and prevention include the emergence of macrolide resistance, the absence of effective therapeutic alternatives to the macrolides, and the absence of highly effective prevention. There also is need to ameliorate specificity of screening methods to maintain sensitivity but increase specificity of testing.

REFERENCES

1. Prescott JF. *Rhodococcus equi*: an animal and human pathogen. Clin Microbiol Rev 1991;4:20–34.
2. Chaffin MK, Cohen ND, Martens RJ. Evaluation of equine breeding farm characteristics as risk factors for development of *Rhodococcus equi* pneumonia in foals. J Am Vet Med Assoc 2003;222:467–75.
3. Chaffin MK, Cohen ND, Martens RJ. Evaluation of equine breeding farm management and preventive health practices as risk factors for development of *Rhodococcus equi* pneumonia in foals. J Am Vet Med Assoc 2003;222:476–85.

4. Cohen ND, O'Conor MS, Chaffin MK, et al. Farm characteristics and management practices associated with *Rhodococcus equi* pneumonia in foals. J Am Vet Med Assoc 2005;226:404–13.
5. Chaffin MK, Cohen ND, Martens RJ, et al. Foal-related risk factors associated with development of *Rhodococcus equi* pneumonia on farms with endemic infection. J Am Vet Med Assoc 2003;223:1791–9.
6. Giguère S, Cohen ND, Chaffin MK, et al. Diagnosis, treatment, control, and prevention of infections caused by *Rhodococcus equi* in foals. J Vet Intern Med 2011;25:1209–20.
7. Chaffin MK, Cohen ND, Blodgett GP, et al. Evaluation of ultrasonographic screening parameters for predicting subsequent onset of clinically apparent *Rhodococcus equi* pneumonia in foals. In: Marr CM, editor. Proceedings of the 59th Annual Convention of the American Association of Equine Practitioners. Lexington (KY): 2013. p. 268–9.
8. Lilienfeld AM, Lilienfeld DE. Selected epidemiologic concepts of disease. In: Lilienfeld AM, Lilienfeld DE, editors. Foundations of epidemiology. New York: Oxford University Press; 1980. p. 46–8.
9. Jain S, Bloom BR, Hondalus MK. Deletion of *vapA*-encoding Virulence Associated Protein A attenuates the intracellular actinonmycete *Rhododoccus equi*. Mol Microbiol 2003;185:2644–52.
10. Giguère S, Hondalus MK, Yager JA, et al. Role of the 85-kilobase plasmid and plasmid-encoded virulence-associated protein A in intracellular survival and virulence of *Rhodococcus equi*. Infect Immun 1999;67:3548–57.
11. Cohen ND, Smith KE, Ficht TA, et al. Epidemiologic study of *Rhodococcus equi* isolates from horses and horse farms using pulsed-field gel electrophoresis. Am J Vet Res 2003;64:153–61.
12. Burton AJ, Giguère S, Sturgill TL, et al. Emergence of widespread macrolide and rifampin resistance in *Rhodococcus equi* isolates from a horse breeding farm. Emerg Infect Dis 2013;19(2):282–5.
13. Morton AC, Baseggio N, Peters MA, et al. Diversity of isolates of *Rhodococcus equi* from Australian Thoroughbred horse farms. Antonie Van Leeuwenhoek 1998;74:21–5.
14. Bolton TA, Kuskie K, Halbert N, et al. Detection of strain variation in isolates of *Rhodococcus equi* from an affected foal using repetitive sequence-based polymerase chain reaction (rep-PCR). J Vet Diagn Invest 2010;22:611–5.
15. Morton AC, Begg AP, Anderson GA, et al. Epidemiology of *Rhodococcus equi* strains on Thoroughbred horse farms. Appl Environ Microbiol 2001;67:2167–75.
16. Giguère S, Lee E, Williams E, et al. Determination of the prevalence of antimicrobial resistance to macrolide antimicrobials or rifampin in *Rhodococcus equi* isolates and treatment outcome in foals infected with antimicrobial-resistant isolates of *R. equi*. J Am Vet Med Assoc 2010;237:74–81.
17. Cohen ND, Carter CN, Scott HM, et al. Association of soil concentrations of *Rhodococcus equi* and incidence of pneumonia attributable to *Rhodococcus equi* in foals on farms in central Kentucky. Am J Vet Res 2008;69:385–95.
18. Grimm MB, Cohen ND, Slovis NM, et al. Evaluation of mares from a Thoroughbred breeding farm as a source of *Rhodococcus equi* for their foals using quantitative culture and a colony immunoblot assay. Am J Vet Res 2007;68:63–71.
19. Buntain S, Carter CN, Kuskie KR, et al. Frequency of *Rhodococcus equi* in feces of mares in central Kentucky. J Equine Vet Sci 2010;30:191–5.

20. Muscatello G, Anderson GA, Gilkerson JR, et al. Associations between the ecology of virulent *Rhodococcus equi* and the epidemiology of *R. equi* pneumonia on Australian Thoroughbred farms. Appl Environ Microbiol 2006;72:6152–60.
21. Muscatello G, Gerbaud S, Kennedy C, et al. Comparison of concentrations of *Rhodocococcus equi* and virulent *R. equi* in air of stables and paddocks on horse breeding farms in a temperate climate. Equine Vet J 2006;38:263–5.
22. Cohen ND, Kuskie KR, Smith JL, et al. Association of airborne concentrations of virulent *Rhodococcus equi* with location (foaling stall versus paddock) and month (January through June) at 30 horse breeding farms in central Kentucky. Am J Vet Res 2012;73:1603–9.
23. Kuskie K, Smith JL, Sinha S, et al. Associations between the exposure to airborne virulent *Rhodococcus equi* and the incidence of *R. equi* pneumonia among individual foals. J Equine Vet Sci 2011;31:463–9.
24. Cohen ND, Chaffin MK, Kuskie KR, et al. Association of perinatal exposure to airborne *Rhodococcus equi* with risk of pneumonia caused by *R. equi* in foals. Am J Vet Res 2013;74:102–9.
25. Malschitzky E, Neves AP, Gregory RM, et al. Reduzir o uso da cocheira a incidencia de infeccoes por *Rhodococcus equi* em potros. A Hora Veterinaria 2005; 24:27–30.
26. Levy O. Innate immunity of the newborn: basic mechanisms and clinical correlates. Nat Rev Immunol 2007;7:379–90.
27. Adkins B, Leclerc C, Marshall-Clarke S. Neonatal adaptive immunity comes of age. Nat Rev Immunol 2004;4:553–64.
28. Boyd NK, Cohen ND, Lim WS, et al. Temporal changes in cytokine expression of foals during the first month of life. Vet Immunol Immunopathol 2003;92:75–85.
29. Breathnach CC, Sturgill-Wright T, Stiltner JL, et al. Foals are interferon gamma-deficient at birth. Vet Immunol Immunopathol 2006;112:199–209.
30. Kachroo P, Ivanov I, Seabury AG, et al. Age-related changes following *in vivo* stimulation with *Rhodococcus equi* of peripheral blood leukocytes from neonatal foals. PLoS One 2013;8:e62879.
31. Ryan C, Giguère S. Equine neonates have attenuated humoral and cell-mediated immune responses to a killed adjuvanted vaccine compared to adult horses. Clin Vaccine Immunol 2010;17:1896–902.
32. Sturgill TL, Giguère S, Berghaus LJ, et al. Comparison of antibody and cell-mediated immune responses of foals and adult horses after vaccination with live *Mycobacterium bovis* BCG. Vaccine 2014;32:1362–7.
33. Jacks S, Giguère S, Crawford PC, et al. Experimental infection of neonatal foals with *Rhodococcus equi* triggers adult-like gamma interferon induction. Clin Vaccine Immunol 2007;14:669–77.
34. Halbert ND, Cohen ND, Slovis NM, et al. Variations in equid *SLC11A1 (NRAMP1)* genes and associations with *Rhodococcus equi* pneumonia in horses. J Vet Intern Med 2006;20:974–9.
35. Mousel MR, Harrison L, Donahue JM, et al. *Rhodococcus equi* and genetic susceptibility: assessing transferrin genotypes from paraffin-embedded tissues. J Vet Diagn Invest 2003;15:470–2.
36. Horín P, Sabakova K, Futas J, et al. Immunity-related gene single nucleotide polymorphisms associated with *Rhodococcus equi* infection in foals. Int J Immunogenet 2010;37:67–71.
37. Horín P, Smola J, Matiasovic J, et al. Polymorphisms in equine immune response genes and their associations with infections. Mamm Genome 2004; 15:843–50.

38. Horín P, Osickova J, Necesankova M, et al. Single nucleotide polymorphisms of interleukin-1 beta related genes and their associations with infection in the horse. Dev Biol (Basel) 2008;132:347–51.
39. Giguère S, Cohen ND, Chaffin MK, et al. *Rhodococcus equi*: clinical manifestations, virulence, and immunity. J Vet Intern Med 2011;25:1221–30.
40. Reuss SM, Chaffin MK, Cohen ND. Extrapulmonary disorders associated with *Rhodococcus equi* infection in foals: 150 cases (1987-2007). J Am Vet Med Assoc 2009;236:855–63.
41. Stratton-Phelps M, Wilson WD, Gardner IA. Risk of adverse effects in pneumonic foals treated with erythromycin versus other antibiotics: 143 cases (1986-1996). J Am Vet Med Assoc 2000;217:68–73.
42. Sellon DC, Besser TE, Vivrette SL, et al. Comparison of nucleic acid amplification, serology, and microbiologic culture for diagnosis of *Rhodococcus equi* pneumonia in foals. J Clin Microbiol 2001;39:1289–93.
43. Martens RJ, Cohen ND, Chaffin MK, et al. Evaluation of 5 serologic assays to detect *Rhodococcus equi* pneumonia in foals. J Am Vet Med Assoc 2002; 221:825–33.
44. Cohen ND, Chaffin MK, Vandenplas M, et al. Study of serum amyloid A (SAA) concentrations as a means of achieving early diagnosis of *Rhodococcus equi* pneumonia in foals. Equine Vet J 2005;37(3):212–6.
45. Pusterla N, Wilson WD, Mapes S, et al. Diagnostic evaluation of real-time PCR in the detection of *Rhodococcus equi* in faeces and nasopharyngeal swabs from foals with pneumonia. Vet Rec 2007;161:272–5.
46. Giguère S, Jacks S, Roberts GD, et al. Retrospective comparison of azithromycin, clarithromycin, and erythromycin for the treatment of foals with *Rhodococcus equi* pneumonia. J Vet Intern Med 2004;18:568–73.
47. Berghaus LJ, Giguère S, Sturgill TL, et al. Plasma pharmacokinetics, pulmonary distribution and *in vitro* activity of gamithromycin in foals. J Vet Pharmacol Ther 2012;35:59–66.
48. Carlson KL, Kuskie KR, Chaffin MK, et al. Antimicrobial activity of tulathromycin and 14 other antimicrobials against virulent *Rhodococcus equi in vitro*. Vet Ther 2010;11:E1–9.
49. Womble A, Giguère S, Murthy YV, et al. Pulmonary disposition of tilmicosin in foals and *in vitro* activity against *Rhodococcus equi* and other common equine bacterial pathogens. J Vet Pharmacol Ther 2006;29:561–8.
50. Prescott JF, Nicholson VM. The effects of combinations of selected antibiotics on the growth of *Corynebacterium equi*. J Vet Pharmacol Ther 1984;7:61–4.
51. Prescott JF, Sweeney CR. Treatment of *Corynebacterium equi* pneumonia of foals: a review. J Am Vet Med Assoc 1985;187:725–8.
52. Hillidge CJ. Use of erythromycin-rifampin combination in treatment of *Rhodococcus equi* pneumonia. Vet Microbiol 1987;14:337–42.
53. Sweeney CR, Sweeney RW, Divers TJ. *Rhodococcus equi* pneumonia in 48 foals: response to antimicrobial therapy. Vet Microbiol 1987;14:329–36.
54. Nordmann P, Kerestedjian JJ, Ronco E. Therapy of *Rhodococcus equi* disseminated infections in nude mice. Antimicrob Agents Chemother 1992;36:1244–8.
55. Berghaus L, Giguère S, Guldbech K. Mutant prevention concentration and mutant selection window for 10 antimicrobial agents against *Rhodococcus equi*. Vet Microbiol 2013;166:670–5.
56. Peters J, Block W, Oswald S, et al. Oral absorption of clarithromycin is nearly abolished by chronic comedication of rifampicin in foals. Drug Metab Dispos 2011;39:1643–9.

57. Peters J, Eggers K, Oswald S, et al. Clarithromycin is absorbed by an intestinal uptake mechanism that is sensitive to major inhibition by rifampicin: results of a short-term drug interaction study in foals. Drug Metab Dispos 2012;40: 522–8.
58. Venner M, Rödiger A, Laemmer M, et al. Failure of antimicrobial therapy to accelerate spontaneous healing of subclinical pulmonary abscesses on a farm with endemic infections caused by *Rhodococcus equi*. Vet J 2012;192: 293–8.
59. Venner M, Astheimer K, Lämmer M, et al. Efficacy of mass antimicrobial treatment of foals with subclinical pulmonary abscesses associated with *Rhodococcus equi*. J Vet Intern Med 2013;27:171–6.
60. Venner M, Credner N, Lämmer M, et al. Comparison of tulathromycin, azithromycin and azithromycin-rifampin for the treatment of mild pneumonia associated with *Rhodococcus equi*. Vet Rec 2013;173:397.
61. Chaffin MK, Cohen ND, Martens RJ. Chemoprophylactic effects of azithromycin against *Rhodococcus equi* pneumonia among foals at endemic equine breeding farms. J Am Vet Med Assoc 2008;232(7):1035–47.
62. Venner M, Reinhold B, Beyerback M, et al. Efficacy of azithromycin in preventing pulmonary abscesses in foals. Vet J 2012;192:293–8.
63. Martens RJ, Martens JG, Fiske RA, et al. *Rhodococcus equi* foal pneumonia: protective effects of immune plasma in experimentally infected foals. Equine Vet J 1989;21:249–55.
64. Madigan JE, Hietala S, Muller N. Protection against naturally acquired *Rhodococcus equi* pneumonia in foals by administration of hyperimmune plasma. J Reprod Fertil Suppl 1991;44:571–8, 571–8.
65. Higuchi T, Arakawa T, Hashikura S, et al. Effect of prophylactic administration of hyperimmune plasma to prevent *Rhodococcus equi* infection on foals from endemically affected farms. Zentralbl Veterinarmed B 1999;46:641–8.
66. Giguère S, Gaskin JM, Miller C, et al. Evaluation of a commercially available hyperimmune plasma product for prevention of naturally acquired pneumonia caused by *Rhodococcus equi* in foals. J Am Vet Med Assoc 2002;220:59–63.
67. Hurley JR, Begg AP. Failure of hyperimmune plasma to prevent pneumonia caused by *Rhodococcus equi* in foals. Aust Vet J 1995;72:418–20.
68. Aleman M, Nieto JE, Carr EA, et al. Serum hepatitis associated with commercial plasma transfusion in horses. J Vet Intern Med 2005;19:120–2.
69. Martens RJ, Martens J, Fiske RA. Failure of passive immunisation by colostrum from immunised mares to protect foals against *Rhodococcus equi* pneumonia. Equine Vet J Suppl 1991;12:19–22.
70. Varga J, Fodor L, Rusvai M, et al. Prevention of *Rhodococcus equi* pneumonia of foals using two different inactivated vaccines. Vet Microbiol 1997;56:205–12.
71. Becu T, Polledo G, Gaskin JM. Immunoprophylaxis of *Rhodococcus equi* pneumonia in foals. Vet Microbiol 1997;56:193–204.
72. Cauchard J, Sevin C, Ballet JJ, et al. Foal IgG and opsonizing anti-*Rhodococcus equi* antibodies after immunization of pregnant mares with a protective VapA candidate vaccine. Vet Microbiol 2004;104:73–81.
73. Prescott JF, Nicholson VM, Patterson MC, et al. Use of *Rhodococcus equi* virulence-associated protein for immunization of foals against *R. equi* pneumonia. Am J Vet Res 1997;58:356–9.
74. Lopez AM, Hines MT, Palmer GH, et al. Analysis of anamnestic immune responses in adult horses and priming in neonates induced by a DNA vaccine expressing the vapA gene of *Rhodococcus equi*. Vaccine 2003;21:3815–25.

75. Mealey RH, Stone DM, Hines MT, et al. Experimental *Rhodococcus equi* and equine infectious anemia virus DNA vaccination in adult and neonatal horses: effect of IL-12, dose, and route. Vaccine 2007;25:7582–97.
76. Lopez AM, Townsend HG, Allen AL, et al. Safety and immunogenicity of a live-attenuated auxotrophic candidate vaccine against the intracellular pathogen *Rhodococcus equi*. Vaccine 2008;26:998–1009.
77. Pei Y, Nicholson V, Woods K, et al. Immunization by intrabronchial administration to 1-week-old foals of an unmarked double gene disruption strain of *Rhodococcus equi* strain 103+. Vet Microbiol 2007;125:100–10.
78. Lohmann KL, Lopez AM, Manning ST, et al. Failure of a VapA/CpG oligodeoxy-nucleotide vaccine to protect foals against experimental *Rhodococcus equi* pneumonia despite induction of VapA-specific antibody and interferon-γ response. Can J Vet Res 2013;77:161–9.
79. Chirino-Trejo JM, Prescott JF, Yager JA. Protection of foals against experimental *Rhodococcus equi* pneumonia by oral immunization. Can J Vet Res 1987;51:444–7.
80. Hooper-McGrevy KE, Wilkie BN, Prescott JF. Virulence-associated protein-specific serum immunoglobulin G-isotype expression in young foals protected against *Rhodococcus equi* pneumonia by oral immunization with virulent *R. equi*. Vaccine 2005;23:5760–7.
81. van der Geize R, Grommen AW, Hessels GI, et al. The steroid catabolic pathway of the intracellular pathogen *Rhodococcus equi* is important for the pathogenesis and a target for vaccine development. PLoS Pathog 2011;7:e1002181.
82. Ryan C, Giguère S, Fultz L, et al. Effects of two commercially available immunostimulants on leukocyte function of foals following ex vivo exposure to *Rhodococcus equi*. Vet Immunol Immunopathol 2010;138:198–205.
83. Sturgill TL, Strong D, Rashid C, et al. Effect of *Propionibacterium acnes*-containing immunostimulant on interferon-gamma (IFNγ) production in the neonatal foal. Vet Immunol Immunopathol 2011;141:124–7.
84. Bordin AI, Liu M, Nerren JR, et al. Neutrophil function of neonatal foals is enhanced in vitro by CpG oligodeoxynucleotide stimulation. Vet Immunol Immunopathol 2012;145:290–7.
85. Liu M, Liu T, Bordin A, et al. Activation of foal neutrophils at different ages by CpG oligodeoxynucleotides and *Rhodococcus equi*. Cytokine 2009;48:280–9.
86. Sturgill TL, Giguère S, Franklin RP, et al. Effects of inactivated parapoxvirus ovis on the cumulative incidence of pneumonia and cytokine secretion in foals on a farm with endemic infections caused by *Rhodococcus equi*. Vet Immunol Immunopathol 2011;140:237–43.
87. Giguère S, Hernandez J, Gaskin JM, et al. Evaluation of WBC concentration, plasma fibrinogen concentration, and an agar gel immunodiffusion test for early identification of foals with *Rhodococcus equi* pneumonia. J Am Vet Med Assoc 2003;222:775–81.
88. Chaffin MK, Cohen ND, Blodgett GP, et al. Evaluation of hematologic screening methods for predicting subsequent onset of clinically apparent *Rhodococcus equi* pneumonia in foals. In: Marr CM, editor. Proceedings of the 59th Annual Convention of the American Association of Equine Practitioners. Lexington (KY): 2013. p. 267.
89. Slovis NM, McCracken JL, Mundy G. How to use thoracic ultrasound to screen foals for *Rhodococcus equi* at affected farms. In: Brokken TD, editor. Proceedings of the 51st Annual Convention of the American Association of Equine Practitioners. Lexington (KY): 2005. p. 274–8.

Managing *Salmonella* in Equine Populations

Brandy A. Burgess, DVM, MSc, PhD[a], Paul S. Morley, DVM, PhD[b],*

KEYWORDS

• Equine • *Salmonella* • Infection control

KEY POINTS

• Veterinary practitioners have an ethical obligation to appropriately manage risks related to *Salmonella* in animal populations and their environments.

• The goal of infection control is to eliminate sources of potentially pathogenic microorganisms and to disrupt infectious disease transmission.

• Congregating animals from multiple sources increases the risk for transmission of infectious agents such as *Salmonella*.

• Practitioners should be aware of the different *Salmonella* testing methods available because this can affect test results and interpretations relative to disease control efforts.

• Managing *Salmonella* in populations can be particularly challenging because of the diversity in clinical consequences of infection and intermittent shedding.

INTRODUCTION

Congregating animals from multiple sources, as occurs at veterinary hospitals, racetracks, equestrian events, and boarding and training facilities, increases the risk for transmission of infectious agents such as *Salmonella*.[1] This article provides equine practitioners with details relevant to effectively managing *Salmonella* in these populations. It begins by focusing on the agent, *Salmonella enterica*, to develop an appreciation of its key features, including the nuances of organism detection and test interpretation. It then considers the fundamentals of veterinary infection control with the intent of developing a foundation that can be applied to both hospital and field settings. In addition, the article discusses how infection control principles and understanding of the epidemiology of *S enterica* can facilitate managing transmission risks related to this organism in hospital populations and field settings. Detailed

a Department of Population Health Sciences, Virginia-Maryland Regional College of Veterinary Medicine, Virginia-Tech, 100 Sandy Hall (MC0395), 210 Drillfield Drive, Blacksburg, VA 24061, USA; b Department of Clinical Sciences, James L. Voss Veterinary Teaching Hospital, Colorado State University, 1678 Campus Delivery, Fort Collins, CO 80523-1678, USA
* Corresponding author.
E-mail address: paul.morley@colostate.edu

Vet Clin Equine 30 (2014) 623–640
http://dx.doi.org/10.1016/j.cveq.2014.08.005
0749-0739/14/$ – see front matter © 2014 Elsevier Inc. All rights reserved.

descriptions of bacteriology, pathophysiology, and treatment are beyond the scope of this article.

IMPORTANCE OF *SALMONELLA* IN EQUINE POPULATIONS

Salmonella is one of the most common causes of epidemic disease in veterinary hospitals[2] and an agent frequently associated with on-farm contamination.[3] Significant efforts are made to control its transmission among animals, especially within equine hospitals. However, these efforts are predominantly based on first principles because many prevention methods have not been critically evaluated in clinical studies. Regardless, outbreaks known to be attributable to *Salmonella* can come at a great cost, not only in terms of morbidity and case fatality to affected animals but also in terms of direct financial costs; they also present a clear risk to veterinary patients and personnel working with these animals.[4,5] Veterinary practitioners have an ethical obligation to appropriately manage risks related to *Salmonella* in animal populations and their environment. There is a recognizable standard of practice with respect to infection control and due effort must be given to control and prevention of infectious disease transmission within animal populations and facilities.[6]

When *Salmonella* spreads among patients, environmental contamination is predictably present, whether as cause or effect.[4,7–9] Although concerns about management are typically focused on clinically affected animals, subclinical infection and shedding in the absence of disease is more common than clinical infections, which can greatly exacerbate environmental contamination before the scope of the problem is recognized.[8,10] However, testing strategies for relevant veterinary samples (ie, fecal and environmental samples) for the presence of *Salmonella* is variable among laboratories and current testing methodology generally lacks in sensitivity, likely because of the intermittent nature and low level of organisms shed in animal feces. Therefore, testing strategies generally require testing of multiple samples and lengthy enrichment steps, and it can often take 3 to 5 days to obtain results. In that time, significant environmental contamination and disease transmission can occur. As a result, risk recognition and the ability to rapidly identify these patients are critical to the effective management of populations and their environments.

SALMONELLA: THE BASICS

S enterica, a member of the family Enterobacteriaceae, is a gram-negative facultative anaerobic bacterium found colonizing the small intestine, cecum, and colon of both cold-blooded and warm-blooded vertebrates. There are more than 2400 serotypes, which are distinguished by the presence of differing O-antigen (polysaccharide portion of lipopolysaccharide) and H-antigen (filamentous portion of flagella or flagellin) on the surface of the bacteria. *S enterica* subspecies *enterica*, the focus of this article, accounts for approximately 59% of all serotypes and is responsible for approximately 99% of clinical and subclinical *Salmonella* infections in warm-blooded animals.[11,12]

S enterica is considered an opportunistic pathogen that is more likely to cause clinical disease in situations of high exposure or patients that have an increased susceptibility, such as neonates and patients with severe systemic illness. Transmission occurs by the fecal-oral route and can result in enterocolitis (ie, diarrhea), bacteremia, or subclinical infection, with infection depending on the infective dose, host susceptibility, and the infecting serotype. As such, identifying subclinical fecal shedding, managing contacts among patients, and practicing effective personal and environmental hygiene are critical for protecting animals and people.

SALMONELLA TESTING AND INTERPRETATION

There are many methods available for the detection of *S enterica* in samples relevant to veterinary medicine, including enriched culture, polymerase chain reaction (PCR), and lateral flow immunoassays (LFIs), all of which require varying levels of expertise, cost, and time to detection. Practitioners should be aware of the different testing methods available, their strengths and limitations, and know which method is being used (eg, the type of enrichments used) by laboratories because this can affect test results and interpretations relative to disease control efforts.[4,13–16]

Culture of Fecal Samples

There are limitations to the detection of *Salmonella* when culturing fecal samples. In experiments, the analytical sensitivity of equine fecal culture has been found to be as few as 4 colony-forming units (cfu) per gram of feces when enriched in tetrathionate broth[17] and 100 cfu/g of feces when enriched in selenite broth.[18] However, in practice, fecal culture is an insensitive detection method, probably because of intermittent shedding of few organisms per gram of feces,[19,20] as well as the heterogeneous distribution of organisms within fecal samples.[21] Because of the need to use 1 or more enrichment steps, it can take up to 3 days to realize test results for a single fecal sample and the limited test sensitivity means that typically 3 to 5 cultures are needed per animal, interpreting tests in parallel, to achieve reasonable sensitivity for the overall diagnostic process.

The reliability of bacterial culture for *S enterica* detection can be affected by the type of sample (feces, swab, or rectal biopsy), heterogeneity of target organism in the sample, sample weight, intermittent shedding, bacterial culture method, and laboratory proficiency. In general, a fecal culture is a more sensitive detection method than a rectal swab; this is likely due to the amount of fecal material that is cultured as larger sample mass generally provides higher test sensitivity.[22] Organisms such as *Salmonella* tend to cluster within a fecal sample rather than being homogeneously distributed, therefore testing of a small aliquot (eg, swabs or <1 g) may result in false-negative test results because there is a higher probability that a single sample does not contain any *Salmonella* organisms even though the animal is actively shedding at low levels.[21] As stated, the relative sensitivity of culture increases with increasing sample weight and this can be improved upon by thoroughly mixing the sample (eg, with a paddle blender).[21,22] As an alternative, culture of a rectal mucosal sample can be performed with a reported greater sensitivity than fecal culture, although given the invasive nature of the sample it may best be reserved for those difficult-to-sample cases that have scant or liquid feces with minimal solid material.[23]

There are many different methods that can be used for aerobic culture of *Salmonella*, which use a wide variety of broth and solid culture media, as well as incubation times and temperatures.[13–16,24,25] These different methodological choices lead to differences in test accuracy and time until results are reported, which should be carefully considered by laboratories, and practitioners should have a general understanding of how methodological choices affect the ability to detect *Salmonella*. A detailed review of culture techniques for *Salmonella* is beyond the scope of this article. In general, using an enrichment step with *Salmonella* selective media (eg, tetrathionate, Rappaport-Vassiliadis) improves overall test sensitivity, allowing *Salmonella* to grow while inhibiting the growth of competing bacteria, thus enabling detection on selective plating media (eg, xylose-lysine-Tergitol 4 or Hektoen enteric agar).[24] Preenrichment of samples with low bacterial burdens (eg, environmental samples) with nonselective media (eg, buffered peptone water [BPW]) can aid in recovery of bacteria that are damaged or stressed because of environmental conditions, but use with samples containing high bacterial burdens (ie, fecal samples) may be counterproductive because this may allow overgrowth of competing bacteria, resulting in a falsely negative test result. In general, samples should be kept refrigerated and processed as soon after collection as possible. However, the proportion of test-positive samples has been shown to not differ significantly when processed the same day, after 6 days of refrigeration (4°C), or after 14 days of freezing (−15°C),[26] suggesting that recovery is not greatly impaired, if at all, when samples are kept cool before cultures are initiated.

We have found, as have others, that the proficiency of laboratories in their ability to detect *Salmonella* in enriched cultures can vary greatly (Paul Morley, personal communication, June, 2014).[14] Some of these differences are attributable to use of suboptimal culture methods (eg, very harsh enrichment media or lower culture temperatures).[13–16,24,25] In addition, some laboratories have substantially lower recovery rates than other laboratories when using the same culture methods, even among laboratories that routinely process fecal samples for *Salmonella* culture (Paul Morley, personal communication, June, 2014).[14,27] These differences highlight the importance of asking laboratories to provide documentation of training and proficiency testing (eg, check tests) when selecting a laboratory to perform *Salmonella* cultures.[14,27]

Culture of Environmental Samples

Salmonella is an organism that is hardy in damp environments that contain organic debris, having the ability to develop biofilms and environmental reservoirs that serve as potential sources for infection. When performing environmental surveillance, the type of sample collection device and testing method should be carefully considered, because the sensitivities of each are likely to differ. For example, electrostatic wipes have been found to be an effective and more sensitive collection method than sterile sponges for detection of *Salmonella* in the hospital environment.[4,28,29] These differences can be attributed to the collection method (the device used and the size of the surface area sampled) as well as the culture method. In general, sampling a larger surface area not only provides a more representative sample but is likely to be a more sensitive method for organism detection. Organisms in the environment may be injured by harsh environmental conditions (eg, drying and ultraviolet light) and by exposure to disinfectants. As such, general practice is to perform a preenrichment step in a nutrient-rich medium (eg, BPW) before performing an enriched culture. Although this extends the lag time required to obtain results, it allows for injured or damaged organisms to repair themselves before being exposed to the harsh enrichment medium, thereby improving overall testing results.

Polymerase Chain Reaction

PCR is generally considered to be a highly sensitive and specific method of *Salmonella* detection.[30] Most PCR assays use primers that target highly conserved bacterial genes, allowing detection of many different *Salmonella* serotypes without cross-reaction with other common bacteria (eg, Enterobacteriaceae).[31] PCR assays have been reported to have an analytical sensitivity of 100 cfu/g of equine feces in testing of overnight broth cultures or 1000 cfu/g of feces in testing of nonenriched samples. They are also generally more rapid than bacterial culture, providing results in 1 to 2 days compared with 2 to 5 days for many enriched culture methods.[18,31–33] As a result, PCR may be particularly useful with samples containing low numbers of organisms and for times when it is important to obtain results quickly (eg, during epidemics). Although PCR may be useful for earlier detection of shedding and environmental contamination compared with culture, it does not necessarily detect viable organisms.

Therefore, a positive PCR result does not necessarily indicate infection risk related to environmental contamination. In addition, PCR does not replace the need for culture because it is important to have more than dichotomous (positive/negative) results to facilitate epidemiologic investigations and ongoing surveillance. It is impossible to determine the likelihood of health care–associated transmission unless additional information is available for strain differentiation, such as antimicrobial susceptibility, serogroup, serotype, or optimally the pulse field gel electrophoresis profile (ie, DNA fingerprint). As such, PCR testing should always be paired with culture of PCR-positive samples. Some laboratories have proposed using PCR for broader initial screening of all samples, which can then be followed by culture-based investigations of the samples that were PCR positive.[30]

PCR is often considered a more sensitive detection method than enriched culture for fecal and environmental samples. However, there is much debate as to the reason for this apparent higher positive detection rate, or even whether this is consistently true. In theory, PCR can detect nonviable organisms as well as degraded DNA, which may account for some of this difference. It is also clear that suboptimal laboratory methods and laboratory proficiency can likewise affect this observation. In addition, low numbers of organisms contained within samples, or poor test specificity of PCR, can also affect apparent test accuracy.[33–35] A caveat to using PCR as a method of detection for environmental samples is that disinfectants target different parts of bacterial organisms. For example, quaternary ammonium and phenolic disinfectants target cytoplasmic membranes, leaving DNA intact, whereas bleach and formaldehyde degrade DNA, which could theoretically lead to differences in PCR detection rates.[36,37]

Lateral Flow Immunoassays

Commercially available LIAs have been developed for use in food safety microbiology, and have shown promise as practical alternatives to traditional culture and PCR methods for detection of *Salmonella* in animals and their environments (**Fig. 1**).[17,38] LFIs have been shown to have an analytical sensitivity of ~4 cfu/g from enriched cultures of experimentally inoculated equine fecal samples, and can reliably detect *S enterica* in 1-g samples after only 18 hours in selective broth culture.[17] The use of these tests does not require any specialized training or equipment; just the purchase of an incubator and premade media are all that are necessary. Although there may be some differences in the ability to detect different strains (serotypes) of *Salmonella*, their low cost, ease of use, and reliability make them an appealing option for point-of-care testing in equine practice.[39] Just as with PCR, it is important to pair LFI testing with follow-up culture of samples that are LFI positive. In addition to characterization of isolates, it also allows epidemiologic investigation and assessment of transmission risks in populations. It should be highlighted that all laboratories, including those that are set up for limited testing of samples in veterinary practices, should have adequate facilities and protocols in place to ensure appropriate and safe handling of infectious materials, especially those that could lead to zoonotic infections if not properly handled.

Testing Strategy and Test Interpretation

Detecting *Salmonella* in equine practice can be challenging because horses frequently shed low numbers of organisms and do so intermittently, except in extreme situations that may or may not be accompanied by clinical disease.[19,20] Regardless of the analytical sensitivity of test methods, this causes the overall detection system (ie, sample type combined with sample processing and detection method) to have poorer

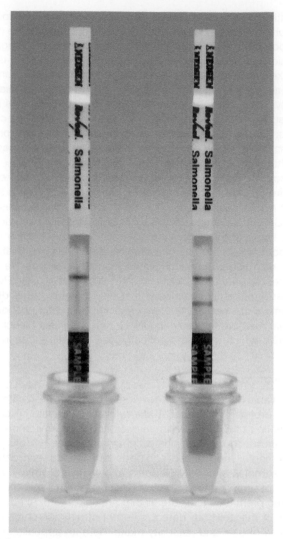

Fig. 1. Commercially available lateral flow immunoassay (Reveal 2.0, Neogen Corporation; see Ref.[38]) used for the detection of *S enterica* in equine fecal and environmental samples (see Refs.[17,39,57]). Test strip on the left indicates a negative test (only the control line is visible); the test strip on the right indicates a positive test (the test line [*lower line*] is as intense in color as the control line [the *top line*]).

epidemiologic sensitivity (ie, lower probability of detecting truly infected/shedding horses). Although testing larger sample volumes improves, up to a limit, test sensitivity,[22] it is also helpful to test multiple samples. Interpreting the results in parallel for multiple tests performed on the same patient has the benefit of greatly improving the overall sensitivity of the testing strategy.

Research suggests that a positive patient is more likely to culture positive with increased number of samples tested.[40] The generally accepted application of this idea is that a minimum of 3 to 5 negative cultures should be obtained in a short time frame (ie, sampling at intervals of 12–24 hours) to be reasonably sure that patients have a low risk of *Salmonella* shedding.[19] Assuming independence of test results, it has been reported that the sensitivities for a series of fecal cultures using selective enrichment were 44% for a single culture, 66% for 2 cultures, 82% for 3 cultures, and 97% for 5 cultures.[41] Thus, by obtaining a series of 3 to 5 negative cultures, practitioners can be reasonably confident that a horse is truly negative.

Regardless of the detection strategy used, many different *Salmonella* serotypes can cause disease and the distribution of serotypes can change over time.[42] Thus it is important to ensure that the test being used can detect many different serotypes, especially those commonly detected in a given geographic or practice location.[16] In addition, when evaluating tests, the way they perform on the bench top may differ from samples relevant to veterinary medicine (ie, fecal and environmental samples), so methods should be appropriately validated and optimized for their intended use on relevant veterinary samples.

FUNDAMENTALS OF VETERINARY INFECTION CONTROL

Many of the practices used in veterinary infection control have not been scientifically evaluated to test their efficacy in applied circumstances. However, veterinarians can learn from infection control strategies applied in human health care. In the Study on the Efficacy of Nosocomial Infection Control (SENIC), conducted in US human health care facilities (1970–1976), the implementation of an infection control program reduced nosocomial infections by an estimated 32%. The minimum components needed for programs to achieve this impressive reduction in infection risk were simply to identify a person to oversee infection control activities, conduct some type of surveillance activity, and maintain a system for reporting.[43] Although similar data are lacking in veterinary medicine, it is realistic to presume that similar measures may be effective. In a recent epidemic of multidrug resistant *Salmonella* Newport, an ineffective infection control program was cited as an important factor in the outbreak, which resulted in patient fatalities, hospital closure, and an estimated financial cost of US$4.1 million.[4]

Infection control is achieved through all efforts used to prevent the introduction and limit the spread of contagious pathogens within a facility or population, with the goal of eliminating sources of potentially pathogenic microorganisms and of disrupting infectious disease transmission. In veterinary hospital settings, this is a challenge because clinicians are purposefully caring for patients with infectious diseases in the midst of animals whose resistance to disease may be compromised; and they are doing so in an environment in which animals from many different farms congregate.

There are several types of preventive measures that can be used to decrease infectious disease transmission risk, including optimizing environmental and personal hygiene and managing patient movement and contacts during hospitalization. Although every equine facility is distinctive with its own physical and operational features, necessitating the tailoring of infection control efforts to each facility's specific needs, all programs are based on these shared infection control principles. Detailed descriptions for program development have been provided elsewhere.[44–46] In addition, there are many available online resources that can facilitate program development.[47–49] Although the structure of specific policies enacted to promote prevention efforts are facility specific, it is important that they are designed with all patients in mind, not just those suspected of harboring an infectious disease. Consideration should be given to establishing distinct, segregated hospital areas to manage neonates, patients with severe disease (eg, colic or systemic illness vs elective surgery), inpatients versus outpatients, and different species (eg, horse vs cattle). Common examples of this include segregating intensive care units, isolation facilities, and having separate equine and livestock hospitals.

MANAGING *SALMONELLA* RISK IN HOSPITAL POPULATIONS
Patient Management

Managing *Salmonella* in populations can be particularly challenging, in part because of the wide diversity in clinical consequences of infection, ranging from asymptomatic, intermittent shedding to acute diarrhea and fever with neutropenia to septicemia and death. In addition, horses recovering from naturally occurring acute salmonellosis can shed for extended periods of time; one-third shed for up to 30 days,[41] and can do so intermittently. Veterinarians have the challenge of caring for the patient standing before them but must consider the population of tomorrow in order to effectively control health care–associated infections (HCAIs).

Factors associated with epidemic disease

Nosocomial outbreaks of salmonellosis, representing a climactic meeting of patient and hospital factors, have repeatedly been shown to be a constant risk in all types of veterinary hospitals, resulting in significant morbidity and mortality among hospitalized patients and zoonotic infections in personnel.[4,7,8,37,50] Environmental hygiene is commonly identified as a contributing factor, including ineffective infection control policies; floor surfaces that allow contamination to accumulate; and use of porous, noncleanable surfaces in other materials such as unsealed concrete and wood.[4,7,37] In addition, contamination of common-use equipment (eg, buckets, nasogastric tubes, and rectal thermometers), and periods of high caseload with limited personnel have been found to affect the occurrence of HCAIs.[7,9,37] In the course of epidemics, horses with severe disease, such as those with colic or undergoing abdominal surgery, are frequently identified as shedding *Salmonella* and likely contribute to ongoing environmental contamination and transmission among hospitalized patients.[7,9,51,52]

Factors associated with endemic disease

During outbreaks, there is typically widespread environmental contamination and it is common for patient and environmental isolates to be phenotypically similar (ie, serotype and antimicrobial susceptibility); this phenomenon has also been identified during times of endemic disease, suggesting animals to be a likely source for this contamination.[4,8,29,53] From experience consulting with different veterinary facilities, disseminated environmental contamination is a ubiquitous feature associated with nosocomial *Salmonella* transmission,[4,7,8] although use of insensitive sampling and culture methods can impair the ability to detect this important feature (Paul Morley, personal communication, June, 2014).[4]

In the past, *Salmonella* shedding among horses was associated with a triad of clinical signs (diarrhea, fever, and leukopenia) based on early studies and observation.[54,55] A recent case-control study supports this observation, finding that horses with acute colic with clinical signs of fever (rectal temperature >39.4°C [103°F]), diarrhea, and abnormal leukocyte count ($\leq$4500 cells/μL or leukocytosis $\geq$12,500 cells/μL) were more likely to shed *Salmonella* in feces and reflux in the first 5 days of hospitalization.[56] This triad of clinical signs can occur infrequently, accounting for only 2.7% of shedding among a hospital population (the population attributable fraction).[57]

A meta-analysis of studies experimentally inoculating healthy animals (horses, cattle, sheep), found that, on average, pyrexia occurred within 1.5 days of infection (95% confidence interval [CI], 1.47, 1.55) and diarrhea occurred within 1.7 days of infection (95% CI, 1.62, 1.83).[58] The 43 studies included in this meta-analysis used inoculating doses from 10^4 to 10^{13}; in natural infection the infective dose is expected to be at least at the low end of this range and is likely to be lower. Thus, the average times to onset reported here are probably more rapid than would be expected in natural infections. This study also reported an average time to shedding of 1.3 days (95% CI, 1.22, 1.39) after inoculation, suggesting that, by the time fever and/or diarrhea are apparent, animals are frequently shedding *Salmonella* in their feces. This finding emphasizes the utility of identifying specific factors or groups of factors associated with shedding that are easily recognizable, thus allowing prevention strategies to be implemented more rapidly, before the situation becomes an epidemic.

The duration from exposure to fecal shedding can be affected by serotype, inoculating dose, as well as the health status of the horse. Time to shedding varies by infecting serotype, ranging from approximately 3 to 5 days among naturally infected horses.[51] This is in contrast with experimental inoculation, which results in shedding within 1.3 days (95% CI, 1.22, 1.39),[58] suggesting that infecting dose plays a role because experimental inoculations are general at much higher doses than would be expected to occur naturally. Not only can time to shedding vary by serotype, it may also be affected by health status. Days from admission to shedding among horses presenting for gastrointestinal disease ranged from 1 day to 3.5 days for serotypes Saint Paul and Java, respectively,[40] likely representing an increased susceptibility in this compromised subgroup of horses, but this may have been attributable to variation in virulence among serotypes and strains.

It has been suggested that horses with severe disease are more likely to shed detectable quantities of *Salmonella* in their feces. In a recent study, horses admitted for acute colic (excluding those presenting with diarrhea) were more likely to shed *Salmonella* with surgical management versus medical management, as were those with more severe disease (eg, inflammatory and vascular compromising conditions) versus those with simple colic (eg, simple obstruction and nonstrangulating lesions) that resolved with minimal medical management.[56] Although the suggestion that horses with more severe disease are more likely to shed makes biological sense, over the years this has not been a consistent finding. Many studies have evaluated shedding risk among horses with gastrointestinal disease, and some studies have reported an increased risk associated with abdominal surgery.[40,56] However, others have not found an association between *Salmonella* shedding and abdominal surgery.[9,59,60] In addition, although it is commonly thought that antimicrobial therapy affects the probability of *Salmonella* shedding, this too has been inconsistently identified as a significant risk factor.[9,40,59-61]

Although horses with severe disease are probably more susceptible to infection than healthy horses, they are also more likely to have fecal samples tested. For this reason, extrapolating findings from studies observing limited patient populations should be done with caution. Studies to determine factors associated with endemic shedding among the general patient population have found that both patient and hospital factors may be important.[57,61-64] Patients with systemic illness, regardless of the body system affected, and those having any of the classic triad of clinical signs (fever, diarrhea, or leukopenia) have a higher likelihood of shedding, but these are not the only animals that shed *Salmonella*.[57] These indicators are specific for identifying shedding, but they are not perfectly sensitive. Patient management factors may also play a role, with transportation distance (patients within 32 km [20 miles] having a greater risk), antimicrobial therapy (specifically being treated with aminoglycosides), and duration of hospitalization affecting the probability of shedding.[57,64] Species or rearing circumstances may be important hospital factors as well, with intensively managed cattle being much more likely to shed than horses; an element that should not be overlooked when managing horses in a multispecies hospital.[57,64] Further, reports consistently show a seasonal occurrence to shedding, generally highest in late summer and early fall, and lowest in the spring.[3,19,40,42,57] Thus, studies evaluating a limited time frame may underestimate risk factor contributions to overall patient shedding. There are also large regional differences in the shedding prevalence that have been found in similar species and rearing conditions; shedding seems to be much more likely to occur in the warmer and wetter regions of North America compared with cooler and dryer regions.[3]

Subpopulations and Salmonella Risk

Managing *Salmonella* in horse populations is challenging because horses can shed intermittently and often in the absence of clinical signs.[10] Patient shedding prevalence can vary markedly from as few as 0.5% up to 7%, with horses tested on admission typically having a lower prevalence than horses tested throughout hospitalization.[3,19,62,63] In contrast, horses admitted for elective procedures (ie, musculoskeletal disease, cryptorchidism) and as hospital companions are less likely to shed[63] and healthy horses in the general equine population have an estimated shedding prevalence of 0.8% (standard error [SE], 0.5).[3] At the Colorado State University Veterinary Teaching Hospital, from 2002 to 2010, culture-positive horses were most commonly admitted with gastrointestinal disease (60.8% [87 of 143]), followed by musculoskeletal disease (34.2% [49 of 143]), and approximately 10% were considered clinically normal by attending clinicians (10.5% [15 of 143]). Thus, differential patient management may be warranted for patient population subgroups identified as being at a high risk for *Salmonella* shedding on admission or throughout hospitalization.

Horses with gastrointestinal disease

Many facilities manage horses with gastrointestinal disease or colic separately from the general patient population because this subgroup has an increased likelihood of shedding, with prevalence ranging from 4.3% up to 13%.[40,60,63] Factors that can be associated with fecal shedding among these patients include transportation distance (travel time >1 hour), abnormal findings on nasogastric intubation, diarrhea, leukopenia ($\leq$5000 white blood cells/μL), previous antimicrobial therapy, abdominal surgery, and duration of hospitalization.[19,40,56,60]

Horses with severe disease

Horses admitted to the critical care unit are also more likely to shed *Salmonella* during hospitalization.[65] This subgroup of horses, along with critical neonates, likely represents patients with greater disease severity (as well as susceptibility to infection) compared with the general hospital population. Equine neonates present a particular challenge. Critically ill foals are typically unable to stand, require intensive management, and those with gastrointestinal disease are at higher risk for shedding *Salmonella* compared with adults.[40] For patients comprising the general inpatient population, approximately 70% of shedding risk can be attributed to systemic illness (ie, the population attributable fraction) regardless of body system affected, with more severe disease having a higher probability of shedding.[57,64]

Salmonella Surveillance Among Patients in Clinical Practice

Routine surveillance by testing fecal samples may be an effective means to identify *Salmonella* shedding among the general inpatient population but careful consideration should be given to how this might be incorporated into an infection control program (including cost and ability to manage positive patients). Targeted surveillance of horses presenting for acute colic or diarrhea or developing diarrhea during hospitalization has been shown to be an effective method for identifying fecal shedding. However, research suggests that many horses can be shedding *Salmonella* in the absence of clinical signs.[8,36,56] A recent case-control study found that most horses presenting for acute colic were identified as shedding *Salmonella* through routine untargeted surveillance of all inpatients (64.4%, excluding isolation patients) rather than on admission (6.8%) or targeted surveillance triggered by the infection control program (28.8%).[56] Therefore, depending on the types of patients seen at a practice, routine patient surveillance may be warranted. **Box 1** shows specific components of the *Salmonella* surveillance program conducted at the James L. Voss Veterinary Teaching Hospital, Colorado State University, as part of long-term infection control efforts. Note that this is but 1 example; infection control programs must be tailored for a particular facility to ensure that they meet those facilities' specific needs and limitations.

A facility may alternatively find it more cost-effective to focus on syndromic surveillance; a method that is effective at detecting adverse events in hospitalized horses.[66] However, applying this technique to horses with *Salmonella* may be a challenge because not all patients shedding *Salmonella* develop clinical signs. As stated earlier, only 2.7% of shedding has been associated with diarrhea, fever, and leukopenia, whereas 70% of shedding has been attributed to either systemic illness or gastrointestinal disease.[64] Given this, practitioners may elect to differentially manage and conduct targeted surveillance of those patients with more severe disease or gastrointestinal disease.

In addition, environmental surveillance for *Salmonella* may also be a cost-effective means for detecting patient shedding because environmental contamination is commonly detected near where positive patients are managed.[29,61] This surveillance could be conducted as routine or periodic surveillance of high-traffic areas such as examination areas or alleyways. If contamination is detected, not only can infection control measures be heightened but more extensive patient testing could be undertaken to facilitate mitigation efforts.

Box 1
Example[a] surveillance program for *S enterica* conducted at the James L. Voss Veterinary Teaching Hospital, Colorado State University

Components	Sample for Culture	Description
Routine surveillance	Patient fecal sample[b]	All large-animal inpatients on admission and twice weekly for the duration of hospitalization
	Environmental swab[c]	Approximately 60 sites throughout the small-animal, equine, and livestock hospitals
Targeted surveillance	Patient fecal sample[b]	All patients with 2 of 3 signs (fever, leukopenia, diarrhea) or developing diarrhea during hospitalization
	Environmental swab[c]	Select locations when an increase (above baseline) in positive patients or positive environmental samples is detected
Passive surveillance	Patient fecal sample[b]	All diagnostic samples culture positive for *Salmonella* from inpatients are reported to biosecurity personnel

[a] Surveillance programs must be tailored to each facility's needs and limitations.
[b] One-gram fecal sample for enriched culture.
[c] Collected using a Swiffer (Proctor & Gamble; see Ref.[29]).

Management of the Hospital Environment

Incorporating environmental surveillance into clinical practice is a common method for managing risks associated with *Salmonella* in populations. Active surveillance of patients and the environment can complement each other to detect endemic shedding among patients and to identify outbreaks early in their course, thereby limiting the overall consequences.[8] Research shows that isolates recovered at times of endemic and epidemic disease can be phenotypically linked (serotype and antimicrobial susceptibility) to animal isolates, suggesting animals as a likely source for environmental contamination and ongoing transmission.[29,53] In addition, recovery of genetically related *Salmonella* isolates during routine patient and environmental surveillance over an extended period of time suggests environmental persistence and nosocomial transmission, despite the implementation of a rigorous infection control program.[67] As such, environmental hygiene and surveillance are critical to eliminating reservoirs for infection within the hospital environment. Again, based on experiences from consulting with a variety of veterinary practices, we have not experienced substantial nosocomial transmission of *Salmonella* without also identifying environmental contamination. Thus, sampling the environment at times of concern can be an important investigative tool for detection of HCAIs related to *Salmonella*. See **Box 1** for specific components of the *Salmonella* surveillance program conducted at the James L. Voss Veterinary Teaching Hospital, Colorado State University, as part of long-term infection control efforts. Note that this is but 1 example; infection control programs must be tailored for a particular facility to ensure that they meet those facilities' specific needs and limitations.

When incorporating environmental surveillance into practice, careful consideration should be given to locations being sampled and type of samples being collected (eg, floor-contact surface, hand-contact surface, or a composite sample of both those surfaces). For example, for mixed-species practices, samples collected in areas used to manage livestock are more likely to be culture positive, as are samples collected from floor-contact surfaces or composite samples (but hand-contact samples may be more important with respect to transmission risk).[68] In addition, sample collection and detection methods, laboratory selection, and available resources (both financial and personnel) should be taken into consideration. Methods should be appropriately validated and optimized for their intended use and practitioners should understand that different collection and testing methodologies can result in different test sensitivities.[4,14,28] In general, sampling a larger surface area provides a more representative sample and is likely to be a more sensitive method for detecting *Salmonella* in the environment.

Environments in veterinary hospitals are frequently contaminated near where positive patients are managed (eg, equine isolation, livestock hospital, calf isolation), with floor samples, floor drains, cracks, and crevices being common sites for contamination.[29,36,69,70] It is imperative to maintain nonporous, cleanable surfaces throughout the hospital environment because epidemics are commonly associated with in-stall matting and surfaces such as unsealed concrete and wood.[4,7,37] Although environmental contamination cannot be completely eliminated, the goal is to reduce contamination of the environment with potential pathogens to a level that becomes biologically irrelevant. To gain meaningful information, environmental testing should be performed regularly to establish a baseline level of environmental contamination with which future findings can be compared. In this way potential environmental reservoirs of *Salmonella* can be detected and cleaning effectiveness can be continually monitored.

MANAGING *SALMONELLA* RISK IN THE FIELD SETTING

In addition to being one of the most common causes of outbreaks of HCAI in equine hospitals,[2] *Salmonella* is also frequently detected on equine operations and farms[3] and is a recognized cause of farm outbreaks and disease in personnel.[71-73] In general, of nonhospitalized horses in the general equine population that are considered healthy, an estimated 0.8% (SE, 0.5) shed *Salmonella* in their feces.[3]

Although much of this article focuses on managing salmonella risk in the hospital setting, the same principles regarding infection control apply to other settings; namely, preventing disease introduction and transmission between facilities and among animals by breaking the cycle of transmission and practicing rigorous hygiene. On-farm infection control practices are largely owner dependent. In a survey of Colorado boarding facilities, only 50% of facility managers reported isolating new horses from resident horses and only 6.6% isolated resident horses returning to the farm after travel.[74] Among US equine operations with at least 5 resident horses, approximately 78% had nonresident horses arriving on farm.[75] Although the risk of exposure to nonresident horses increased with operation size, so too did the likelihood of implementing some biosecurity measures such as entry requirements for personnel. Advising owners and managers regarding implementation of best practices for infection control remains an excellent opportunity for veterinarians to provide service and strengthen productive veterinarian-client relationships.

It is clearly important for practitioners to maintain a minimum standard of infection control, whether in the clinic or in the field. As ambulatory practitioners move from farm to farm, it is critically important to maintain a high level of hygiene within practice vehicles, with respect to multiuse equipment, and with outer attire worn on an individual farm. There are many online resources available to help facilitate on-farm infection control program development[47-49] as well as published resources on program development[44,45] and outbreak investigation and control.[76]

SUMMARY

An international panel of infection control experts recently identified critical needs for infection control in equine populations. One of the issues specifically identified was the need to expand knowledge about the epidemiology and control of *Salmonella* infections in equine populations, along with improving methods for detection.[6] Recognizing the challenges faced by practitioners in managing this agent is the first step to improving its control. Despite the way this organism is shed, intermittently, at low levels, and often subclinically, due effort must be made to mitigate associated risks, whether in the hospital or field setting. Veterinary practitioners have an ethical responsibility to appropriately manage risks related to S enterica in animal populations and their environments.

REFERENCES

1. Christley RM, French NP. Small-world topology of UK racing: the potential for rapid spread of infectious agents. Equine Vet J 2003;35(6):586-9.
2. Benedict KM, Morley PS, Van Metre DC. Characteristics of biosecurity and infection control programs at veterinary teaching hospitals. J Am Vet Med Assoc 2008;233(5):767-73.
3. Traub-Dargatz JL, Barber LP, Fedorka-Cray PJ, et al. Fecal shedding of *Salmonella spp* by horses in the United States during 1998 and 1999 and detection of

Salmonella spp in grain and concentrate sources on equine operations. J Am Vet Med Assoc 2000;217(2):226–30.

4. Dallap Schaer BL, Aceto H, Rankin SC. Outbreak of salmonellosis caused by *Salmonella enterica* serovar Newport MDR-AmpC in a large animal veterinary teaching hospital. J Vet Intern Med 2010;24(5):1138–46.

5. Weaver DR, Newman LS, Lezotte DC, et al. Perceptions regarding workplace hazards at a veterinary teaching hospital. J Am Vet Med Assoc 2010;237(1):93–100.

6. Morley P, Anderson ME, Burgess BA, et al. Report of the third Havemeyer workshop on infection control in equine populations. Equine Vet J 2012;45(2):131–6.

7. Tillotson K, Savage CJ, Salman MD, et al. Outbreak of *Salmonella* Infantis infection in a large animal veterinary teaching hospital. J Am Vet Med Assoc 1997; 211(12):1554–7.

8. Steneroden KK, Van Metre DC, Jackson C, et al. Detection and control of a nosocomial outbreak caused by *Salmonella* Newport at a large animal hospital. J Vet Intern Med 2010;24(3):606–16.

9. Hird DW, Pappaioanou M, Smith BP. Case-control study of risk factors associated with isolation of *Salmonella* Saintpaul in hospitalized horses. Am J Epidemiol 1984;120(6):852–64.

10. Palmer JP, Benson CE, Whitlock RH. Subclinical salmonellosis in horses with colic. In Equine Colic Research Symposium. University of Georgia, Athens, 1982; 180–6.

11. Lan R, Reeves PR, Octavia S. Population structure, origins and evolution of major *Salmonella enterica* clones. Infect Genet Evol 2009;9(5):996–1005.

12. Brenner FW, Villar RG, Angulo FJ, et al. *Salmonella* nomenclature. J Clin Microbiol 2000;38(7):2465–7.

13. Rostagno MH, Gailey JK, Hurd HS, et al. Culture methods differ on the isolation of *Salmonella enterica* serotypes from naturally contaminated swine fecal samples. J Vet Diagn Invest 2005;17(1).80–3.

14. Voogt N, Nagelkerke NJD, van de Giessen AW. Differences between reference laboratories of the European community in their ability to detect *Salmonella* species. Eur J Clin Microbiol Infect Dis 2002;21(6):449–54.

15. Love BC, Rostagno MH. Comparison of five culture methods for *Salmonella* isolation from swine fecal samples of known infection status. J Vet Diagn Invest 2008;20(5):620–4.

16. Singer RS, Mayer AC, Hanson TE. Do microbial interactions and cultivation media decrease the accuracy of *Salmonella* surveillance systems and outbreak investigations? J Food Prot 2009;72(4):707–13.

17. Burgess BA, Noyes NR, Bolte DS, et al. Rapid *Salmonella* detection in experimentally-inoculated equine feces and veterinary hospital environmental samples using commercially available lateral flow antigen detection systems. Equine Vet J 2014.

18. Cohen ND, Neibergs HL, Wallis DE, et al. Genus-specific detection of salmonellae in equine feces by use of the polymerase chain reaction. Am J Vet Res 1994;55(8):1049–54.

19. Smith BP, Reina-Guerra M, Hardy AJ. Prevalence and epizootiology of equine salmonellosis. J Am Vet Med Assoc 1978;172(3):353–6.

20. Smith BP, Reina-Guerra M, Hardy AJ, et al. Equine salmonellosis: experimental production of four syndromes. Am J Vet Res 1979;40(8):1072–7.

21. Cannon RM, Nicholls TJ. Relationship between sample weight, homogeneity, and sensitivity of fecal culture for *Salmonella enterica*. J Vet Diagn Invest 2002;14(1):60–2.

22. Funk JA, Davies PR, Nichols MA. The effect of fecal sample weight on detection of *Salmonella enterica* in swine feces. J Vet Diagn Invest 2000;12(5): 412–8.
23. Palmer JE, Witlock RH, Benson CE, et al. Comparison of rectal mucosal cultures and fecal cultures in detecting *Salmonella* infection in horses and cattle. Am J Vet Res 1985;46(3):697–8.
24. Davies PR, Turkson PK, Funk JA, et al. Comparison of methods for isolating *Salmonella* bacteria from faeces of naturally infected pigs. J Appl Microbiol 2000; 89(1):169–77.
25. Waltman WD, Mallinson ET. Isolation of *Salmonella* from poultry tissue and environmental samples: a nationwide survey. Avian Dis 1995;39:45–54.
26. O'Carroll JM, Davies PR, Correa MT, et al. Effects of sample storage and delayed secondary enrichment on detection of *Salmonella spp* in swine feces. Am J Vet Res 1999;60(3):359–62.
27. Kuijpers A, Mooijman KA. EU Interlaboratory comparison study veterinary XV (2012): detection of *Salmonella* in pig faeces. RIVM Report 330604028. 2013. Available at: http://hdl.handle.net/10029/313961. Accessed September 18, 2014.
28. Ruple-Czerniak A, Bolte DS, Burgess BA, et al. Comparison of two sampling and culture systems for detection of *Salmonella enterica* in the environment of a large animal hospital. Equine Vet J 2014;46(4):499–502.
29. Burgess BA, Morley PS, Hyatt DR. Environmental surveillance for *Salmonella enterica* in a veterinary teaching hospital. J Am Vet Med Assoc 2004;225(9): 1344–8.
30. Malorny B, Hoorfar J. Toward standardization of diagnostic PCR testing of fecal samples: lessons from the detection of salmonellae in pigs. J Clin Microbiol 2005;43(7):3033–7.
31. Cohen ND, Neibergs HL, McGruder ED, et al. Genus-specific detection of salmonellae using the polymerase chain reaction (PCR). J Vet Diagn Invest 1993;5(3):368–71.
32. Kurowski PB, Traub-Dargatz JL, Morley PS, et al. Detection of *Salmonella spp* in fecal specimens by use of real-time polymerase chain reaction assay. Am J Vet Res 2002;63(9):1265–8.
33. Ward MP, Alinovi CA, Couetil LL, et al. Evaluation of a PCR to detect *Salmonella* in fecal samples of horses admitted to a veterinary teaching hospital. J Vet Diagn Invest 2005;17(2):118–23.
34. Cohen ND, Martin LJ, Simpson RB, et al. Comparison of polymerase chain reaction and microbiological culture for detection of salmonellae in equine feces and environmental samples. Am J Vet Res 1996;57(6):780–6.
35. Pusterla N, Byrne BA, Hodzic E, et al. Use of quantitative real-time PCR for the detection of *Salmonella spp.* in fecal samples from horses at a veterinary teaching hospital. Vet J 2010;186(2):252–5.
36. Ewart SL, Scott HC 2nd, Robinson RL, et al. Identification of sources of *Salmonella* organisms in a veterinary teaching hospital and evaluation of the effects of disinfectants on detection of *Salmonella* organisms on surface materials. J Am Vet Med Assoc 2001;218(7):1145–51.
37. Schott HC 2nd, Ewart SL, Walker RD, et al. An outbreak of salmonellosis among horses at a veterinary teaching hospital. J Am Vet Med Assoc 2001;218(7): 1152–9, 1100.
38. Bird CB, Miller RL, Miller BM. Reveal for *Salmonella* test system. J AOAC Int 1999;82(3):625–33.

39. Burgess BA, Bolte DS, Hyatt DR, et al. Rapid *Salmonella* detection in fecal and veterinary hospital environmental samples using commercially available lateral flow antigen detection systems. In American College of Veterinary Internal Medicine Forum. Seattle, June 12–15, 2013.

40. Ernst NS, Hernandez JA, MacKay RJ, et al. Risk factors associated with fecal *Salmonella* shedding among hospitalized horses with signs of gastrointestinal tract disease. J Am Vet Med Assoc 2004;225(2):275–81.

41. Palmer JE, Benson CE. *Salmonella* shedding in the equine. In International Symposium on *Salmonella*. New Orleans, July 19–20, 1984.

42. Carter JD, Hird DW, Farver TB, et al. Salmonellosis in hospitalized horses: seasonality and case fatality rates. J Am Vet Med Assoc 1986;188(2):163–7.

43. Haley RW, Culver DH, White JW, et al. The efficacy of infection surveillance and control programs in preventing nosocomial infections in US hospitals. Am J Epidemiol 1985;121(2):182–205.

44. Morley PS. Biosecurity of veterinary practices. Vet Clin North Am Food Anim Pract 2002;18(1):133–55, vii.

45. Traub-Dargatz JL, Dargatz DA, Morley PS, et al. An overview of infection control strategies for equine facilities, with an emphasis on veterinary hospitals. Vet Clin North Am Equine Pract 2004;20(3):507–20, v.

46. Morley PS, Weese JS. Biosecurity and infection control for large animal practices. In: Smith BP, editor. Large animal internal medicine. 5th edition. New York: Elsevier; 2015. p. 1407–31.

47. Anonymous. Equine biosecurity policies and best practices guide. 2011. Available at: http://www.albertaequestrian.com/Biosecurity. Accessed September 18, 2014.

48. Flynn K, Wilson EM, Traub-Dargatz J, et al. Biosecurity toolkit for equine events. 2012. Available at: http://www.cdfa.ca.gov/ahfss/animal_health/pdfs/Biosecurity_Toolkit_Full_Version.pdf. Accessed September 18, 2014.

49. Guelph E. Equine biosecurity risk calculator. 2011. Available at: http://www.equineguelph.ca/Tools/biosecurity_2011.php. Accessed September 18, 2014.

50. Wright J, Tengelsen LA, Smith KE, et al. Multidrug-resistant *Salmonella* Typhimurium in four animal facilities. Emerg Infect Dis 2005;11(8):1235–41.

51. House JK, Mainer-Jaime RC, Smith BP, et al. Risk factors for nosocomial *Salmonella* infection among hospitalized horses. J Am Vet Med Assoc 1999;214(10):1511–6.

52. Ekiri AB, MacKay RJ, Gaskin JM, et al. Epidemiologic analysis of nosocomial *Salmonella* infections in hospitalized horses. J Am Vet Med Assoc 2009;234(1):108–19.

53. Castor ML, Wooley RE, Shotts EB, et al. Characteristics of *Salmonella* isolated from an outbreak of equine salmonellosis in a veterinary teaching hospital. J Equine Vet Sci 1989;9(5):236–41.

54. Dorn CR, Coffman JR, Schmidt DA, et al. Neutropenia and salmonellosis in hospitalized horses. J Am Vet Med Assoc 1975;166(1):65–7.

55. Owen R, Fullerton JN, Tizard IR, et al. Studies on experimental enteric salmonellosis in ponies. Can J Comp Med 1979;43(3):247–54.

56. Dallap Schaer BL, Aceto H, Caruso MA, et al. Identification of predictors of *Salmonella* shedding in adult horses presented for acute colic. J Vet Intern Med 2012;26(5):1177–85.

57. Burgess BA. Epidemiology and prevention of *Salmonella enterica* in veterinary hospitals. Colorado State University, Libraries Fort Collins, CO, PhD Dissertation; 2014.

58. Aceto H, Miller SA, Smith G. Onset of diarrhea and pyrexia and time to detection of *Salmonella enterica* subsp *enterica* in feces in experimental studies of cattle,

horses, goats, and sheep after infection per os. J Am Vet Med Assoc 2011; 238(10):1333–9.

59. Hird DW, Casebolt DB, Carter JD, et al. Risk factors for salmonellosis in hospitalized horses. J Am Vet Med Assoc 1986;188(2):173–7.

60. Kim LM, Morley PS, Traub-Dargatz JL, et al. Factors associated with *Salmonella* shedding among equine colic patients at a veterinary teaching hospital. J Am Vet Med Assoc 2001;218(5):740–8.

61. Dunowska M, Patterson G, Traub-Dargatz JL, et al. Recent progress in controlling *Salmonella* in veterinary hospitals. In 50th Annual Convention of the American Association of Equine Practitioners. Lexington, December 4-8, 2004:350–3.

62. Traub-Dargatz JL, Salman MD, Jones RL. Epidemiologic study of salmonellae shedding in the feces of horses and potential risk factors for development of the infection in hospitalized horses. J Am Vet Med Assoc 1990;196(10):1617–22.

63. Alinovi CA, Ward MP, Couetil LL, et al. Risk factors for fecal shedding of *Salmonella* from horses in a veterinary teaching hospital. Prev Vet Med 2003;60(4): 307–17.

64. Burgess, BA, Morley PS. Factors associated with large animal inpatient shedding of *Salmonella enterica* in a veterinary teaching hospital. In 94th Annual Conference of Research Workers in Animal Diseases. Chicago, December 9-10, 2013.

65. Mainar-Jaime RC, Atashparvar N, Chirino-Trejo M. Influence of fecal shedding of *Salmonella* organisms on mortality in hospitalized horses. J Am Vet Med Assoc 1998;213(8):1162–6.

66. Ruple-Czerniak AA, Aceto HW, Bender JB, et al. Syndromic surveillance for evaluating the occurrence of healthcare-associated infections in equine hospitals. Equine Vet J 2014;46(4):435–40.

67. Dunowska M, Morley PS, Traub-Dargatz JL, et al. Comparison of *Salmonella enterica* serotype Infantis isolates from a veterinary teaching hospital. J Appl Microbiol 2007;102(6):1527–36.

68. Burgess BA, Morley PS. Hospital risk factors for environmental contamination with *Salmonella enterica*. In 93rd Annual Conference of Research Workers in Animal Diseases. Chicago, December 3-4, 2012.

69. Pandya M, Wittum T, Tadesse DA, et al. Environmental *Salmonella* surveillance in the Ohio State University Veterinary Teaching Hospital. Vector Borne Zoonotic Dis 2009;9(6):649–54.

70. Alinovi CA, Ward MP, Couetil LL, et al. Detection of *Salmonella* organisms and assessment of a protocol for removal of contamination in horse stalls at a veterinary teaching hospital. J Am Vet Med Assoc 2003;223(11):1640–4.

71. Hartmann FA, Callan RJ, McGuirk SM, et al. Control of an outbreak of salmonellosis caused by drug-resistant *Salmonella* Anatum in horses at a veterinary hospital and measures to prevent future infections. J Am Vet Med Assoc 1996; 209(3):629–31.

72. Jay-Russell MT, Madigan JE, Bengson Y, et al. *Salmonella* Oranienburg isolated from horses, wild turkeys and an edible home garden fertilized with raw horse manure. Zoonoses Public Health 2014;61(1):64–71.

73. Walker RL, Madigan JE, Hird DW, et al. An outbreak of equine neonatal salmonellosis. J Vet Diagn Invest 1991;3(3):223–7.

74. Kirby AT, Traub-Dargatz JL, Hill AE, et al. Development, application, and validation of a survey for infectious disease control practices at equine boarding facilities. J Am Vet Med Assoc 2010;237(10):1166–72.

75. Traub-Dargatz J, Kopral C, Wagner B. Relationship of biosecurity practices with the use of antibiotics for the treatment of infectious disease on U.S. equine operations. Prev Vet Med 2012;104(1–2):107–13.

76. Kane AJ, Morley PS. How to investigate a disease outbreak. In Annual Convention of the American Association of Equine Practitioners. Albuquerque, December 5-8, 1999.

Lawsonia intracellularis and Equine Proliferative Enteropathy

Allen E. Page, DVM, PhD[a], Nathan M. Slovis, CHT, CHT-V[b,*], David W. Horohov, MS, PhD[a]

KEYWORDS

- Equine proliferative enteropathy • Lawsonia intracellularis • EPE

KEY POINTS

- *Lawsonia intracellularis* is the etiologic agent for equine proliferative enteropathy (EPE), which typically affects weanling and yearling horses.
- In North America, EPE cases often occur between August and January, although cases outside of this time frame have been reported.
- Clinical signs of EPE are usually nonspecific and include lethargy, pyrexia, anorexia, peripheral edema, weight loss, colic, and diarrhea.
- Diagnosis is based on the presence of hypoproteinemia and hypoalbuminemia along with clinical signs and positive commercial serologic and/or molecular testing.
- Treatment of EPE requires the use of antimicrobials with good intracellular penetration as well as supportive care to prevent or decrease secondary complications.

INTRODUCTION

Lawsonia intracellularis is an obligate, intracellular, gram-negative bacterium that is associated with proliferative enteropathy (PE) in a variety of species. An economically devastating disease of commercial pig production worldwide, *L. intracellularis* has been shown to have a detrimental effect on average daily gain and market weight in pigs.[1,2] *L. intracellularis* is also the etiologic agent for equine PE (EPE) which is now an emerged pathogen that has been reported worldwide and typically affects young horses, with those between 4 and 9 months of age particularly susceptible to disease.[3–5] The pathogenesis of *L. intracellularis*–induced PE involves an initial colonization of the mitotically active enterocytes of the crypts resulting in crypt hyperplasia. This hyperplasia leads to adenomatous thickening of the mucosa (commonly noted

[a] Department of Veterinary Science, Maxwell H. Gluck Equine Research Center, University of Kentucky, Lexington, KY 40546, USA; [b] McGee Medicine Center, Hagyard Equine Medical Institute, 4250 Iron Works Pike, Lexington, KY 40511, USA
* Corresponding author.
E-mail address: nslovis@hagyard.com

Vet Clin Equine 30 (2014) 641–658
http://dx.doi.org/10.1016/j.cveq.2014.08.001
0749-0739/14/$ – see front matter © 2014 Elsevier Inc. All rights reserved.

in the ileum), with later involvement of other intestinal segments possible.[6] In horses, EPE results in hypoproteinemia and hypoalbuminemia,[3] among other signs, with some horses ultimately dying of the disease despite aggressive care.[7]

EPIDEMIOLOGY

The epidemiology of L. intracellularis remains poorly understood in the horse, although it is thought that transmission occurs through the ingestion of fecal material from wild or domestic animals.[8] Because of the significant impact of L. intracellularis on the swine industry, progress in understanding porcine PE (PPE) epidemiology is much more evolved than it is with EPE. It has been hypothesized that PPE persists and is transmitted within swine operations via poor/inadequate disinfection techniques as well as subclinical shedders of the bacterium. Indeed, work has shown that subclinically infected pigs can efficiently spread the bacterium among cohorts.[9] Although a study with bimonthly fecal polymerase chain reaction (PCR) testing did identify several weanling horses that shed the bacterium in the absence of clinical signs,[10] the role, if any, subclinically infected horses play in transmission remains to be determined. In one study, clinically affected horses were shown to potentially play a role in the transmission of L. intracellularis.[11] It is, therefore, currently recommended that horses with documented EPE not be allowed to comingle with the rest of the herd until after at least 1 week of antimicrobial therapy.

Exposure to L. intracellularis is widespread, with reports of EPE cases occurring worldwide.[12,13] In the United States, regional exposure varies greatly, with farm-specific seroprevalence ranging from 14% to 100%.[5,10,14,15] Only 11% of exposed young horses will develop a form of EPE (5% clinical EPE and 6% subclinical EPE).[5] With EPE, the most commonly affected age groups are weanling and young yearlings, with those between 4 and 9 months of age appearing to be most susceptible to infection.[3,15] EPE has also, on occasion, been diagnosed in older horses up to 17 years of age at one of the author's clinic (NMS); these older horses typically have an additional underlying disease process (Slovis, 2009). In North America, the disease is often detected between August and January,[3,10,15] although cases outside of this time frame have been reported.[5]

It was once hypothesized that exposure to pig feces is a potential source of infection for horses. However, in most cases of EPE, no history or evidence of exposure to pigs or pig feces has been reported.[16] Further, molecular typing of equine isolates using variable number tandem repeat (VNTR) sequencing has demonstrated a clear distinction between the isolates obtained from porcine and equine species.[17] A recent study also revealed evidence of L. intracellularis host adaptation in horses and pigs using different isolates.[18] Fecal shedding and serologic responses were higher and longer in foals infected with the equine isolate compared with foals infected with the porcine isolate. Similarly, reduced average daily weight gain and diarrhea were observed in pigs with the porcine isolate. This species specificity for equine and porcine isolates of L. intracellularis is also noted in other animal models of the disease. For example, hamsters challenged with an equine isolate of L. intracellularis do not develop infection, whereas hamsters challenged with a pig isolate can develop disease.[19] Conversely, rabbits challenged with an equine isolate develop lesions, whereas they do not develop typical intestinal lesions when challenged with the pig isolate.[19]

Since lagomorphs may represent an effective reservoir/amplifier host due to their large population, close contact with horses, short reproductive cycle, and worldwide distribution, recent work has examined a possible role of rabbits in the epidemiology of EPE. When nasogastrically intubated with feces from rabbits that had been experimentally challenged with an equine strain of *L. intracellularis*, foals were noted to seroconvert and shed the bacterium in their feces, however, clinical signs of EPE were noted.[20]

A role for rodents, rats in particular, with respect to the transmission of *L. intracellularis* warrants additional investigation as work has shown a proportion of rats on PPE-endemic farms can shed up to 10^{10} *L. intracellularis* organisms per gram of feces.[21] This finding is of particular importance as experimental challenge studies in pigs have induced PPE at bacterial doses as low as 10^5 per pig,[22] whereas EPE has been induced in horses using doses of 10^{10} per horse.[11,23] Further, it has been shown that the bacterium may be infective for up to 2 weeks in the environment at temperatures of 5°C to 15°C,[24] raising the possibility of a prolonged period during which there is a risk of exposure. Raccoons can be particularly pervasive on horse farms; although *L. intracellularis* has been found previously in raccoon feces on an EPE-endemic farm in central Kentucky (unpublished data, Page, Slovis, and Dr. Nicola Pusterla, 2008), VNTR comparisons of the raccoon and equine-strains showed that they were genetically unrelated (unpublished data from Dr Connie Gebhart, University of Minnesota, 2008).

In addition to the studies mentioned earlier, several have revealed the presence of *L. intracellularis* in a variety of other species, including black-tailed jackrabbits, cottontail rabbits, cats, striped skunks, Virginia opossums, coyotes, guinea pigs, mice, hamsters, hedgehogs, ferrets, rabbits, wild pigs, dogs, foxes, calves, wolves, deer, ostriches, emus, monkeys, and giraffes[6,25–27]; however, none have been successfully implicated in the induction of clinical EPE. Although there is evidence that *L. intracellularis* variants may have evolved to be adapted to more than one host,[28] it seems likely that susceptibilities to the bacterium are driven by the origin of the isolate[28]; thus, the role that each carrier species plays, if any, in the epidemiology of EPE is unknown. It is important to note that *L. intracellularis* is not currently considered a zoonotic disease.

CLINICAL SIGNS

As noted previously, EPE is generally seen in weaned horses less than 1 year of age. Clinical signs of EPE are usually nonspecific and include lethargy, pyrexia (>38.5°C), anorexia, peripheral edema (**Fig. 1**), weight loss (**Fig. 2**), colic, and diarrhea.[3,4,16] Because of the nonspecific nature of the clinical signs, diagnostic testing may be

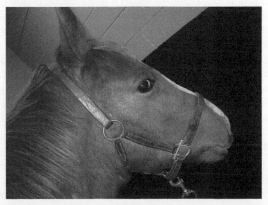

Fig. 1. A 5-month-old Thoroughbred with EPE displaying marked edema of the head and throatlatch region.

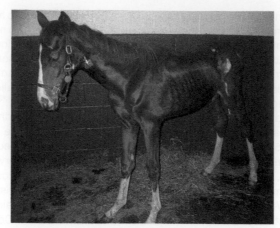

Fig. 2. Severe weight loss in a 4-month-old Thoroughbred with EPE.

necessary to rule out protein loss in the urine as well as peritoneal and pleural cavities. For those horses that recover, the recovery period can take weeks to months before they regain the appearance of unaffected cohorts.

DIAGNOSTIC TESTS

Although the definitive diagnosis of EPE requires direct observation of *L. intracellularis* within enterocytes of the hyperplastic small intestine at necropsy, a presumptive, antemortem diagnosis can generally be made based on the age of the affected animal and clinical signs as well as the presence of hypoproteinemia/hypoalbuminemia, thickened small intestinal loops on abdominal ultrasound, and concurrent positive commercially available diagnostic tests for *L. intracellularis*.

Abdominal Ultrasonography

Proliferative enteropathy caused by *L. intracellularis* results in small intestinal mucosal hyperplasia; as a result, abdominal ultrasonography can be a useful diagnostic in horses. The use of a 2.5- to 5.0-mHz ultrasonographic probe is typically needed in order to obtain a depth of 8 to 20 cm. Although a linear rectal probe may provide sufficient depth to detect thickened small intestine, a negative result using such a probe should not rule out EPE. By itself, small intestinal wall thickness greater than 3 mm is not pathognomonic for EPE[10]; but increased thickness (**Fig. 3**) accompanied by compatible clinical and clinicopathologic signs is highly suspicious. Practitioners should avoid relying solely on abdominal ultrasonography for EPE diagnosis because EPE cases can have normal small intestinal wall thickness[3]; other pathologic conditions can cause small intestine and colonic serosal edema, including salmonellosis, *Clostridium difficile,* and peritonitis.

Total Protein/Albumin/Clinicopathologic Changes

Hypoproteinemia and hypoalbuminemia, which cause the dependent edema seen in clinical EPE cases, are the most consistent laboratory finding associated with EPE.[3–5,8] The pathophysiology of hypoproteinemia and hypoalbuminemia is still under debate. Replication of *L. intracellularis* results in the proliferation and hyperplasia of the rapidly dividing cells of the crypts, leading to an overpopulation of

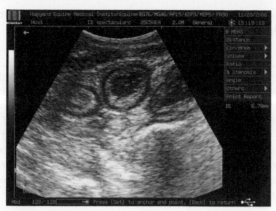

Fig. 3. Ultrasound image revealing thickened sections of small intestine serosa in a 6-month-old Thoroughbred filly. The wall thickness measured 6.78 mm (normal <3 mm).

immature epithelial cells lacking microvilli.[29] These immature epithelial cells, with the capability to be secretory,[30] replace mature epithelial cells lining small intestinal villi, likely resulting in a malabsorptive state and subsequent hypoproteinemia.[31] A malabsorptive state is further supported by evidence that EPE-affected horses experience a diminished ability to absorb glucose.[32] Recent evidence for a protein-losing component of EPE exists based on case reports of acute death following enterocyte infection with *L. intracellularis*.[7,33] The horses in these reports experienced secondary bacteremia/septicemia and necrotizing enteritis, suggesting that pathogenic bacteria were able to penetrate the mucosal epithelial layer in areas with concurrent *L. intracellularis* infection.[7] It stands to reason that if pathogenic bacteria were able to penetrate through this layer into the blood stream, protein could be exuded into the lumen of the gastrointestinal tract via those same damaged areas.

According to Starling's law, the hypoproteinemia seen with EPE results in lower plasma oncotic pressure and a net movement of free fluid from the circulation into tissues. It is important to note that total protein and albumin values drop rapidly in clinical EPE cases as previous work has shown a total protein drop of 3 g/dL can occur over the span of 4 to 7 days.[23] Although the actual values depend on the laboratory used, total protein concentrations are generally less than 5.0 to 5.2 g/dL with albumin concentrations less than 3.0 to 3.1 g/dL.[3,5] There are several conditions that can also result in decreased total protein and albumin levels, including renal disease, peritonitis, pleuritis, salmonellosis, colitis, and intestinal parasites; therefore, it is imperative that a thorough physical examination along with other confirmatory diagnostics be performed before a diagnosis of EPE is made.

Because *L. intracellularis* infections are located in the intestinal enterocytes and clinical cases of EPE usually lack an intestinal inflammatory response,[6] other clinicopathologic tests, such as complete blood counts and fibrinogen levels, are not typically considered useful for an EPE diagnosis.[10] Metabolic abnormalities are unusual except in cases with severe diarrhea, chronic cases, or in cases with concurrent disease.[3,34] Necrotizing EPE (N-EPE) cases were found to have varying degrees of leukocyte count abnormalities; although coagulation diagnostics were not performed, these cases exhibited signs of disseminated intravascular coagulation.[7] Infarctions of the small intestine and kidneys associated with EPE have also been documented by one of the authors (NMS) **(Fig. 4)**.

Fecal Polymerase Chain Reaction

Fecal PCR for *L. intracellularis* is a highly specific test that detects sequences of bacterium-specific DNA.[6,35] However, the sensitivity of *L. intracellularis*–specific fecal PCR testing is variable[35–38] as there are a variety of PCR inhibitors in feces[39] and it is thought that the bacterium is only intermittently shed in the feces of infected horses. Another problem with fecal PCR diagnostics is that fecal shedding stops after 4 to 6 days of antimicrobial administration.[8] With respect to EPE sample collection, a study concluded that feces and rectal swabs yielded similar PCR results for *L. intracellularis*, demonstrating that rectal swabs can be considered as an alternative sample type for patients with decreased or no fecal output.[40]

Serologic Testing

Several *L. intracellularis*–specific serologic assays currently exist for use in horses. The first assay to be developed, the immunoperoxidase monolayer assay (IPMA), was initially used in pigs[9] but has since been adapted for commercial use in horses. Additional tests are also available for use in horses, including a modified version of the IPMA, a blocking enzyme-linked immunosorbent assay (ELISA) (outside of the United States), and a new indirect ELISA.[15] All of the serologic tests, with the exception of the blocking ELISA, seem to be highly specific for *L. intracellularis* exposure.[41]

All of these tests rely on the detection of *L. intracellularis*–specific antibodies, which indicate exposure, but do not necessarily indicate clinical EPE or ongoing infection. It is important for practitioners to note that the severity of exposure and infection cannot be inferred from the titer because the antibody response of an individual to the bacterium depends on multiple factors. Seroconversion in the horse has been documented to occur approximately 14 days following large-dose experimental challenges, whereas most begin showing clinical signs of EPE by day 19 to 21 **(Fig. 5)**.[11,23] It is essential to combine both molecular and serologic testing because these modalities have high analytical specificity but may have variable sensitivity, especially early in the course of disease. To the authors' knowledge, there are

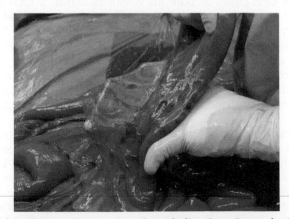

Fig. 4. Infarcted bowel secondary to thromboembolism in a 5-month-old Thoroughbred with EPE. A resection and anastomosis of the affected region was required.

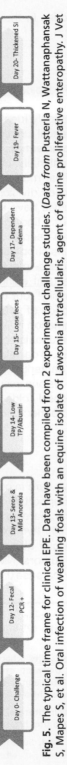

Fig. 5. The typical time frame for clinical EPE. Data have been compiled from 2 experimental challenge studies. (*Data from* Pusterla N, Wattanaphansak S, Mapes S, et al. Oral infection of weanling foals with an equine isolate of Lawsonia intracellularis, agent of equine proliferative enteropathy. J Vet Intern Med 2010;24:622–7; and Page AE, Loynachan AT, Bryant U, et al. Characterization of the interferon gamma response to Lawsonia intracellularis using an equine proliferative enteropathy challenge (EPE) model. Vet Immunol Immunopathol 2011;143:55–65.)

Day 0- Challenge

Day 12- Fecal PCR +

Day 13- Sero+ & Mild Anorexia

Day 14- Low TP/Albumin

Day 15- Loose feces

Day 17- Dependent edema

Day 19- Fever

Day 20- Thickened SI

only 4 commercial diagnostic laboratories in the United States that offer serologic testing for *L. intracellularis.*[1–4]

PATHOLOGY/PATHOPHYSIOLOGY

The pathologic features of EPE and PPE typically identified on postmortem examination of affected animals are fairly similar, namely, small intestinal mucosal hyperplasia. *L. intracellularis* in horses is most commonly identified in enterocytes of the terminal ileum, immediately proximal to the ileocecal junction. The bacterium has been shown to enter enterocytes within 3 hours of infection,[42] and its uptake into enterocytes depends on host-cell function.[42,43] Additionally, cytosolic bacteria are present within several hours after infection.[42] Intestinal mucosal hyperplasia, a hallmark of this disease, results from rapid and unchecked division of the crypt cells by an unknown mechanism. Genomic sequencing studies have identified type III secretion system components in *L. intracellularis.*[44,45] This finding is important as type III secretion systems in other enteric pathogens have been shown to contribute to apoptosis perturbations, cellular invasion, and immune suppression.[44]

Histologically (**Fig. 6**A, B), *L. intracellularis*–infected regions of small intestine exhibit crypt epithelial hyperplasia with subsequent elongation and branching of the crypts and villi and decreased goblet cell density[6] but typically lack evidence of a cellular inflammatory process,[6] with the exception of N-EPE (and, similarly, porcine hemorrhagic enteropathy) whereby the inflammation is likely secondary to mucosal necrosis (**Fig. 7**A, B).[7] The use of specific (immunohistochemistry) (**Fig. 8**) and nonspecific stains (ie, Warthin-Starry silver stain) (**Fig. 9**) can aid in the diagnosis of *L. intracellularis* by demonstrating the presence of the bacterium, typically in the apical cytoplasm of enterocytes. Grossly, small intestinal lesions result in a thickened appearance on cross-section and an increase in mucosal folds (**Fig. 10**). In cases of N-EPE, the mucosal surface may appear reddened or necrotic, with only mild mucosal hyperplasia apparent.[7]

TREATMENT

Treatment of EPE consists of supportive care in combination with specific antimicrobials directed against *L. intracellularis.* Supportive care includes the use of intravenous (IV) fluids, colloids, plasma transfusions, parenteral nutrition, and antiulcer medications. Colloids typically used include 6% hydroxyethyl starch 130/0.4 (Vetastarch) administered at 10 mL/kg IV. Plasma can also be given after the Vetastarch at a rate of 4 to 10 mL/kg IV. One of the authors (NMS) has noted that, in an average 250-kg weanling, the albumin level may increase 0.1 to 0.3 g/dL for every 1 L of plasma

[1] Veterinary Diagnostic Laboratory, College of Veterinary Medicine, University of Minnesota, 1333 Gortner Avenue, St. Paul, MN 55108. Phone: (612) 625-8787; fax: (612) 624-8707; e-mail: vdl@umn.edu; Web site: www.vdl.umn.edu.

[2] Real-time PCR Research and Diagnostics Core Facility, School of Veterinary Medicine, Department of Medicine and Epidemiology, 3110 Tupper Hall, University of California, One Shields Avenue, Davis, CA 95616. Phone: (530) 752-7991; fax: (530) 754-6862; e-mail: carjohnson@ucdavis.edu; Web site: www.vetmed.ucdavis.edu/vme/taqmanservice/diagnosics.html.

[3] Hagyard Laboratory, Hagyard Equine Medical Institute, 4250 Iron Works Pike, Lexington, KY 40511. Phone: (859) 259-3685; fax: (859) 258-9652; Web site: http://hagyard.com/divisions/laboratory.

[4] Equine Diagnostic Services, 1501 Bull Lea Road, Suite 104, Lexington, KY 40511. Phone: (859) 288-5255; Web site: www.edslabky.com/.

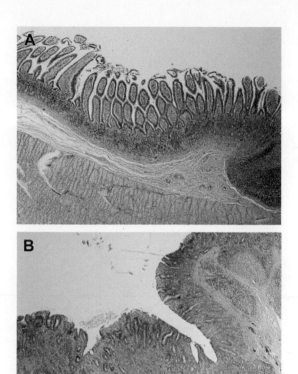

Fig. 6. (*A*) Normal, equine ileum (H&E Stain, original magnification ×4). (*B*) EPE-affected ileum with characteristic mucosal hyperplasia and crypt elongation (H&E Stain, original magnification ×4). (*Courtesy of* Dr Alan Loynachan, University of Kentucky.)

administered. Clinical patients with a protein-losing enteropathy, like EPE, may also have decreased antithrombin levels, increasing the risk of a hypercoagulable state. Thus, the use of medications to aid in preventing platelet aggregation may be of some benefit. These medications may include heparin (40–80 IU/kg subcutaneously or IV 3 times a day), clopidogrel (4 mg/kg by mouth once a day loading dose then 2 mg/mL by mouth once a day)[46] or aspirin (10 mg/kg by mouth once a day or 17 mg/kg by mouth every other day).

The use of antimicrobials that are able to reach therapeutic concentrations within the cytoplasm of the infected enterocyte is required because of the intracellular nature of *L. intracellularis*. Although successful treatment of *L. intracellularis* has been documented with the use of the macrolides (azithromycin [10 mg/kg by mouth once a day] or clarithromycin [7.5 mg/kg by mouth twice a day]), the authors do not recommend the use of macrolide antibiotics in adults or animals greater than 500 pounds because of the increased risk for colitis. Other antimicrobial treatment options include tetracycline-class drugs (oxytetracycline [6.6 mg/kg IV twice a day for 5 days followed by an oral antimicrobial for 7–10 days], doxycycline [10 mg/kg by mouth twice a day for 10–14 days] or minocycline [4 mg/kg by mouth twice a day for 10–14 days]) or chloramphenicol (44–50 mg/kg by mouth 3–4 times a day for 7–14 days). Although some clinical improvement (eg, appetite and fever) can occur rapidly following

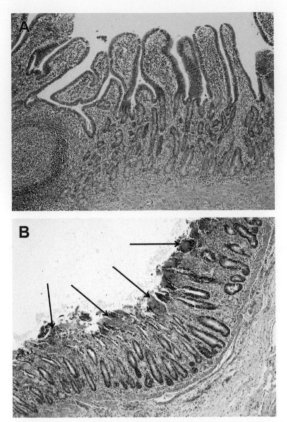

Fig. 7. (*A*) Normal, equine ileum (H&E Stain, original magnification ×4). (*B*) N-EPE–affected ileum with mucosal necrosis (*arrows*) (H&E Stain, original magnification ×4). (*Courtesy of* Dr Alan Loynachan, University of Kentucky.)

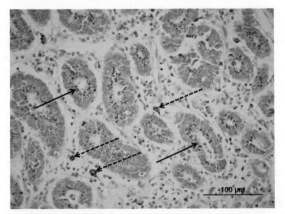

Fig. 8. *L. intracellularis*–specific immunohistochemistry of EPE-affected ileum section (original magnification ×40). Bacteria stain dark and are present primarily within the apical cytoplasm of enterocytes (*solid arrows*) and within the lamina propria macrophages (*hatched arrows*). (*Courtesy of* Dr Alan Loynachan, University of Kentucky.)

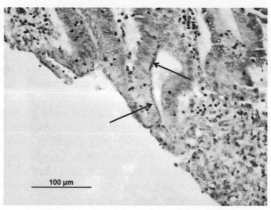

Fig. 9. Warthin-Starry silver stain of EPE-affected ileum section (original magnification ×40). Bacteria stain dark and are present primarily within the apical cytoplasm of enterocytes (*arrows*). (*Courtesy of* Dr Alan Loynachan, University of Kentucky.)

treatment, it can take weeks for total protein and albumin levels to normalize. Additionally, in horses with noticeable weight loss, it can take several months before their appearance matches that of unaffected horses the same age. It is important to note that although previously affected EPE horses sold for 68% less at public auction as yearlings than unaffected horses by the same stallion,[3] no negative effect of EPE was noted on monetary earnings from racing.[47] Generally, EPE is regarded as having a favorable prognosis; however, cases that present with fever and/or complete blood count (CBC) derangements (possibly indicating N-EPE) should be treated aggressively in an attempt to prevent the complications associated with this severe form as the prognosis for N-EPE is poor.[7]

PREVENTION
Monitoring of Herd Status Following Diagnosis of Initial Index Case

Multiple seroprevalence studies have now shown that the number of *L. intracellularis* seropositive horses on a farm is significantly higher than the number of EPE cases on that same farm.[5,10,14,15] In fact, some farms will have up to 100% seroprevalence, and yet the EPE attack rate will only be 10% to 11% of those young horses exposed to *L. intracellularis*.[5] Despite this, and based on recent work showing that exposure on a farm likely occurs within a relatively short window of time,[5] repeat cases of EPE on farms are typical.[15] Therefore, it is advisable to test the herd mates of EPE-affected horses to determine their exposure and clinical status. Doing so will help

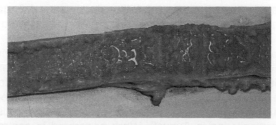

Fig. 10. Gross necropsy picture of the typical mucosal hyperplasia and resulting prominent mucosal folds noted with clinical EPE cases. (*Courtesy of* Dr Alan Loynachan, University of Kentucky.)

the farm determine their exposure level and may help to decrease the number and/or severity of EPE cases.[10] This testing is best achieved by collecting serum to determine the levels of L. intracellularis–specific antibodies and to measure total protein or albumin concentrations. A more expensive alternative is to measure both total protein and albumin concentrations by chemical analysis because there have been cases of false positives (low concentrations) when only one of the parameters was examined.[5] EPE cases will be those with concurrent hypoproteinemia (<5.0 g/dL) and hypoalbuminemia (<3.0 g/dL), although these parameters should be used as a rough guide since actual values will be laboratory dependent.[5] A positive antibody titer (≥60) in a healthy horse with no hypoproteinemia or hypoalbuminemia should be viewed as an exposed horse free of disease. Seropositive or seronegative clinically healthy herd mates with hypoproteinemia and hypoalbuminemia should undergo further diagnostic testing (abdominal ultrasound examination and fecal PCR ± CBC) to determine if the horse has EPE. PCR testing of feces from healthy herd mates is not generally advised because of the costs of testing and issues regarding the test's sensitivity. Daily monitoring of all herd mates may be one of the most effective and cost-efficient means of detecting early EPE. This monitoring is best achieved via daily physical examinations, including rectal temperature and appetite assessment, along with regular body weight measurements, which will allow the determination of daily weight gain.

Treating young horses with suspected EPE should be based on clinical findings and, at the very least, concurrent hypoproteinemia and hypoalbuminemia, given the risks associated with antimicrobial use. Ideally, an L. intracellularis–specific antibody assay would also be used to support an EPE diagnosis. Healthy herd mates should continue to be monitored daily for clinical signs of EPE and monthly for total protein or albumin levels and/or detectable antibodies to L. intracellularis. Foals with EPE should be separated from the rest of the herd for at least 1 week after the initiation of treatment in order to decrease environmental contamination. This separation is particularly important when the weather is cooler as L. intracellularis can survive in the environment for up to 2 weeks.[24] Further, it has been previously shown that clinically affected horses are capable of exposing healthy herd mates to the bacterium.[11]

Monitoring the Herd with Endemic Status

Monitoring endemic herds should follow similar guidelines as for herds with diagnosed cases. This monitoring includes regular physical evaluation and regular monthly assessment of the serologic status of resident foals along with determining the total protein and/or albumin concentrations once or twice a month. Herds with valuable livestock may consider evaluating total protein and/or albumin more frequently (every 1–2 weeks) to decrease the chances of missing an early EPE case. Data including total protein and/or albumin concentrations, as well as weight gains, should be evaluated for each horse and compared with previous time points in order to detect trends potentially associated with early disease. Additionally, average daily gain comparisons between individual horses and the farm average may help with the detection of subclinical cases.

Recent data have shown that the time frame for exposure varies by year and geographic region.[5] Therefore, it is impossible to state exactly when a farm should begin monitoring its foals/weanlings for EPE. Initiation of monitoring for hypoproteinemia and exposure to L. intracellularis should begin at least 4 weeks before the historical first detection of clinical cases (ie, if the first cases have previously been seen in September, begin monitoring in August). Work performed in central Kentucky has shown a seasonal occurrence of EPE cases, with peak cases recorded in November and December.[3] Although year-to-year variations can be expected, most of the EPE cases are seen between August and January in the northern hemisphere. While most of central Kentucky EPE cases occur in the fall and early winter months (October–January), there are published[5] and unpublished data indicating that cases are possible during the spring and summer.

Considering the cost of treating and/or potentially losing a horse with EPE, the monitoring programs outlined earlier, although not inexpensive, can be cost-effective, especially if total protein concentrations are performed by farm personnel via refractometry. Because of an increasing demand for herd monitoring, several laboratories now offer screening tests at competitive prices, especially when bulk samples are submitted.[1,2,3,4]

The lack of epidemiologic data regarding potential natural reservoir hosts and the epidemiology of *L. intracellularis* preclude the institution of any management changes on endemic farms. Given the number of species shown to shed the bacterium, good pest control and preventing nonequine domestic and wild animals access to feed and feeding areas may potentially minimize the risk of disease spread. Additionally, early recognition of clinical cases along with appropriate isolation and biosecurity techniques should help to decrease the bacterial burden in the environment.

Prevention and Vaccination

In piglets, large group size, weaning, transportation, diet change, and mixing have been associated with increased susceptibility to clinical disease.[48] Suggested predisposing factors for the development of EPE in foals include the stress of weaning, parasitism, and other underlying disease.[3] It is, therefore, advisable to minimize stress and control heavy parasite burdens in susceptible animals. Prevention strategies have been best described in pigs using in-feed antimicrobials and a commercially available *L. intracellularis* vaccine.[49–52] Recent work with horses using an avirulent live *L. intracellularis* vaccine (Enterisol Ileitis) has shown that detectable humoral and cellular responses can be measured in foals following vaccination.[53,54] The vaccine protocol that yielded the strongest immunologic responses was intrarectal administration of 30 mL of either the lyophilized (100-mL [50 dose] vial) or the frozen-thawed formulation of the avirulent *L. intracellularis* vaccine (Enterisol Ileitis) given twice, 30 days apart (**Fig. 11**). The *L. intracellularis* vaccine is safe, and

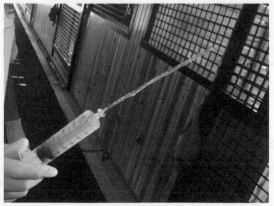

Fig. 11. The use of a nasal applicator for intranasal vaccines is used by one of the authors (NMS) for intrarectal administration of a modified-live *L. intracellularis* vaccine (Enterisol Ileitis). The same applicator is used for all foals housed in the same barn.

the administration is well tolerated by horses. Further, the vaccine has not been associated with the induction of clinical disease in pigs or horses, though fecal shedding up to 12 days has been documented following intrarectal vaccine administration in foals.[53]

Using the aforementioned protocols, vaccine efficacy has been evaluated under field and experimental conditions. A field trial performed on EPE endemic farms in central Kentucky in 2008 showed that vaccinated horses maintained higher daily weight gains and higher total protein concentrations when compared with nonvaccinated naturally exposed seropositive horses.[55] Because of the low incidence of disease reported on the study farms, no difference in the disease rate between vaccinated and nonvaccinated horses could be determined. Under experimental conditions, weanlings vaccinated intrarectally with an avirulent live vaccine against L. intracellularis were protected against clinical EPE following exposure to an equine isolate of the bacterium.[56] This protective effect in the vaccinated group was determined by a lack of clinical disease, lack of hypoproteinemia, and absence of ultrasonographic abnormalities compatible with EPE. Additionally, there was a significant reduction in L. intracellularis fecal shedding in vaccinated versus nonvaccinated horses. Lastly, average daily weight gains from the vaccinated foals over the entire study period were similar to the control foals and significantly higher when compared with the nonvaccinated challenged horses.[56]

It is important to note that the avirulent L. intracellularis vaccine is approved for use only in pigs, and the use in horses is considered extralabel. Therefore, the use of the vaccine should be restricted to endemic farms in an attempt to reduce or prevent EPE. Currently, the cost of vaccination can be a limiting factor for its routine use on endemic farms given that, depending on the formulation (lyophilized vs frozen-thawed), the price per vaccine milliliter ranges from $1.00 to $1.50 (veterinarian cost is $30–$45 per dose per horse). Future studies will be needed in order to refine the vaccine protocol and determine if a single dose and/or a lower vaccine volume confers adequate protection.

Timing of vaccine administration should be synchronized with historical disease occurrence. For example, if foals have been diagnosed with EPE previously in September, it would be recommended to start intrarectal vaccination in August (30 days before the anticipated disease occurrence), and then administer a booster 30 days later. Work in horses has shown that there is a cell-mediated response to stimulation with the bacterium at 180 days after vaccination,[57] suggesting that vaccination before historical disease occurrence should protect young horses long enough to last through the normal exposure time frame. One of the authors (NMS) has been using the 2-dose vaccine protocol on several EPE-endemic farms (~10% clinical disease) since 2009 and has noted no clinical disease from EPE since initiating vaccination. Given the extralabel status of this vaccine, routine monitoring for clinical signs and hypoproteinemia/hypoproteinemia is still recommended (antibody testing is not considered useful in vaccinated animals).

FUTURE DIRECTIONS

There remain a large number of questions regarding L. intracellularis and equine proliferative enteropathy. Of the most pressing would be where the bacterium is maintained in the environment and how it is transmitted to and/or among horses. Additionally, a better understanding of the reasons for the sporadic nature of clinical EPE in exposed animals would likely improve strategies to prevent and/or lessen the effect of this disease on the horse industry.

REFERENCES

1. McOrist S, Smith SH, Green LE. Estimate of direct financial losses due to porcine proliferative enteropathy. Vet Rec 1997;140:579–81.
2. McOrist S. Defining the full costs of endemic porcine proliferative enteropathy. Vet J 2005;170:8–9.
3. Frazer ML. *Lawsonia intracellularis* infection in horses: 2005-2007. J Vet Intern Med 2008;22:1243–8.
4. Lavoie JP, Drolet R, Parsons D, et al. Equine proliferative enteropathy: a cause of weight loss, colic, diarrhoea and hypoproteinaemia in foals on three breeding farms in Canada. Equine Vet J 2000;32:418–25.
5. Page AE, Stills HF, Horohov DW. The effect of passively-acquired antibodies on Lawsonia intracellularis infection and immunity in the horse. Equine Vet J 2014. [Epub ahead of print].
6. Lawson GH, Gebhart CJ. Proliferative enteropathy. J Comp Pathol 2000;122:77–100.
7. Page AE, Fallon LH, Bryant UK, et al. Acute deterioration and death with necrotizing enteritis associated with Lawsonia intracellularis in 4 weanling horses. J Vet Intern Med 2012;26:1476–80.
8. Dauvillier J, Picandet V, Harel J, et al. Diagnostic and epidemiological features of *Lawsonia intracellularis* enteropathy in 2 foals. Can Vet J 2006;47:689–91.
9. Guedes RM, Gebhart CJ, Deen J, et al. Validation of an immunoperoxidase monolayer assay as a serologic test for porcine proliferative enteropathy. J Vet Diagn Invest 2002;14:528–30.
10. Page AE, Slovis NM, Gebhart CJ, et al. Serial use of serologic assays and fecal PCR assays to aid in identification of subclinical *Lawsonia intracellularis* infection for targeted treatment of Thoroughbred foals and weanlings. J Am Vet Med Assoc 2011;238:1482–9.
11. Pusterla N, Wattanaphansak S, Mapes S, et al. Oral infection of weanling foals with an equine isolate of Lawsonia intracellularis, agent of equine proliferative enteropathy. J Vet Intern Med 2010;24:622–7.
12. Wuersch K, Huessy D, Koch C, et al. Lawsonia intracellularis proliferative enteropathy in a filly. J Vet Med A Physiol Pathol Clin Med 2006;53:17–21.
13. Feary DJ, Gebhart CJ, Pusterla N. Lawsonia intracellularis proliferative enteropathy in a foal. Schweiz Arch Tierheilkd 2007;149:129–33.
14. Pusterla N, Higgins JC, Smith P, et al. Epidemiological survey on farms with documented occurrence of equine proliferative enteropathy due to Lawsonia intracellularis. Vet Rec 2008;163:156–8.
15. Page AE, Stills HF, Chander Y, et al. Adaptation and validation of a bacteria-specific enzyme-linked immunosorbent assay for determination of farm-specific *Lawsonia intracellularis* seroprevalence in central Kentucky Thoroughbreds. Equine Vet J 2011;43(Suppl 40):25–31.
16. Pusterla N, Gebhart C. Lawsonia intracellularis infection and proliferative enteropathy in foals. Vet Microbiol 2013;167:34–41.
17. Gebhart CJ, Kelley MR, Chander Y. Molecular typing of equine *Lawsonia intracellularis* isolates. J Equine Vet Sci 2012;32:S32–3.
18. Vannucci FA, Pusterla N, Mapes SM, et al. Evidence of host adaptation in Lawsonia intracellularis infections. Vet Res 2012;43:53.
19. Sampieri F, Vannucci FA, Allen AL, et al. Species-specificity of equine and porcine Lawsonia intracellularis isolates in laboratory animals. Can J Vet Res 2013;77:261–72.

20. Pusterla N, Sanchez-Migallon Guzman D, Vannucci FA, et al. Transmission of Lawsonia intracellularis to weanling foals using feces from experimentally infected rabbits. Vet J 2013;195:241–3.
21. Collins AM, Fell S, Pearson H, et al. Colonisation and shedding of Lawsonia intracellularis in experimentally inoculated rodents and in wild rodents on pig farms. Vet Microbiol 2011;150:384–8.
22. Collins AM, Love RJ. Re-challenge of pigs following recovery from proliferative enteropathy. Vet Microbiol 2007;120:381–6.
23. Page AE, Loynachan AT, Bryant U, et al. Characterization of the interferon gamma response to Lawsonia intracellularis using an equine proliferative enteropathy challenge (EPE) model. Vet Immunol Immunopathol 2011;143:55–65.
24. Collins A, Love RJ, Pozo J, et al. Studies on the ex vivo survival of Lawsonia intracellularis. Swine Health Prod 2000;8:211–5.
25. Herbst W, Willems H, Baljer G. Distribution of Brachyspira hyodysenteriae and Lawsonia intracellularis in healthy and diarrhoeic pigs. Berl Munch Tierarztl Wochenschr 2004;117:493–8 [in German].
26. Pusterla N, Mapes S, Rejmanek D, et al. Detection of Lawsonia intracellularis by real-time PCR in the feces of free-living animals from equine farms with documented occurrence of equine proliferative enteropathy. J Wildl Dis 2008;44: 992–8.
27. Pusterla N, Mapes S, Gebhart C. Further investigation of exposure to Lawsonia intracellularis in wild and feral animals captured on horse properties with equine proliferative enteropathy. Vet J 2012;194:253–5.
28. Vannucci FA, Gebhart CJ. Recent advances in understanding the pathogenesis of Lawsonia intracellularis Infections. Vet Pathol 2014;51:465–77.
29. Boutrup TS, Boesen HT, Boye M, et al. Early pathogenesis in porcine proliferative enteropathy caused by Lawsonia intracellularis. J Comp Pathol 2010;143: 101–9.
30. Cunningham J. Digestion and absorption: the non-fermentative processes. In: Cunningham J, editor. The text book of veterinary physiology. Philadelphia: W.B. Saunders; 1997. p. 301–30.
31. Cooper DM, Gebhart CJ. Comparative aspects of proliferative enteritis. J Am Vet Med Assoc 1998;212:1446–51.
32. Wong DM, Alcott CJ, Sponseller BA, et al. Impaired intestinal absorption of glucose in 4 foals with Lawsonia intracellularis infection. J Vet Intern Med 2009;23:940–4.
33. Arroyo LG, Ter Woort F, Baird JD, et al. Lawsonia intracellularis-associated ulcerative and necro-hemorrhagic enteritis in 5 weanling foals. Can Vet J 2013;54:853–8.
34. McGurrin MK, Vengust M, Arroyo LG, et al. An outbreak of Lawsonia intracellularis infection in a standardbred herd in Ontario. Can Vet J 2007;48:927–30.
35. Jacobson M, Aspan A, Konigsson MH, et al. Routine diagnostics of Lawsonia intracellularis performed by PCR, serological and post mortem examination, with special emphasis on sample preparation methods for PCR. Vet Microbiol 2004;102:189–201.
36. Herbst W, Hertrampf B, Schmitt T, et al. Diagnosis of Lawsonia intracellularis using the polymerase chain reaction (PCR) in pigs with and without diarrhea and other animal species. Dtsch Tierarztl Wochenschr 2003;110:361–4 [in German].
37. Knittel JP, Jordan DM, Schwartz KJ, et al. Evaluation of antemortem polymerase chain reaction and serologic methods for detection of Lawsonia intracellularis-exposed pigs. Am J Vet Res 1998;59:722–6.

38. Moller K, Jensen TK, Jorsal SE, et al. Detection of Lawsonia intracellularis, Serpulina hyodysenteriae, weakly beta-haemolytic intestinal spirochaetes, Salmonella enterica, and haemolytic Escherichia coli from swine herds with and without diarrhoea among growing pigs. Vet Microbiol 1998;62:59–72.

39. Machiels BM, Ruers T, Lindhout M, et al. New protocol for DNA extraction of stool. Biotechniques 2000;28:286–90.

40. Pusterla N, Mapes S, Johnson C, et al. Comparison of feces versus rectal swabs for the molecular detection of Lawsonia intracellularis in foals with equine proliferative enteropathy. J Vet Diagn Invest 2010;22:741–4.

41. Gebhart CJ, Page AE, Kelly M, et al. Comparative study of serology assays for equine proliferative enteropathy. Proceedings of the 58th Annual Convention of the American Association of Equine Practitioners, Anaheim, California, USA, 2-5 December 2009. p. 502–3.

42. McOrist S, Jasni S, Mackie RA, et al. Entry of the bacterium ileal symbiont intracellularis into cultured enterocytes and its subsequent release. Res Vet Sci 1995;59:255–60.

43. Lawson GH, Mackie RA, Smith DG, et al. Infection of cultured rat enterocytes by Ileal symbiont intracellularis depends on host cell function and actin polymerisation. Vet Microbiol 1995;45:339–50.

44. Alberdi MP, Watson E, McAllister GE, et al. Expression by Lawsonia intracellularis of type III secretion system components during infection. Vet Microbiol 2009;139:298–303.

45. Sait M, Aitchison K, Wheelhouse N, et al. Genome sequence of Lawsonia intracellularis strain N343, isolated from a sow with hemorrhagic proliferative enteropathy. Genome Announc 2013;1.

46. Brooks MB, Divers TJ, Watts AE, et al. Effects of clopidogrel on the platelet activation response in horses. Am J Vet Res 2013;74:1212–22.

47. Frazer ML. Sale price and race performance in horses previously diagnosed with Lawsonia intracellularis infection. In: White N II, editor. Proceedings of the 55th Annual Convention of the American Association of Equine Practitioners, Las Vegas, Nevada, USA, 5-9 December. 2009. p. 35.

48. Wattanaphansak S, Asawakarn T, Gebhart CJ, et al. Development and validation of an enzyme-linked immunosorbent assay for the diagnosis of porcine proliferative enteropathy. J Vet Diagn Invest 2008;20:170–7.

49. Guedes RM, Gebhart CJ. Onset and duration of fecal shedding, cell-mediated and humoral immune responses in pigs after challenge with a pathogenic isolate or attenuated vaccine strain of Lawsonia intracellularis. Vet Microbiol 2003;91:135–45.

50. Kroll JJ, Roof MB, McOrist S. Evaluation of protective immunity in pigs following oral administration of an avirulent live vaccine of Lawsonia intracellularis. Am J Vet Res 2004;65:559–65.

51. Almond PK, Bilkei G. Effects of oral vaccination against Lawsonia intracellularis on growing-finishing pig's performance in a pig production unit with endemic porcine proliferative enteropathy (PPE). Dtsch Tierarztl Wochenschr 2006;113:232–5.

52. McOrist S, Smits RJ. Field evaluation of an oral attenuated Lawsonia intracellularis vaccine for porcine proliferative enteropathy (ileitis). Vet Rec 2007;161:26–8.

53. Pusterla N, Jackson R, Mapes SM, et al. Lawsonia intracellularis: humoral immune response and fecal shedding in weanling foals following intra-rectal administration of frozen-thawed or lyophilized avirulent live vaccine. Vet J 2010;186:110–2.

54. Pusterla N, Collier J, Mapes SM, et al. Effects of administration of an avirulent live vaccine of Lawsonia intracellularis on mares and foals. Vet Rec 2009;164: 783–5.

55. Nogradi N, Slovis NM, Gebhart CJ, et al. Evaluation of the field efficacy of an avirulent live Lawsonia intracellularis vaccine in foals. Vet J 2012;192:511–3.

56. Pusterla N, Vannucci FA, Mapes SM, et al. Efficacy of an avirulent live vaccine against Lawsonia intracellularis in the prevention of proliferative enteropathy in experimentally infected weanling foals. Am J Vet Res 2012;73:741–6.

57. Pusterla N, Mapes S, Gebhart C. Lawsonia intracellularis-specific interferon gamma gene expression by peripheral blood mononuclear cells in vaccinated and naturally infected foals. Vet J 2012;192:249–51.

Equine Protozoal Myeloencephalitis

Daniel K. Howe, PhD[a],*, Robert J. MacKay, BVSc, PhD[b], Stephen M. Reed, DVM[a,c]

KEYWORDS

- *Sarcocystis* • *Neospora* • Opossum • Protozoa • EPM • Central nervous system

KEY POINTS

- Equine protozoal myeloencephalitis is an infectious neurologic disease of horses in North, Central, and South America. The disease is caused by the coccidian parasite *Sarcocystis neurona* and less frequently by the related pathogen *Neospora hughesi*.
- Horses are infected with *Sarcocystis neurona* by ingesting food or water that has been contaminated with feces from an infected opossum. The mode of transmission remains uncertain for *Neospora hughesi*.
- In many geographic areas of the Americas, infection is common, as evidenced by the proportion of horses exhibiting antibodies against the parasites. However, clinical disease is uncommon (<1% of seropositive horses).
- Anticoccidial drugs will halt infection, but early diagnosis and treatment are critical to minimize immune-mediated damage in the central nervous system.

 A video of the horse with EPM, acute ataxia caused by equine protozoal myeloencephalitis accompanies this article.

INTRODUCTION

An unusual neurologic condition of horses termed *segmental myelitis* was first observed by Rooney in Kentucky in 1964.[1] Rooney renamed the syndrome *focal encephalitis-myelitis* because of brain involvement, and Prickett, Rooney and others reported on 44 cases at the annual meeting of American Association of Equine Practitioners in 1968[2] and on 52 cases in 1970.[1] In 1974, protozoa were first seen in association with characteristic lesions,[3] and the disease was given its current name, equine protozoal myeloencephalitis (EPM) by Mayhew and colleagues,[4] who reported on 45 cases at the American Association of Equine Practitioners meeting in 1976. Over the

[a] Department of Veterinary Science, M.H. Gluck Equine Research Center, University of Kentucky, Lexington, KY 40546-0099, USA; [b] Department of Large Animal Clinical Sciences, College of Veterinary Medicine, University of Florida, 2015 Southwest 16th Avenue, Room VH-136, PO Box 100136, Gainesville, FL 32610-0125, USA; [c] Rood and Riddle Equine Hospital, PO Box 12070, Lexington, KY 40580, USA
* Corresponding author.
E-mail address: daniel.howe@uky.edu

Vet Clin Equine 30 (2014) 659–675
http://dx.doi.org/10.1016/j.cveq.2014.08.012   vetequine.theclinics.com
0749-0739/14/$ – see front matter © 2014 Elsevier Inc. All rights reserved.

years, a better understanding of EPM etiology and epidemiology has been obtained. However, EPM pathogenesis remains uncertain.

ETIOLOGIC AGENTS

Sarcocystis neurona[5] and *Neospora hughesi*[6–10] are the 2 known causative agents of EPM, although most cases are caused by infection with *S neurona*. Both are protozoan parasites in the phylum, Apicomplexa, which is a broad and important group of obligate intracellular pathogens that cause significant disease in humans and animals.

All species of *Sarcocystis* have a 2-host life cycle that alternates between definitive and intermediate hosts. The opossum (*Didelphis virginiana*) is the definitive host for *S neurona* in North America.[11] As well, South American opossums can act as definitive hosts for *S neurona*.[12] The parasite undergoes sexual reproduction in the intestinal epithelium of the infected opossum, resulting in the production of sporozoite-containing sporocysts that are passed in the feces and are infectious for the intermediate hosts. Skunks,[13] raccoons,[14] armadillos,[15] and cats[16] have been identified as intermediate hosts for *S neurona*. In the natural intermediate hosts, *S neurona* forms latent sarcocysts in the muscle tissue, which is the source of infection for the opossum definitive hosts. Opossums are commonly infected with *S neurona*,[17] so there can be significant contamination of the environment in locations in which opossums are frequently observed.

Horses become infected with *S neurona* when they ingest food or water contaminated with feces from an infected opossum. Horses are considered incidental/dead-end hosts that do not contribute to the parasite's life cycle, because *S neurona* sarcocysts are not found routinely in these animals. However, *S neurona* sarcocysts were described in 1 case of a 4-month-old foal with clinical signs of EPM.[18] Although it remains unlikely that horses play a major role in the life cycle of *S neurona*, this finding suggests that the parasite has the capacity to establish long-term latent infection in these animals. It is important to note that *S neurona* cannot be transmitted horizontally between horses nor can it be transmitted to horses from the intermediate hosts.

The complete lifecycle of *N hughesi* is unknown, so the mode(s) of transmission of this parasite to horses remains uncertain. Canids are known to be a definitive host for the related species *Neospora caninum*,[19] but it has not been established that *N hughesi* use dogs as a definitive host. Vertical transmission of *N caninum* is efficient in cattle, and several studies now suggest that transplacental passage of *N hughesi* can occur in horses.[20,21]

EPIDEMIOLOGY

The first national epidemiologic survey of EPM used postmortem data gathered retrospectively from 10 diagnostic centers throughout the United States and Canada.[22] Most horses (61.8%) were 4 years of age or less and, 19.8% were 8 years of age or older. Although Thoroughbreds, Standardbreds, and Quarter Horses were most commonly affected, no breed, gender, or seasonal bias was established. In a smaller retrospective study, 82 horses with histologic lesions compatible with EPM were reviewed.[23] Disease risk was highest among male Standardbred horses compared with the gender and breed distributions of the attendant hospital population. The mean age of affected horses was 3.6 ± 2.8 years, similar to the findings of Fayer and colleagues.[22]

The prevalence of *S neurona*–specific serum antibodies in horses from the United States has varied widely, ranging from as low as 15% to a high of 89%, depending on geographic location.[24–28] Seroprevalences of 35.6% and 35.5% were reported in horses in Brazil and Argentina, respectively,[29,30] thus, showing that horses in South America are commonly exposed to the parasite.

In general, horses are less likely to exhibit serum antibodies against *N hughesi*. Seroprevalence greater than 10% has been reported in some geographic regions,[6,31–35] whereas other studies found antibodies against *N hughesi* in much lower proportions of horses (less than 3%).[29,30,36–39] Some of the seroprevalence variation may be caused by geographic differences, but studies that used Western blot to confirm serologic results have suggested that seroprevalence to *N hughesi* is commonly overestimated.[34,36,39]

A survey conducted by the National Animal Health Monitoring System (NAHMS) estimated that the average annual incidence of EPM in horses 6 months of age or older was 14 ± 6 cases per 10,000 horses.[40] Although it is apparent that equine neosporosis caused by *N hughesi* can manifest as a neurologic disease,[6–10] it remains unclear what proportion of EPM cases are attributable to this parasite species.

Many clinical reports of EPM suggest that the disease occurs sporadically and seldom involves more than 1 horse on an operation.[4,41] Clusters of cases can occur, however.[42,43] A retrospective study conducted at The Ohio State University found that young horses (1–5 years) and older horses (>13 years) had a higher risk of EPM development than did other horses.[44] The number of cases was lowest in the winter, with the risk 3 times higher in spring and summer and 6 times higher in the fall. Other factors associated with increased risk on a given premises were presence of opossums (2.5-fold), previous diagnosis of EPM (2.5-fold), and presence of woods (2-fold). In contrast, the likelihood of EPM was reduced by one-third by preventing wildlife access to feed and by one-half by the presence of a creek or river as a water source for wildlife.

Stress or advanced age may predispose to development of EPM via immune suppression.[45] A strong dose-response relationship was found between various stressful events (eg, heavy exercise, transport, injury, surgery, or parturition) and the risk of EPM.[44] After such an event, the risk of manifesting the disease increased with time. Racehorses and show horses had a higher risk of EPM development compared with breeding and pleasure horses. Not surprisingly, horses with EPM that were treated were 10 times more likely to improve than were untreated horses.[45]

From the National Animal Health Monitoring System equine study,[40] EPM was found more likely to occur on premises where opossums were identified. Interestingly, the presence of mice or rats also was associated with increased risk for EPM develop in horses. High population density also increased the risk of EPM development, which may be related to the encroachment of humans on opossum habitats.

PATHOGENESIS

Although all horses are thought to be susceptible, it is apparent that infection with *S neurona* or *N hughesi* does not equate with EPM, with clinical disease developing in only a small proportion of seropositive horses. Unfortunately, it is not clear what can cause a simple, asymptomatic infection to progress to severe neurologic disease; this has confounded EPM diagnosis in the past and continues to hamper efforts to prevent and control the disease. As mentioned, factors such as parasite inoculum and stress-induced immune suppression have been implicated in the occurrence of EPM.[45–47] However, efforts to increase stress by use of a second transport and treatment with immunosuppressive steroids did not exacerbate disease,[48,49] so it is apparent that the interplay between immune suppression and infection is more complex than currently understood. Modest genetic and antigenic diversity exist among strains of *S neurona* that have been isolated,[50–52] and there is some suggestion that particular parasite genotypes may be more virulent than others.[53] This finding was based on a large collection of S neurona isolates from marine mammals, however, and the association between parasite genotype and disease was not apparent in the more limited sample set of isolates from horses suffering from EPM. Consequently, further work is needed to assess whether some strains of S neurona have a greater capacity to cause neurologic disease in horses.

Experimental Infections

Resistance to many intracellular pathogens is dependent on a generation of a normal T helper cell 1 cellular immune response, including the expression of cytokines such as interferon gamma and interleukin 12. Consistent with the importance of cell-mediated immunity, protozoal encephalitis with S neurona has been induced in athymic nude mice, interferon gamma knockout mice, and CD8+ knockout mice by subcutaneous or intraperitoneal injection of cultured merozoites or by gavage with sporocysts.[54–56] Immunocompetent mice (C57BL/6 and BALB/c) are seemingly resistant to S neurona infection, even after corticosteroid treatment. Paradoxically, severe combined immunodeficient mice and horses, which completely lack adaptive immune systems but have a population of natural killer cells, do not get neurologic disease when infected with S neurona, despite persistent, low-level infection.[55,57,58]

Initial work aimed at reproducing EPM in horses used as challenge inoculum a mixture of uncharacterized sporocysts collected from 10 feral opossums.[59] When molecular markers were identified that were able to differentiate the various Sarcocystis spp sporocysts found in opossums,[60] it became possible to use challenge inocula containing known quantities of S neurona sporocysts.[46,48] In all of these studies, serum and cerebrospinal fluid (CSF) antibodies to S neurona developed in horses, and mild to moderately severe neurologic signs were observed in some but not all challenged horses. In many cases, signs were progressive initially and then stabilized or even improved. Evidence of mild to moderate subacute to chronic multifocal changes was generally found in the central nervous system (CNS), but protozoa were not observed in blood or CNS tissue nor were they detected by immunohistochemical staining, polymerase chain reaction, culture, or mouse inoculation. Immunosuppression by dexamethasone administration reduced the time to the appearance of antibodies in the CSF, and clinical signs and histologic lesions were equivalent or even milder than those observed in the challenged control horses.[48]

With establishment of the S neurona lifecycle in the laboratory, it became possible to infect horses with a homogeneous inoculum of parasite sporocysts.[47] This study found that a large inoculum (10^5–10^6 sporocysts) was needed to consistently obtain evidence of CNS infection (antibodies in CSF). Similar to the prior challenge studies, mild to moderate clinical signs were observed, but organisms were not seen histologically.

In vitro infection of buffy coat cells and intravenous inoculation of the infected cells back into horses has been used as a challenge model for EPM.[61] Similar to the prior studies using a natural route of infection, challenged horses had moderate clinical signs, and antibodies were detected in serum and CSF. Although parasites were not observed histologically within CNS lesions, culture isolation of organisms from tissues was described.

The collective results from the various experimental horse infection studies indicate that horses are resistant S neurona infection and development of neurologic disease, and the role of the immune response in the progression from simple infection to acute EPM is complicated. Whereas severe immunosuppression may promote CNS invasion by S neurona, components of the immune response are seemingly required for development of EPM (**Box 1**).

> **Box 1**
> **Etiology and epidemiology of EPM**
>
> • EPM is caused primarily by the protozoan parasite *S neurona*, although some cases have been associated with the related pathogen *N hughesi*.
>
> • *S neurona* is transmitted to horses via food or water contamination with feces from infected opossums. The complete life cycle of *N hughesi* is uncertain, but this parasite may be transmitted in the feces of dogs.
>
> • Infection of horses is fairly common, but EPM is rare. The factors influencing disease susceptibility remain unknown.

CLINICAL SIGNS

EPM is often a progressive debilitating disease affecting the CNS of horses (Video 1). Clinical signs vary from acute to chronic with insidious onset of focal or multifocal signs of neurologic disease involving the brain, brainstem, or spinal cord.[41] Affected horses may initially exhibit unusual signs such as dysphagia, evidence of abnormal upper airway function, unusual or atypical lameness, or even seizures.[62] Severely affected horses may have difficulty standing, walking, or swallowing, and the disease may progress very rapidly. In other cases, the clinical signs appear to stabilize, only to relapse days or weeks later.

The variability of clinical signs is caused by the parasite's ability to infect both white and gray matter randomly at multiple sites along the CNS. Signs of gray matter involvement include focal muscle atrophy (**Fig. 1**) and severe muscle weakness, whereas damage to white matter frequently results in ataxia and weakness in limbs caudal to the site of damage. The early signs of the disease, such as stumbling and frequent interference between limbs, can be confused easily with lameness. Horses affected with EPM commonly experience a gradual progression in the severity and range of clinical signs, including ataxia. In some cases, however, a gradual onset may give way to a sudden exacerbation in the severity of clinical illness, resulting in recumbency.

The vital signs in affected horses are usually normal and animals appear bright and alert. Some horses with EPM may appear thin and mildly depressed. Neurologic examination often finds asymmetric ataxia, weakness, and spasticity involving all 4

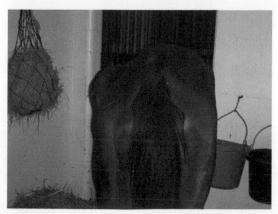

Fig. 1. Asymmetric gluteal muscle atrophy in a horse with EPM.

limbs. Areas of hyporeflexia, hypalgesia, or complete sensory loss are frequently present. The most commonly observed signs of brain/brainstem disease include depression, head tilt, facial nerve paralysis, and difficulty in swallowing. Signs are not necessarily limited to these areas.[63] Gait abnormalities most often result from lesions in the spinal cord and may be variable in severity, depending on the location and extent of tissue damage.

PATHOLOGY

On necropsy examination of cases of EPM, lesions may be grossly visible on cut surfaces of the CNS; these may vary from clearly demarcated discoloration (usually of gray matter) to massive lesions that destroy large portions of the brain or multiple segments of the spinal cords.[64] Histologically, parasites are seen in less than 50% of cases. When present, they can be difficult to detect using standard staining procedures (eg, hematoxylin and eosin), but may be more apparent after immunohistochemical staining (**Fig. 2**). Histologic lesions are remarkably consistent regardless of the presence of associated organisms. Typically, there is cuffing of blood vessels by mononuclear cells, necrosis of parenchyma with phagocytosis and gitter cell formation, astrocyte proliferation, and gemistocyte formation. Eosinophils are seen commonly as are multinucleated cells, which may be giant in size. Lesions may extend to produce a nonsuppurative meningitis. Lesions may vary from peracute to chronic with prominent lymphoid vascular cuffing with minimal tissue destruction in the former case and marked tissue loss, prominent astrocyte proliferation, and minimal inflammatory response in chronic cases. The amount of fiber degeneration in ascending and descending pathways below and above the lesions is dependent on the chronicity of the condition.

DIAGNOSIS

EPM should always be considered in any horse exhibiting signs of CNS disease. Horses displaying such signs should be subjected to a thorough neurologic examination and appropriate laboratory tests undertaken to support a diagnosis of EPM and to exclude other likely diagnoses. Laboratory testing should be considered ancillary and not a substitute for an in-depth clinical examination. In many cases of EPM, there is asymmetry of gait and focal muscle atrophy; when present, EPM should be high on

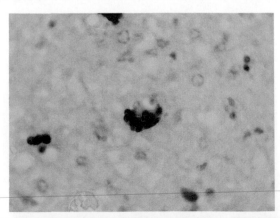

Fig. 2. Immunohistochemical labeling with anti–*S neurona* rabbit serum shows multiple stained parasites in equine CNS tissue.

the list of possible causes. This combination of signs has proved to be a useful distinguishing feature of the disease and is helpful in clinically differentiating EPM from similar neurologic conditions affecting the horse.

Differential Diagnoses

Virtually any neurologic disease of horses can produce clinical signs that mimic those associated with cases of EPM. Cervical vertebral stenotic myelopathy (CVSM) is a frequently encountered disease that results from compression of the cervical spinal cord. CVSM signs usually are symmetric, and, typically, the pelvic limbs are more severely affected than the thoracic limbs. Focal muscle atrophy is not a clinical feature of CVSM. In horses with clinical signs that localize neuroanatomically to the cervical spinal cord, radiographs of the cervical vertebrae should be taken to determine the intervertebral and intravertebral sagittal ratios (**Fig. 3**). Trauma also can cause spinal cord damage at any level, potentially causing abnormal neurologic signs in one to all limbs.

A history of respiratory disease or an outbreak of abortion is a common prelude to the occurrence of equine herpesvirus–1–associated neurologic disease. Affected horses may be febrile shortly before or at the onset of neurologic signs. Neurologic signs most commonly are symmetric with primary pelvic limb weakness and ataxia, bladder distention (usually without incontinence), and, more rarely, perineal hypalgesia, tail paralysis, and fecal retention. Signs of brain involvement are seen rarely.

Equine motor neuron disease also produces signs that initially may be confused with those observed in horses affected with EPM. Severe limb weakness with muscle fasciculations and tremors are typical, early signs of equine motor neuron disease. With chronicity, there is widespread, profound, muscle atrophy.

Other causes of spinal cord disease that may result in similar clinical signs include extradural and spinal cord tumors, epidural abscess, migrating metazoan parasites, rabies, West Nile viral encephalomyelitis, equine degenerative myeloencephalopathy, lead poisoning, creeping indigo toxicity, vascular malformations, and discospondylopathies. Any of the many equine diseases of the brain or cranial nerves must be considered as potential rule-outs in cases of EPM showing signs attributable to dysfunction of the brain or cranial nerves. This list includes viral encephalitides, neoplasia, head trauma, brain abscess, migrating parasites, temporohyoid osteoarthropathy, polyneuritis equi, cholesterol granuloma, metabolic derangement, and hepatoencephalopathy.

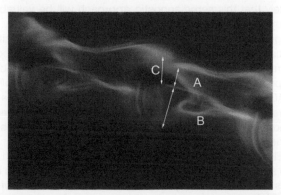

Fig. 3. Radiograph of the cervical vertebrae to assess intervertebral and intravertebral sagittal ratios. A/B is the intravertebral sagittal ratio and A/C is the intervertebral sagittal ratio.

Postmortem Diagnosis

Confirmation of EPM on postmortem examination is based on demonstration of protozoa in CNS lesions, although the diagnosis frequently is made presumptively even when parasites are not detected, if the characteristic inflammatory changes are found. In 2 reported series, organisms were seen in hematoxylin and eosin sections of CNS tissue in 10% to 36% of suspected cases.[23,65] Sensitivity was increased from 20% to 51% by immune staining with antibody against S neurona.[65] The likelihood of finding organisms is reduced by prior treatment with antiprotozoal drugs and may be increased by treatment with corticosteroids.

Immunodiagnostic Testing

As described, EPM occurs only in a small proportion of horses infected with either S neurona or N hughesi.[40] As a consequence, the simple detection of antibodies against these parasites has minimal diagnostic value. Even the presence of antibodies in the CSF is not a definitive indicator of EPM, as there will be normal passive transfer of antibody across an intact blood-brain barrier (BBB).[66] Therefore, immunodiagnostic testing was eschewed for many years by some veterinary practitioners because of lack of confidence in the test results.

Immunodiagnosis of EPM has improved greatly in recent years because of the development of semiquantitative assays and the utilization of diagnostic methodologies that detect intrathecal antibody production, indicating active parasite infection in the CNS. The Goldman-Witmer coefficient (C-value) and the antigen-specific antibody index are tests of proportionality that assess whether there is a greater amount of pathogen-specific antibody in the CSF than would be present owing to normal passive transfer across the BBB. Application of these tests to a sample set of 29 clinical cases showed the value of this methodology for accurate EPM diagnosis.[67] Moreover, many EPM cases have antibody titers in CSF that far exceed what would be present owing to passive transfer across the BBB. Two studies examining an extensive collection of horses with neurologic disease found that a simple ratio of serum/CSF titers was sufficient to reveal intrathecal antibody production and an accurate diagnosis of EPM caused by S neurona.[68,69] Therefore, the use of the more expensive and laborious C value or antibody index can be limited to cases that have uncompelling ELISA titer results (ie, the serum/CSF ratio equals the cutoff) or when a condition that compromises the BBB is suspected.

Although use of serum/CSF titer ratios has not been investigated for N hughesi infection, it is likely that this serodiagnostic approach will be valuable for diagnosis of EPM caused by this parasite.

Several serologic assays are available that measure antibodies against S neurona or N hughesi and can be used, therefore, to assess intrathecal antibody production. Enzyme-linked immunosorbent assays (ELISAs) have been developed based on parasite antigens expressed as recombinant proteins in Escherichia coli.[39,70–72] Specifically, the SnSAG and NhSAG surface antigens from S neurona or N hughesi, respectively, have been used as the serologic targets in the ELISAs, as these proteins are abundant and typically elicit robust immune responses in horses that have been infected with either of these 2 parasite species.[73–75]

The SnSAG2 ELISA and the SnSAG4/3 ELISA have been validated extensively and found to provide accurate detection of antibodies against S neurona in equine serum and CSF samples.[71,72] These 2 assays were used to show the value of intrathecal antibody production[68,69] and are currently offered commercially for EPM diagnostic testing (Equine Diagnostic Solutions, LLC).

An ELISA based on the SnSAG1 surface protein has been described.[70] However, it has been found that this protein is not expressed by all strains of *S neurona*,[52] thereby reducing the utility of this antigen for antibody detection[71] and EPM diagnosis.[76] Assays that combine SnSAG1 with 2 additional SnSAGs (SnSAG5 and SnSAG6) are currently offered commercially (Pathogenes, Inc; Prota, LLC), but no published reports describe validation of the assays, so it is uncertain whether these tests reliably detect antibodies to *S neurona*.

For immunodiagnosis of EPM caused by *N hughesi*, an ELISA based on the NhSAG1 surface protein yields high sensitivity and specificity when compared with the gold standard for detecting antibodies against this parasite (Western blot).[39] The NhSAG1 ELISA is offered commercially by Equine Diagnostic Solutions.

The *S neurona* indirect fluorescent antibody test (IFAT) uses whole, culture-derived *S neurona* merozoites as the antigen source. Like ELISA, this assay yields an endpoint antibody titer and can be used to detect intrathecal antibody production. The *S neurona* IFAT was optimized and validated at the University of California–Davis[77,78] and is currently offered by their Veterinary Diagnostic Laboratory. Additionally, the University of California–Davis facility offers an IFAT based on *N hughesi* tachyzoites to detect antibodies against this alternative EPM parasite. Although serum titers obtained with the IFAT have been used to estimate the probability of EPM, seemingly obviating the need for CSF collection and testing, studies that have used diverse collections of neurologic disease cases have shown that a serum titer alone is a poor predictor of EPM (**Box 2**).[68,69]

TREATMENT
Folate-Inhibiting Drugs

A combination of sulfadiazine and pyrimethamine (SDZ/PYR), which block successive steps in protozoal folate synthesis, was one of the initial therapies for treatment of EPM. A dosage regimen of PYR, 1 mg/kg, and SDZ, 20 mg/kg, administered once daily for at least 3 months is considered the standard treatment for EPM. Because dietary folate can interfere with the uptake of diaminopyrimidine drugs like PYR,[79] hay should not be fed for 2 hours before or after treatment. PYR given orally to horses at 1 mg/kg/d achieves a concentration of approximately 0.02 to 0.10 µg/mL in the CSF 4 to 6 hours after administration.[80] Interestingly, these experimental horses were allowed free access to prairie hay, potentially reducing the bioavailability of the drug.[79] Additionally, because PYR is concentrated in CNS tissue relative to plasma,[81] the concentration at the desired site of action may be greater than 0.1 µg/mL. Mean peak CSF concentrations of sulfonamide after single or multiple dosing (22–44 mg/kg) are reported to be approximately 2 to 8 µg/mL.[82,83] These drugs are available as a US Food and Drug Administration (FDA)-approved product (ReBalance; PRN Pharmacal).

Box 2
Achieving an accurate diagnosis of EPM

- Confirm the presence of clinical signs consistent with EPM by conducting a thorough neurologic examination.
- Rule out other potential causes using available tools (eg, cervical radiography).
- Use immunodiagnostic testing to assess intrathecal antibody production against *S neurona* or *N hughesi*.

The toxic effects of these drugs relate to the inhibition of folate synthesis and fortunately are rarely serious, even when the drug is given at twice the standard dose. Typically, there is progressive mild anemia (packed cell volume in the low 20s) over a 6-month treatment period, and neutropenia may be seen in some cases. Pyrimethamine is considered teratogenic and causes both abortions and birth of malformed pups in treated rats.[84] At least 4 cases of a fatal syndrome have been observed in neonatal foals born to mares that were given these drugs during the latter stages of pregnancy (R. MacKay, unpublished observations, 1979).[85] Three of the mares had been given folic acid as a supplement. Evidence from other species would suggest that supplementation with folic acid (a synthetic nonreduced form of folate) either will not prevent PYR-induced toxicity[86] or may even exacerbate it.[84] In light of these observations, the supplemental use of folic acid in SDZ/PYR-treated horses cannot be justified.

Triazines

Over the last 10 or more years, 2 members of the triazine group of compounds, diclazuril and toltrazuril, have been approved for treatment of EPM. These drugs are found to have broad-spectrum anticoccidial activity in many avian and mammalian species and are thought to target the parasite's apicoplast organelle.[87] The activity of triazine compounds against *S neurona* was initially shown in vitro.[88,89] In horses, pharmacokinetic studies have established that therapeutic steady-state concentrations of both diclazuril and ponazuril are achieved by day 7 using labeled doses.[90,91] Moreover, use of a loading dose of ponazuril at 15 mg/kg resulted in steady-state concentrations in blood and CSF by day 2.[92]

The formulations of these drugs adapted for clinical use in horses are Protazil (1.56% diclazuril; Merck Animal Health, Kansas City, KS) and Marquis (15% ponazuril; Bayer Inc, Kansas City, KS).

Anti-inflammatory Therapy

Nonsteroidal anti-inflammatory drugs such as flunixin meglumine are frequently given to moderately or severely affected horses during the first 3 to 7 days of antiprotozoal therapy. In the case of horses in danger of falling down or those that exhibit signs of brain involvement, the additional use of corticosteroids (0.1 mg/kg of dexamethasone twice daily) and dimethyl sulfoxide (1 g/kg as a 10% solution intravenously or by nasogastric tube twice daily) for the first several days may control the inflammatory response and associated clinical signs. Because the damaged CNS is susceptible to oxidant injury, it has become common practice to use pharmacologic doses of the antioxidant vitamin E (eg, 20 IU/kg/d orally) throughout the treatment period. Although vitamin E therapy may not significantly alter the course of recovery, it is unlikely to cause harm.

Biological Response Modifiers

Based on the assumption that horses that have EPM may be immune compromised, immunomodulators have been included by some in treatment of the disease. The drugs used include levamisole (1 mg/kg orally twice a day for the first 2 weeks of antiprotozoal therapy and for the first week of each month thereafter), killed *Propionibacterium acnes* (Eqstim; Neogen, Lansing, MI), mycobacterial wall extract (Equimune IV; Bioniche Animal Health Vetoquinol, Belville, Ontario, Canada), and transfer factor (4Life Transfer Factor, 4LifeResearch, Sandy, UT). No study has been published to date to evaluate the efficacy of these adjuvant treatments (**Box 3**).

Box 3
Treatment of EPM

- Use one of the FDA-approved anticoccidial drugs to halt infection.
  - Ponazuril (Marquis, Bayer Animal Health)
  - Diclazuril (Protazil, Merck Animal Health)
  - Sulfadiazine/Pyrimethamine (eg, ReBalance, PRN Pharmacal)
- Give supportive anti-inflammatory therapy, as needed

PREVENTION

The prevention of EPM is difficult because of the widespread distribution of the etiologic agents in many parts of the United States. Methods for effective control of this disease have not been delineated; however, it is prudent to attempt to eliminate known risk factors.

Access of opossums and other wildlife or pests to feed and water should be eliminated. Cereal grains should be kept in rodent-proof containers, and forages should be protected from wildlife access by use of enclosed facilities. Although it remains unconfirmed whether insects such as flies and cockroaches can serve as biological vectors that transport *S neurona* sporocysts, controlling the insect population on farms is advisable.

The case histories of EPM-affected horses frequently indicate recent adverse health events.[44] Close monitoring is warranted of heavily pregnant or lactating mares and of horses that have recently experienced a major illness, injury, or been transported a considerable distance or under arduous conditions.

Protective immunization against *S neurona* and *N hughesi* would be the ideal approach to prevent EPM. However, difficulties experienced in developing vaccines against other protozoan pathogens suggest that this approach may take many years to achieve. A conditional license was given for a killed *S neurona* vaccine, but this product has been withdrawn since efficacy was not demonstrated.

Perhaps of more immediate value would be the use of antiprotozoal drugs given according to a protocol that would allow initial infection and short-term immunity (metaphylaxis) but prevent spread to the CNS. Any of the therapeutic drugs that are thought to inhibit *S neurona* growth would be logical candidates for this intermittent preventative approach.

SUMMARY

Since EPM was initially described in the 1960s, diagnosis, treatment and prevention have improved through advances in the understanding of the parasite and the disease. Epidemiologic studies have identified numerous risk factors associated with development of the disease. Despite generally high seroprevalence of *S neurona* in horses in the Americas, the annual incidence of EPM is less than 1%, thus, demonstrating that infection does not equate with disease. Therefore, further studies are needed to gain a better understanding of the pathogenesis of parasite infection and the occurrence of EPM. Moreover, the mode of transmission for *N hughesi* and the contribution of this parasite species to EPM incidence is not certain, so additional work is needed in this area. Challenge studies have confirmed that horses can be experimentally infected with *S neurona*. However, severe and persistent clinical signs and abnormal CNS histology are not seen consistently. Several FDA-approved EPM treatments are now available. Development of an effective EPM vaccine remains a long-term goal, whereas prophylactic treatment with an antiprotozoal drug may be a viable preventative.

SUPPLEMENTARY DATA

Supplementary data related to this article can be found online at http://dx.doi.org/10.1016/j.cveq.2014.08.012.

REFERENCES

1. Rooney JR, Prickett ME, Delaney FM, et al. Focal myelitis-encephalitis in horses. Cornell Vet 1970;60:494–501.
2. Prickett ME. Equine spinal ataxia. Paper presented at: 14th Annual Convention of the American Association of Equine Practitioners. Philadelphia (PA), December 9–11, 1968.
3. Cusick PK, Sells DM, Hamilton DP, et al. Toxoplasmosis in two horses. J Am Vet Med Assoc 1974;164(1):77–80.
4. Mayhew IG, De Lahunta A, Whitlock RH, et al. Equine protozoal myeloencephalitis. Proc Annu Conv Am Assoc Equine Pract 1976;22d:107–14.
5. Dubey JP, Davis SW, Speer CA, et al. *Sarcocystis neurona* n. sp. (Protozoa: Apicomplexa), the etiologic agent of equine protozoal myeloencephalitis. J Parasitol 1991;77(2):212–8.
6. Cheadle MA, Lindsay DS, Rowe S, et al. Prevalence of antibodies to *Neospora* sp. in horses from Alabama and characterisation of an isolate recovered from a naturally infected horse [corrected]. Int J Parasitol 1999;29(10):1537–43.
7. Dubey JP, Liddell S, Mattson D, et al. Characterization of the Oregon isolate of *Neospora hughesi* from a horse. J Parasitol 2001;87(2):345–53.
8. Hamir AN, Tornquist SJ, Gerros TC, et al. *Neospora caninum*-associated equine protozoal myeloencephalitis. Vet Parasitol 1998;79(4):269–74.
9. Marsh AE, Barr BC, Madigan J, et al. Neosporosis as a cause of equine protozoal myeloencephalitis. J Am Vet Med Assoc 1996;209(11):1907–13.
10. Lindsay DS, Steinberg H, Dubielzig RR, et al. Central nervous system neosporosis in a foal. J Vet Diagn Invest 1996;8(4):507–10.
11. Fenger CK, Granstrom DE, Langemeier JL, et al. Identification of opossums (*Didelphis virginiana*) as the putative definitive host of *Sarcocystis neurona*. J Parasitol 1995;81(6):916–9.
12. Dubey JP, Lindsay DS, Kerber CE, et al. First isolation of *Sarcocystis neurona* from the South American opossum, *Didelphis albiventris*, from Brazil. Vet Parasitol 2001;95(2–4):295–304.
13. Cheadle MA, Yowell CA, Sellon DC, et al. The striped skunk (*Mephitis mephitis*) is an intermediate host for *Sarcocystis neurona*. Int J Parasitol 2001;31(8):843–9.
14. Dubey JP, Saville WJ, Stanek JF, et al. *Sarcocystis neurona* infections in raccoons (*Procyon lotor*): evidence for natural infection with sarcocysts, transmission of infection to opossums (*Didelphis virginiana*), and experimental induction of neurologic disease in raccoons. Vet Parasitol 2001;100(3–4):117–29.
15. Cheadle MA, Tanhauser SM, Dame JB, et al. The nine-banded armadillo (*Dasypus novemcinctus*) is an intermediate host for *Sarcocystis neurona*. Int J Parasitol 2001;31(4):330–5.
16. Dubey JP, Saville WJ, Lindsay DS, et al. Completion of the life cycle of *Sarcocystis neurona*. J Parasitol 2000;86(6):1276–80.
17. Dubey JP. Prevalence of *Sarcocystis* species sporocysts in wild-caught opossums (*Didelphis virginiana*). J Parasitol 2000;86(4):705–10.

18. Mullaney T, Murphy AJ, Kiupel M, et al. Evidence to support horses as natural intermediate hosts for *Sarcocystis neurona*. Vet Parasitol 2005;133(1):27–36.
19. McAllister MM, Dubey JP, Lindsay DS, et al. Dogs are definitive hosts of *Neospora caninum*. Int J Parasitol 1998;28(9):1473–8.
20. Antonello AM, Pivoto FL, Camillo G, et al. The importance of vertical transmission of *Neospora* sp. in naturally infected horses. Vet Parasitol 2012;187(3–4): 367–70.
21. Pusterla N, Conrad PA, Packham AE, et al. Endogenous transplacental transmission of *Neospora hughesi* in naturally infected horses. J Parasitol 2011; 97(2):281–5.
22. Fayer R, Mayhew IG, Baird JD, et al. Epidemiology of equine protozoal myeloencephalitis in North America based on histologically confirmed cases. J Vet Intern Med 1990;4(2):54–7.
23. Boy MG, Galligan DT, Divers TJ. Protozoal encephalomyelitis in horses: 82 cases (1972–1986). J Am Vet Med Assoc 1990;196(4):632–4.
24. Bentz BG, Granstrom DE, Stamper S. Seroprevalence of antibodies to *Sarcocystis neurona* in horses residing in a county of southeastern Pennsylvania. J Am Vet Med Assoc 1997;210(4):517–8.
25. Bentz BG, Ealey KA, Morrow J, et al. Seroprevalence of antibodies to *Sarcocystis neurona* in equids residing in Oklahoma. J Vet Diagn Invest 2003;15:597–600.
26. Blythe LL, Granstrom DE, Hansen DE, et al. Seroprevalence of antibodies to *Sarcocystis neurona* in horses residing in Oregon. J Am Vet Med Assoc 1997; 210(4):525–7.
27. Saville WJ, Reed SM, Granstrom DE, et al. Seroprevalence of antibodies to *Sarcocystis neurona* in horses residing in Ohio. J Am Vet Med Assoc 1997;210(4): 519–24.
28. Tillotson K, McCue PM, Granstrom DE, et al. Seroprevalence of antibodies to *Sarcocystis neurona* in horses residing in northern Colorado. J Equine Vet Sci 1999;19(2):122–6.
29. Dubey JP, Kerber CE, Granstrom DE. Serologic prevalence of *Sarcocystis neurona, Toxoplasma gondii*, and *Neospora caninum* in horses in Brazil. J Am Vet Med Assoc 1999;215(7):970–2.
30. Dubey JP, Venturini MC, Venturini L, et al. Prevalence of antibodies to *Sarcocystis neurona, Toxoplasma gondii* and *Neospora caninum* in horses from Argentina. Vet Parasitol 1999;86(1):59–62.
31. Bartova E, Sedlak K, Syrova M, et al. *Neospora* spp. and *Toxoplasma gondii* antibodies in horses in the Czech Republic. Parasitol Res 2010;107(4):783–5.
32. Dubey JP, Mitchell SM, Morrow JK, et al. Prevalence of antibodies to *Neospora caninum, Sarcocystis neurona*, and *Toxoplasma gondii* in wild horses from central Wyoming. J Parasitol 2003;89(4):716–20.
33. Pitel PH, Pronost S, Romand S, et al. Prevalence of antibodies to *Neospora caninum* in horses in France. Equine Vet J 2001;33(2):205–7.
34. Vardeleon D, Marsh AE, Thorne JG, et al. Prevalence of *Neospora hughesi* and *Sarcocystis neurona* antibodies in horses from various geographical locations. Vet Parasitol 2001;95(2–4):273–82.
35. Villalobos EM, Furman KE, Lara Mdo C, et al. Detection of *Neospora* sp. antibodies in cart horses from urban areas of Curitiba, Southern Brazil. Rev Bras Parasitol Vet 2012;21(1):68–70.
36. Dangoudoubiyam S, Oliveira JB, Viquez C, et al. Detection of antibodies against *Sarcocystis neurona, Neospora* spp., and *Toxoplasma gondii* in horses from Costa Rica. J Parasitol 2011;97(3):522–4.

37. Gupta GD, Lakritz J, Kim JH, et al. Seroprevalence of *Neospora, Toxoplasma gondii* and *Sarcocystis neurona* antibodies in horses from Jeju island, South Korea. Vet Parasitol 2002;106(3):193–201.

38. Hoane JS, Gennari SM, Dubey JP, et al. Prevalence of *Sarcocystis neurona* and *Neospora* spp. infection in horses from Brazil based on presence of serum antibodies to parasite surface antigen. Vet Parasitol 2006;136(2):155–9.

39. Hoane JS, Yeargan MR, Stamper S, et al. Recombinant NhSAG1 ELISA: a sensitive and specific assay for detecting antibodies against *Neospora hughesi* in equine serum. J Parasitol 2005;91(2):446–52.

40. NAHMS. Equine protozoal myeloencephalitis (EPM) in the U.S. USDA: APHIS:VS, Centers for Epidemiology and Animal Health, National Animal Health Monitoring System. Fort Collins, CO; 2001.

41. MacKay RJ, Davis SW, Dubey JP. Equine protozoal myeloencephalitis. Compend Contin Educ Pract Vet 1992;14(10):1359–67.

42. Fenger CK, Granstrom DE, Langemeier JL, et al. Epizootic of equine protozoal myeloencephalitis on a farm. J Am Vet Med Assoc 1997;210(7):923–7.

43. Granstrom DE, Alvarez O Jr, Dubey JP, et al. Equine protozoal myelitis in Panamanian horses and isolation of *Sarcocystis neurona*. J Parasitol 1992;78(5): 909–12.

44. Saville WJ, Reed SM, Morley PS, et al. Analysis of risk factors for the development of equine protozoal myeloencephalitis in horses. J Am Vet Med Assoc 2000;217(8):1174–80.

45. Saville WJ, Morley PS, Reed SM, et al. Evaluation of risk factors associated with clinical improvement and survival of horses with equine protozoal myeloencephalitis. J Am Vet Med Assoc 2000;217(8):1181–5.

46. Saville WJ, Stich RW, Reed SM, et al. Utilization of stress in the development of an equine model for equine protozoal myeloencephalitis. Vet Parasitol 2001; 95(2–4):211–22.

47. Sofaly CD, Reed SM, Gordon JC, et al. Experimental induction of equine protozoan myeloencephalitis (EPM) in the horse: effect of *Sarcocystis neurona* sporocyst inoculation dose on the development of clinical neurologic disease. J Parasitol 2002;88(6):1164–70.

48. Cutler TJ, MacKay RJ, Ginn PE, et al. Immunoconversion against *Sarcocystis neurona* in normal and dexamethasone-treated horses challenged with *S. neurona* sporocysts. Vet Parasitol 2001;95(2–4):197–210.

49. Saville WJ, Sofaly CD, Reed SM, et al. An equine protozoal myeloencephalitis challenge model testing a second transport after inoculation with *Sarcocystis neurona* sporocysts. J Parasitol 2004;90(6):1406–10.

50. Asmundsson IM, Dubey JP, Rosenthal BM. A genetically diverse but distinct North American population of *Sarcocystis neurona* includes an overrepresented clone described by 12 microsatellite alleles. Infect Genet Evol 2006;6(5):352–60.

51. Elsheikha HM, Schott HC 2nd, Mansfield LS. Genetic variation among isolates of *Sarcocystis neurona*, the agent of protozoal myeloencephalitis, as revealed by amplified fragment length polymorphism markers. Infect Immun 2006;74(6): 3448–54.

52. Howe DK, Gaji RY, Marsh AE, et al. Strains of *Sarcocystis neurona* exhibit differences in their surface antigens, including the absence of the major surface antigen SnSAG1. Int J Parasitol 2008;38(6):623–31.

53. Wendte JM, Miller MA, Lambourn DM, et al. Self-mating in the definitive host potentiates clonal outbreaks of the apicomplexan parasites Sarcocystis neurona and Toxoplasma gondii. PLoS Genet 2010;6(12):e1001261.

54. Dubey JP, Lindsay DS. Isolation in immunodeficient mice of *Sarcocystis neurona* from opossum (*Didelphis virginiana*) faeces, and its differentiation from *Sarcocystis falcatula*. Int J Parasitol 1998;28(12):1823–8.
55. Marsh AE, Barr BC, Lakritz J, et al. Experimental infection of nude mice as a model for *Sarcocystis neurona*-associated encephalitis. Parasitol Res 1997;83(7):706–11.
56. Witonsky SG, Gogal RM Jr, Duncan RB Jr, et al. Prevention of meningo/encephalomyelitis due to *Sarcocystis neurona* infection in mice is mediated by CD8 cells. Int J Parasitol 2005;35(1):113–23.
57. Sellon DC, Knowles DP, Greiner EC, et al. Depletion of natural killer cells does not result in neurologic disease due to *Sarcocystis neurona* in mice with severe combined immunodeficiency. J Parasitol 2004;90(4):782–8.
58. Sellon DC, Knowles DP, Greiner EC, et al. Infection of immunodeficient horses with *Sarcocystis neurona* does not result in neurologic disease. Clin Diagn Lab Immunol 2004;11(6):1134–9.
59. Fenger CK, Granstrom DE, Gajadhar AA, et al. Experimental induction of equine protozoal myeloencephalitis in horses using *Sarcocystis* sp. sporocysts from the opossum (*Didelphis virginiana*). Vet Parasitol 1997;68(3):199–213.
60. Tanhauser SM, Yowell CA, Cutler TJ, et al. Multiple DNA markers differentiate *Sarcocystis neurona* and *Sarcocystis falcatula*. J Parasitol 1999;85(2):221–8.
61. Ellison SP, Greiner E, Brown KK, et al. Experimental infection of horses with culture-derived *Sarcocystis neurona* merozoites as a model for equine protozoal myeloencephalitis. Int J Appl Res Vet Med 2004;2(2):79–89.
62. Dunigan CE, Oglesbee MJ, Podell M, et al. Seizure activity associated with equine protozoal myeloencephalitis. Progr Vet Neurol 1995;6(2):50–4.
63. Reed SM, Granstrom DE. Equine protozoal encephalomyelitis. Paper presented at: 11th Annual Veterinary Medical Forum of the American College of Veterinary Internal Medicine. Washington, DC. May 22, 1993.
64. Mayhew IG, deLahunta A, Whitlock RH, et al. Spinal cord disease in the horse. Cornell Vet 1978;68(Suppl 6):1–207.
65. Hamir AN, Moser G, Galligan DT, et al. Immunohistochemical study to demonstrate *Sarcocystis neurona* in equine protozoal myeloencephalitis. J Vet Diagn Invest 1993;5(3):418–22.
66. Furr M. Antigen-specific antibodies in cerebrospinal fluid after intramuscular injection of ovalbumin in horses. J Vet Intern Med 2002;16(5):588–92.
67. Furr M, Howe D, Reed S, et al. Antibody coefficients for the diagnosis of equine protozoal myeloencephalitis. J Vet Intern Med 2011;25(1):138–42.
68. Johnson AL, Morrow JK, Sweeney RW. Indirect fluorescent antibody test and surface antigen ELISAs for antemortem diagnosis of equine protozoal myeloencephalitis. J Vet Intern Med 2013;27(3):596–9.
69. Reed SM, Howe DK, Morrow JK, et al. Accurate antemortem diagnosis of equine protozoal myeloencephalitis (EPM) based on detecting intrathecal antibodies against *Sarcocystis neurona* using the SnSAG2 and SnSAG4/3 ELISAs. J Vet Intern Med 2013;27(5):1193–200.
70. Ellison SP, Kennedy T, Brown KK. Development of an ELISA to detect antibodies to rSAG1 in the horse. J Appl Res Vet Med 2003;1(4):318–27.
71. Hoane JS, Morrow J, Saville WJ, et al. Enzyme-linked immunosorbent assays for detection of equine antibodies specific to *Sarcocystis neurona* surface antigens. Clin Diagn Lab Immunol 2005;12(9):1050–6.
72. Yeargan MR, Howe DK. Improved detection of equine antibodies against *Sarcocystis neurona* using polyvalent ELISAs based on the parasite SnSAG surface antigens. Vet Parasitol 2011;176(1):16–22.

73. Ellison SP, Omara-Opyene AL, Yowell CA, et al. Molecular characterisation of a major 29 kDa surface antigen of *Sarcocystis neurona*. Int J Parasitol 2002;32(2): 217–25.

74. Howe DK, Gaji RY, Mroz-Barrett M, et al. *Sarcocystis neurona* merozoites express a family of immunogenic surface antigens that are orthologues of the *Toxoplasma gondii* surface antigens (SAGs) and SAG-related sequences. Infect Immun 2005;73(2):1023–33.

75. Marsh AE, Howe DK, Wang G, et al. Differentiation of *Neospora hughesi* from *Neospora caninum* based on their immunodominant surface antigen, SAG1 and SRS2. Int J Parasitol 1999;29(10):1575–82.

76. Johnson AL, Burton AJ, Sweeney RW. Utility of 2 immunological tests for antemortem diagnosis of equine protozoal myeloencephalitis (*Sarcocystis neurona* infection) in naturally occurring cases. J Vet Intern Med 2010;24(5):1184–9.

77. Duarte PC, Daft BM, Conrad PA, et al. Comparison of serum indirect fluorescent antibody test with two Western blot tests for the diagnosis of equine protozoal myeloencephalitis. J Vet Diagn Invest 2003;15(1):8–13.

78. Duarte PC, Daft BM, Conrad PA, et al. Evaluation and comparison of an indirect fluorescent antibody test for detection of antibodies to *Sarcocystis neurona*, using serum and cerebrospinal fluid of naturally and experimentally infected, and vaccinated horses. J Parasitol 2004;90(2):379–86.

79. Bogan JA, Galbraith A, Baxter P, et al. Effect of feeding on the fate of orally administered phenylbutazone, trimethoprim and sulphadiazine in the horse. Vet Rec 1984;115(23):599–600.

80. Clarke CR, MacAllister CG, Burrows GE, et al. Pharmacokinetics, penetration into cerebrospinal fluid, and hematologic effects after multiple oral administrations of pyrimethamine to horses. Am J Vet Res 1992;53(12):2296–9.

81. Cavallito JC, Nichol CA, Brenckman WD Jr, et al. Lipid-soluble inhibitors of dihydrofolate reductase. I. Kinetics, tissue distribution, and extent of metabolism of pyrimethamine, metoprine, and etoprine in the rat, dog, and man. Drug Metab Dispos 1978;6(3):329–37.

82. Brown CM, Morrow JK, Carleton CL, et al. Persistence of serum antibodies to *Sarcocystis neurona* in horses moved from North America to India. J Vet Intern Med 2006;20(4):994–7.

83. Green SL, Mayhew IG, Brown MP, et al. Concentrations of trimethoprim and sulfamethoxazole in cerebrospinal fluid and serum in mares with and without a dimethyl sulfoxide pretreatment. Can J Vet Res 1990;54(2):215–22.

84. Chung MK, Han SS, Roh JK. Synergistic embryotoxicity of combination pyrimethamine and folic acid in rats. Reprod Toxicol 1993;7(5):463–8.

85. Toribio RE, Bain FT, Mrad DR, et al. Congenital defects in newborn foals of mares treated for equine protozoal myeloencephalitis during pregnancy. J Am Vet Med Assoc 1998;212(5):697–701.

86. Castles TR, Kintner LD, Lee CC. The effects of folic or folinic acid on the toxicity of pyrimethamine in dogs. Toxicol Appl Pharmacol 1971;20(4):447–59.

87. Hackstein JH, Mackenstedt U, Mehlhorn H, et al. Parasitic apicomplexans harbor a chlorophyll a-D1 complex, the potential target for therapeutic triazines. Parasitol Res 1995;81(3):207–16.

88. Lindsay DS, Dubey JP. Determination of the activity of diclazuril against *Sarcocystis neurona* and *Sarcocystis falcatula* in cell cultures. J Parasitol 2000;86(1): 164–6.

89. Lindsay DS, Dubey JP, Kennedy TJ. Determination of the activity of ponazuril against *Sarcocystis neurona* in cell cultures. Vet Parasitol 2000;92(2):165–9.

90. Dirikolu L, Lehner F, Nattrass C, et al. Diclazuril in the horse: its identification and detection and preliminary pharmacokinetics. J Vet Pharmacol Ther 1999;22(6): 374–9.
91. Furr M, Kennedy T. Cerebrospinal fluid and serum concentrations of ponazuril in horses. Vet Ther 2001;2(3):232–7.
92. Reed SM, Wendel M, King S, et al. Pharmacokinetics of ponazuril in horses. Paper presented at: 58th Annual Convention of the American Association of Equine Practitioners. Anaheim (CA), December 1–5, 2012.

Equine Piroplasmosis

L. Nicki Wise, DVM, MS[a],*, Angela M. Pelzel-McCluskey, DVM[b],
Robert H. Mealey, DVM, PhD[c], Donald P. Knowles, DVM, PhD[d]

KEYWORDS

- *Theileria equi* • *Babesia caballi* • Erythrocytic parasite • Tick-borne disease
- Anemia

KEY POINTS

- The disease equine piroplasmosis is caused by tick-transmitted, intraerythrocytic parasites *Theileria equi* and *Babesia caballi*.
- Clinical signs of acute infection generally include those related to intravascular hemolysis and thrombocytopenia. All infected animals that survive become subclinical carriers and are reservoirs for transmission.
- The United States and Canada are considered nonendemic for equine piroplasmosis, yet recent outbreaks in the United States have elucidated challenges with control and prevention.
- Control of infection and disease in nonendemic areas is provided by import surveillance and can only be completed by a certified laboratory.
- Alleviation of clinical symptoms and clearance of the parasite can be accomplished with imidocarb diproprionate.

INTRODUCTION

Equine piroplasmosis is an infectious, tick-borne disease caused by the hemoprotozoan parasites *Theileria* (previously *Babesia*) *equi* and *Babesia caballi*. Piroplasmosis affects all wild and domestic equids and clinical presentation is related to intravascular hemolysis and associated systemic illness. Infection with either parasite can lead to a

Funding: USDA ARS CRIS # 5348-32000-034-00D (Drs L.N. Wise and D.P. Knowles); United States Department of Agriculture-National Institute of Food and Agriculture-Agriculture and Food Research Initiative Grant Number 2013-01149.
Conflicts of Interest: None.
[a] Department of Large Animal Medicine and Surgery, St. George's University, USDA ARS ADRU, True Blue PO Box 7, St. George's, Grenada, West Indies; [b] Surveillance, Preparedness, and Response Services, USDA APHIS Veterinary Services, 2150 Centre Avenue, Building B, Mailstop 3E113, Fort Collins, CO 80526, USA; [c] Department of Veterinary Microbiology and Pathology, College of Veterinary Medicine, Washington State University, PO Box 647040, Pullman, WA 99164–7040, USA; [d] Department of Veterinary Microbiology and Pathology, USDA ARS ADRU, Washington State University, PO Box 46630, Pullman, WA 99164, USA
* Corresponding author.
E-mail address: lwise1@sgu.edu

similar clinical presentation yet *T equi* and *B caballi* are distinct in terms of disease severity, life cycle, infection dynamics, persistence in the horse, and drug susceptibility. Although most horses recover from the initial phase of the disease, infection can be fatal. Horses that survive acute disease inevitably become inapparent carriers and exhibit no clinical signs of infection yet can serve as reservoirs for transmission to naive horses.[1] Carriers represent challenges in diagnosis, eradication, and control measures. The parasites and their natural tick vectors are endemic to most countries with tropical and subtropical climates yet the United States and Canada, and a small number of other nations, are considered "free" or nonendemic.[2,3] Goals of infection and disease control vary tremendously between endemic and nonendemic nations, and as demonstrated by the "silent" re-emergence of *T equi* in 2009 on a ranch in Texas, endeavors to control transmission especially in areas that wish to remain nonendemic must continue.[4]

ETIOLOGY

Theileria equi and *B caballi* are obligate intraerythrocytic apicomplexan parasites that infect only equids. Taxonomy of the causative agents of piroplasmosis has been in question since their discovery and remains controversial for *T equi*.[5,6] It was recognized in 1998 that *T equi* did not fit into "babesia" taxonomy given its size and an extra-erythrocytic stage within equine peripheral blood mononuclear cells (PBMCs). Molecular phylogenetic investigations and recent genomic analyses support both babesia and theileria lineages, possibly placing it between the two, perhaps in a new genus.

The recent analysis of the genome for the laboratory or "Florida" strain of *T equi*, which was isolated in the 1970s, has also allowed more detailed insight into the parasite's molecular pathways and genetic structure.[5] These genomic data and additional research further confirmed the assumption that geographic isolates of *T equi* can genetically differ greatly from one another.[7] Globally, it is recognized that *T equi* causes more disease in some areas than others. For example, *T equi* is recognized as a common reason for a horse to be admitted to an equine intensive care unit in South Africa, whereas only mild clinical disease was reported in one horse during the US outbreak that affected more than 400 horses.[4,8] Genomic differences have not yet been correlated with virulence. Recently, a *T equi* variant was isolated from a Mexican-origin stray horse intercepted in south Texas and data collected thus far indicate that the parasite is genetically distinct from the *T equi* found in the Texas outbreak, being much more closely related to parasites identified in South African horses and zebras.[7] The impact this information will have on diagnostic testing, therapeutics, and vaccine development is currently under investigation.

Transmission of infection can occur via an infected tick or through iatrogenic blood transfer. The precise tick-vector-parasite-host requirements for infection or clinical disease are not fully understood. Clinically inapparent infection can occur and data indicate that the risk of life-threatening clinical disease increases with the presence of factors, such as immunologic naivety and increased density of infected ticks and horses.[9] Ticks competent for transmission are biologic vectors and therefore incredibly efficient. Competent tick vectors are found in almost all climates globally. Only hard ticks, or ixodid ticks, are capable of transmitting *T equi* and *B caballi* naturally, and in North America, there are five species of ticks that are known to act as competent vectors (**Box 1**).[1,10–14] Other species have been implicated as potential vectors, but confirmation requires additional research.

> **Box 1**
> **Ticks capable of naturally transmitting equine piroplasmosis in North America**
>
> *Theileria equi*
>
> *Dermacentor variabilis*: American dog tick
>
> *Boophilus (Rhiphicephalus) microplus*: Cattle tick
>
> *Amblyomma cajennense*: Cayenne tick
>
> *Babesia caballi*
>
> *Dermacentor nitens*: Tropical horse tick
>
> *Dermacentor albipictus*: Winter or moose tick

The life cycle of a tick includes four stages (egg, larva, nymph, and adult) and transmission of the parasites can occur in three distinct forms: (1) intrastadially, (2) transtadially, or (3) transovarially (**Fig. 1**). Although the specific transmission events for *T equi* and *B caballi* vary from one tick species to another, it is of utmost importance to recognize that because of transovarial transmission of *B caballi*, infected ticks can act as reservoirs of infection within a population.[15] The presence of competent tick vectors and infected horses within the same area does not always lead to further infection or disease. Many factors must be considered including season, climate, host specificity, and the particulars of the competent tick's life cycle.

Recent discoveries support that species of ticks in North America, previously unidentified as vectors, are likely involved in transmission. Tick surveillance that occurred during the *T equi* outbreak in Texas allowed identification of two novel vectors, *Amblyomma cajennense* and *Dermacentor varibilis*, capable of transmitting *T equi*.[12] *A cajennense* is present in the Southern most parts of Texas and Mexico and is a vector of *T equi*. *D variabilis* has a much more widespread distribution within North America yet its prevalence and efficiency as a natural vector of *T equi* remain undefined.

Both parasites can be efficiently iatrogenically transmitted. This can occur during transfusions of infected blood to naive horses, as was the case in a recent Florida outbreak where blood doping (prerace blood transfusions) practices were being used commonly before unsanctioned racing events.[16] Likewise, infections can be accidental when using an untested, inapparent carrier as a blood donor. Transfer of the parasites can also occur through the use of any blood-contaminated equipment, such as needles or dental tools. There is no evidence that infection can be transmitted during routine breeding practices.

In utero transmission of both parasites has been reported, but the specific mechanisms for this process and its prevalence remain unclear.[17–19] Abortions and stillbirths have been reported commonly in some areas of Africa. Foals can be born infected and may develop severe disease within a few days after parturition.[20,21] Not all infected mares transmit the parasite to their offspring as evidenced by the data collected from the outbreak on the Texas ranch where no transplacental transmissions were detected by comparing foal and mare blood by serial polymerase chain reaction (PCR).

EPIDEMIOLOGY

Piroplasmosis is a globally significant disease and is considered endemic in most countries worldwide that have an equine population plus competent tick vectors.[22]

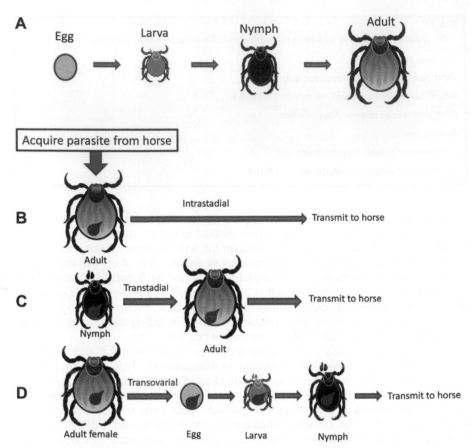

Fig. 1. Tick life stages and tick transmission forms. (*A*) The four life stages. (*B*) Intrastadial transmission, when acquisition and transmission of the parasite occurs entirely within one life stage. (*C*) Transtadial transmission, where acquisition occurs in one stage and the same tick to transmit the infection during subsequent life stages. (*D*) Transovarial transmission, when the female acquires parasites that enter ovaries and are transmitted to offspring, allowing maintenance of the parasites across tick generations.

These ticks are found in tropical, subtropical, and some temperate climates. In general, *T equi* is more prevalent that *B caballi* but surveillance to specifically compare the prevalence of these parasites worldwide has not been performed. The global distribution of the parasites follows that of the ticks with *B caballi* being identified in more temperate climates than *T equi*.[3] Numerous studies have been published regarding epidemiology and distribution of these parasites within equid populations of specific countries and regions. In general, these publications should be interpreted with caution given the profound variation in experimental design, sample population, and detection methods used.

According to the Office International des Epizooties/The World Organization for Animal Health (OIE), most of the equid-inhabited regions of the world are considered endemic for infection and disease.[23] Cases are reported consistently from Central and South America (with the exception of the Southern regions of Chile and Argentina), Cuba, Southern Europe, Asia, and Africa. Infection prevalence in the Caribbean is ill defined but disease has been reported on several islands including Trinidad. Presently, countries are not required to report all infected horses to the OIE meaning that there are several countries and regions where an accurate and current status is unclear because of lack of reporting. The import and export regulations and testing requirements differ for each country making standardized surveillance of global piroplasmosis and confirmation of nonendemic regions difficult. **Fig. 2** depicts a general overview of current global equine piroplasmosis disease distribution. The most current disease status for all reporting countries can be found on the OIE Web site (www.OIE.int).

In general, Canada is considered nonendemic with only sporadic reports of infections. Mexico does not report cases routinely to the OIE, yet literature published in that region indicates that the disease is endemic at least in some areas of the country.[24] Horses presented for import from Mexico and Mexican-origin stray horses identified at the US- Mexico border often test positive for *T equi* and/or *B caballi*. Although detection of infection within the United States in recent years has placed its "piroplasmosis free" status under scrutiny, intensive active surveillance for piroplasmosis since 2009 has confirmed that the United States is nonendemic. An extensive surveillance program to eliminate piroplasmosis from a previously endemic region in South Florida identified in the 1960s resulted in declaration of the United States "free" status in 1988. To maintain this status, US Department of Agriculture Animal and Plant Health Inspection Service (USDA APHIS) improved restrictions on importation of horses from endemic areas. Consequently, only sporadic cases (generally a result of illegal importation) were identified until 2008. In 2008, 20 *T equi*–infected horses were identified on seven epidemiologically linked premises in Florida. All affected horses were associated with horses imported from Mexico and all were engaged in unsanctioned horse racing.[16] Inappropriate management practices including needle sharing and blood doping were the most likely modes of transmission. No tick vectors were identified despite aggressive surveillance.

In 2009, an outbreak of *T equi* was identified on a ranch in southern Texas involving approximately 400 horses.[4] All infected horses resided on the premises or had been at some time associated with the ranch. Importantly, tick transmission was found to be responsible for this outbreak. Intense surveillance of the US horse population has thus far resulted in the testing of more than 245,000 horses with only 219 being positive for either *T equi* (209) or *B caballi* (10). The 219 cases were unrelated to the Texas ranch outbreak and involve only two distinct high-risk populations of horses: sanctioned racehorses (mostly Quarter Horses) with epidemiologic links to unsanctioned racing and horses imported to the United States before 2005 when the complement fixation test (CFT) was the official import test. Positive horses in the United States are quarantined and are either (1) enrolled in an approved treatment program to eliminate infection and transmission risk, (2) maintained under life-long quarantine, or (3) euthanized. Surveillance of horses within the United States, especially in Texas and in horses involved in sanctioned racing, continues to ensure containment of the infection.

PATHOGENESIS AND IMMUNITY

The life cycles of *B caballi* and *T equi* involve distinct phases that occur in the horse and tick, the details of which vary depending on the species of tick (**Fig. 3**).[25,26] Regardless, both parasites progress through three life stages: (1) sporozoite, (2) merozoite, and (3) gamete. Infectious sporozoites are transmitted through the tick saliva to the equid host. As **Fig. 3** indicates, the sporozoite pathway once inside the horse varies between *B caballi* and *T equi*. *B caballi* sporozoites directly invade erythrocytes where they develop first into trophozoites and then into merozoites. Merozoites asexually reproduce leading to erythrocyte rupture, which then allows the merozoites to be

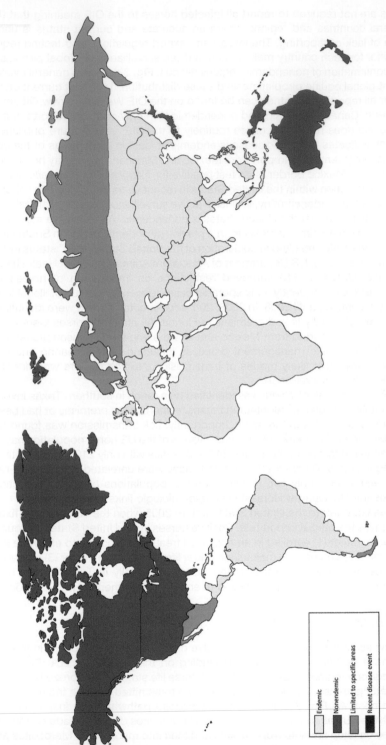

Fig. 2. General representation of the global distribution of equine piroplasmosis.

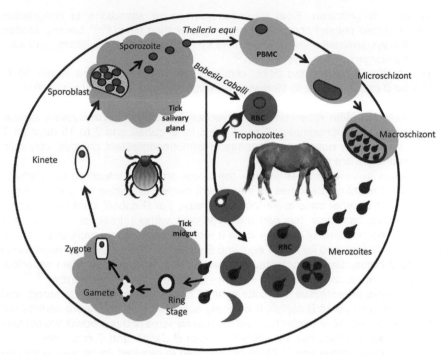

Fig. 3. Life cycle of *Babesia caballi* and *Theileria equi* during tick transmission. RBC, red blood cells.

released into the circulation to invade other erythrocytes. *T equi*'s initial invasion is different in that sporozoites first enter PBMCs. Recent in vitro data indicate that *T equi* sporozoites can invade T and B lymphocytes, and monocytes and macrophages.[27] Inside PBMCs, *T equi* sporozoites develop into large schizonts and then merozoites, which are released to invade erythrocytes. There is no evidence that PBMCs continue to be used after establishment of the intraerythrocytic phase of infection. Continued asexual reproduction results in an escalating population of merozoites and parasitized erythrocytes. Some merozoites develop into gamete forms within peripheral blood. On ingestion of merozoites (and/or gametes) by a tick, the parasites undergo sexual reproduction, with gametes combining to form zygotes within the tick midgut. Continued development results in sporoblasts within the salivary gland of the tick and production of infective sporozoites within tick saliva.[28,29] Data suggest that the merozoite is the persistent life stage present in inapparent infections of *T equi* and *B caballi*, although the exact role of PBMCs remains unclear, especially in *T equi*. With iatrogenic transmission, merozoites present in the infected horse blood are transferred to the blood of the naive host where they invade new erythrocytes and begin asexual replication. The mechanisms involved during in utero transmission are unknown but most likely result in transfer of merozoites from the dam to the fetus.

Although some specifics of disease pathogenesis remain unknown, infection with either *T equi* or *B caballi* causes erythrocyte lysis resulting in varying degrees of hemolytic anemia. Intravascular hemolytic anemia ensues upon the physical rupture of erythrocytes during the release of merozoites. The anemia is exacerbated by the removal of infected erythrocytes by splenic macrophages (extravascular). Nonparasitized erythrocytes are also removed from circulation but the cause for this phenomenon is unknown. Both parasites can cause alterations in coagulation including reduced platelet counts and prolonged clotting times.[30,31] Severe disease can result in systemic inflammatory response syndrome, hypercoagulability, and subsequent multiorgan system dysfunction.[32]

After infestation by infected ticks, clinical signs typically develop within 10 to 30 days for B caballi and 12 to 19 days for T equi. The time to clinical signs after iatrogenic transmission likely depends on parasite dose, immune status of the horse, and route of infection. With experimental intravenous inoculation of merozoites, clinical signs can occur in approximately 5 to 16 days for B caballi and 7 to 15 days for T equi.[2] Often with low doses of merozoites in immunocompetent animals, very mild or no clinical signs are noted.

In all cases in which horses survive the acute phase of infection, the parasite persists and the animal becomes an inapparent carrier, exhibiting no obvious signs of infection. The carrier state is life-long for T equi. For B caballi, data indicate that infected horses can clear the parasite over time without treatment.[2,3] Although defining the mechanisms of persistence is a focus of ongoing research, one mechanism commonly assumed for both T equi and B caballi is physical sequestration within the infected horse. Several potential sequestration locations have been reported, including capillaries, central nervous system vasculature, and bone marrow.[33–35]

The correlates of protective immunity against T equi are not fully understood, and even less is known about B caballi. It is widely accepted that inapparent carriers are protected from disease or reinfection, but the mechanisms of this process are not fully defined. Because horses can be coinfected with B caballi and T equi, there is no evidence for cross-protection.[34] Although a spleen is required for horses to survive infection with T equi, infection of splenectomized horses with B caballi may or may not result in terminal disease.[36–38] Regardless, an intact spleen and functioning innate immune system is not adequate to confer protection against T equi infection. Foals with severe combined immunodeficiency (SCID) lack functional B and T lymphocytes, and therefore lack the ability to mount antigen-specific immune responses.[39] Experimental infection of SCID foals with T equi invariably results in fulminant infection and terminal disease.[40] Therefore, adaptive immune responses are required to control T equi parasitemia but are not required for lysis of erythrocytes. B caballi infection of SCID foals has not been documented.

Theileria equi–infected horses produce high titered antibody responses that are associated with control of parasitemia.[41] Antibodies are produced against immunodominant merozoite proteins termed equi merozoite antigens (EMAs), which are surface expressed on merozoites. Horses seroconvert within 7 to 11 days after natural infection and levels peak at 30 to 45 days. The exact role of antibody responses in immunity and persistence remains unclear.

Even less is known about the immune responses against B caballi infection. Infected horses produce antibodies to the apical merozoite protein rhoptry associated protein (RAP) 1, which is used in serologic diagnosis of infection.[42] Additional research is needed to define the protective roles of antibody and cellular adaptive immune responses against both parasites.

CLINICAL SIGNS

Clinical disease can manifest in several different forms as summarized in **Table 1**. In general, infection with T equi results in more severe clinical disease than B caballi and as previously discussed, the signs and severity can vary significantly from one region to another.[34]

Table 1
Clinical presentation and diagnosis of equine piroplasmosis

	Acute *Theileria equi*	Chronic *Theileria equi*	Carrier *Theileria equi*	Acute *Babesia caballi*	Chronic/Carrier *Babesia caballi*
Clinical signs, physical examination findings	Fever, lethargy, petechiations, edema → pale mucous membranes, icterus, pigmenturia	Nonspecific signs of chronic infection, splenomegaly	None	Fever, lethargy, petechiations, edema → pale mucous membranes, icterus, pigmenturia	None
Clinical path	Anemia Thrombocytopenia	+/− Mild anemia	None	Anemia Thrombocytopenia	None
Blood smear	Smaller, pyriform bodies (maltese cross) measuring 2–3 μm	No parasites	No parasites	Larger, pyriform bodies, measuring 2–5 μm	No parasites
Parasitemia (%)	1–5	0	0	1–0.1	0
Preferred diagnostic test	Blood smear IFA CFT	cELISA IFA	cELISA IFA	Blood smear IFA CFT	cELISA WB

Abbreviations: cELISA, competitive enzyme-linked immunosorbent assay; CFT, complement fixation test; IFA, immunofluorescent antibody test; WB, Western blot.

Acute infection initially presents with nonspecific signs of a high fever, lethargy, anorexia, peripheral edema, and petechiations of the mucous membranes. As the infection progresses, the horse may exhibit signs of hemolysis including icteric or pale mucous membranes, tachycardia, tachypnea, weakness, and pigmenturia.[43] Other systemic complications may arise as other body systems are impacted including the gastrointestinal tract (colic, diarrhea), respiratory system (pulmonary edema, pneumonia), renal system (pigment nephropathy), and central nervous system (ataxia, myalgia, seizures).[44] With *T equi* infection, severe clinical signs and fatalities are most commonly related to hemolysis and anemia. Rare cases of acute death from *B caballi* infection are reportedly a result of multiple organ dysfunction related to systemic formation of microthrombi and disseminated intravascular coagulation.

Peracute disease, characterized by fulminant onset of signs with or without collapse and sudden death, has been documented. Although uncommon, this has been reported to occur on introduction of naive horses into a *T equi*–endemic region, or can be diagnosed in neonatal foals infected in utero.[9,20,21] These foals may exhibit clinical signs at birth or become ill at 2 to 3 days of age. Clinical signs are often nonspecific, such as weakness and decreased suckling, but progress to resemble those of an infected adult.

Chronic *T equi* or *B caballi* infection may result in nonspecific signs of chronic inflammation or infection including lethargy, partial anorexia, weight loss, poor hair coat, and poor performance. Mild anemia may be present and the spleen might be enlarged on rectal palpation.[2,45]

The most common clinical presentation of horses infected with either *T equi* or *B caballi* in both endemic and nonendemic regions is that of the inapparent carrier with no obvious signs of disease. Because inapparent carriers serve as reservoirs for transmission by a variety of routes, these horses represent the greatest challenge to nonendemic nations attempting to remain free of those parasites. Inapparent *T equi* carriers have exhibited relapses of clinical disease associated with stress, strenuous exercise, immunosuppression, and steroid administration.[46,47] Similar relapses have not been reported for *B caballi*.

DIAGNOSIS

Routine laboratory analyses may aid in confirming clinical findings. Most horses regardless of clinical syndrome exhibit some degree of anemia characterized by decreased packed cell volume, hemoglobin, and erythrocyte count. Although acutely infected horses can have profound anemia with a packed cell volume as low as 10%, the packed cell volume rarely decreases lower than 20%.[43,45,48] Thrombocytopenia is common and clotting times can be prolonged or normal.[43] The leukogram and fibrinogen levels can vary depending on infection stage and severity.[49] Hyperbilirubinemia is often observed and the liver enzymes, alkaline phosphatase, aspartate aminotransferase, and γ-glutamyl transferase can be elevated.[43] Infected erythrocytes can be identified in sternal bone marrow aspirates of asymptomatic horses but the use of this test as a diagnostic tool is limited.[35] Gross and histopathologic findings at necropsy vary depending on the severity of disease and associated systemic complications.[44]

Definitive diagnosis of infection is most often accomplished with serologic testing performed at a certified laboratory under the guidance of the regulatory officials involved. In North America, these diagnoses are most often made during surveillance and import/export testing. Various diagnostic modalities are available and can be used alone or in combination to diagnose infection. Management of suspect and confirmed infected horses in nonendemic countries, such as Canada and the United States, requires involvement of the appropriate regulatory agencies so that the confirmatory diagnostic methods and immediate infection control strategies (ie, quarantine) can be applied.

Light microscopy can be used to identify the organisms within the erythrocytes during the acute stage of infection (see **Table 1**). A thin blood smear can reveal organisms, but smears must be thoroughly examined because even during severe infection, the percent parasitemia remains quite low. In cases of chronic or inapparent infection, parasite numbers are too low for reliable detection on blood smears.

Several serologic tests were developed to increase diagnostic sensitivity especially in those carrier horses exhibiting no clinical signs. These tests include the complement fixation test (CFT), indirect immunofluorescence assay (IFA), Western blot (WB), and competitive enzyme-linked immunosorbent assay (cELISA).

The CFT depends on activation of complement during specific interaction of antibody and antigen. Infected horses seroconvert on the CFT approximately 8 to 11 days after infection with titers beginning to decline at 2 to 3 months.[46–48,50] The CFT is a very specific test yet lacks sensitivity in chronic or inapparent phases of infection mainly because some antibodies produced during these phases of infection do not fix complement.[41,51,52] Cross-reactivity between *T equi* and *B caballi* antibodies when using the CFT has been documented.[53] The CFT should only be used in acute cases of infection; results in a nonclinical carrier should be interpreted with caution.

The IFAT is considered to be more sensitive than the CFT during chronic infection.[50] However, the need to dilute serum to improve specificity in IFAT performance reduces sensitivity. Experimentally infected *T equi* and *B caballi* horses are positive on the IFAT at 3 to 20 days postinfection.[54] The IFAT is often used as an adjunct test to aid in analysis of CFT and cELISA results, and it remains one of the prescribed tests for equine piroplasmosis recommended by the OIE.[23]

The cELISA, the other regulatory test approved by the OIE for international horse transport, is considered to be the most sensitive test for chronic or inapparent *T equi* infection. The cELISA, which detects antibody responses to EMA 1 and 2, is validated for detection of antibodies against numerous isolates of *T equi* found globally.[51] The *B caballi* cELISA is also routinely used for detection of chronic infection or inapparent carriers.[42] The currently available *B caballi* cELISA relies on the recognition of epitopes on RAP-1 that are not conserved across all isolates. For this reason, the cELISA is unable to detect infected horses in South Africa because of differences between the recombinant RAP-1 used in the test and South African isolates of *B caballi*.[55] Both cELISA kits are marketed by VMRD (Pullman, WA) and are not available to general practitioners.

Diagnostics historically used only in a research setting have recently become a part of routine diagnosis and surveillance. A WB, or immunoblot test, is currently offered by the National Veterinary Services Laboratory in Ames, Iowa as an adjunct diagnostic tool for detection of *B caballi* infection. A WB test is also under validation to be used as a means of clearance confirmation in *T equi*–infected horses treated with imidocarb diproprionate (ID). PCR relies on the amplification and detection of parasite DNA isolated from the peripheral blood of an infected horse. It is an exquisitely sensitive test that when performed as a nested PCR can detect a positive result in an animal with *T equi* parasitemia as low as 0.000006%.[56] However, the genetic variation reported between isolates of *T equi* make the use of this test on a global scale challenging. The validity of the *T equi* EMA-based nested PCR used in the United States has been questioned in other countries like South Africa.[57] Given the variation in PCR methodology, isolate inconsistencies, and the inherent nature of the test, it is unlikely in the near future that PCR will be standardized and used commercially for detection of T equi or B caballi. Because of the sensitivity of PCR, it is currently being used as one of several tests to confirm clearance of T equi horses enrolled in the USDA treatment program.

The research conducted to validate the USDA treatment program has raised questions regarding positive cELISA results. Despite apparent clearance of T equi, as evidenced by serial negative PCR results and transmission studies, the cELISA can remain positive for up to 24 months in some horses.[4] The reason for the continued presence of antibodies in these horses despite removal of the parasite remains unclear, but it is well documented that nonspecific bystander activation of long-lived human memory B cells can result in measurable antibody production long after an infection has been eliminated.[58]

THERAPEUTIC STRATEGIES

The goals of treatment vary tremendously between nonendemic and endemic regions. In endemic countries, the goals of therapy are to reduce clinical signs and accelerate recovery from acute infection caused by either parasite. It is widely assumed that parasite persistence during an inapparent infection results in life-long protection from super-infection (ie, new infection in the face of current infection) and clinical disease. Therefore, clearing the parasite from such a horse in an endemic region would be detrimental to their long-term survival. The opposite is true in nonendemic areas wishing to remain free of T equi and B caballi (eg, the United States and Canada). To eliminate all transmission risk, treatment is directed at complete clearance of the parasite. Numerous drugs have reported efficacy against these parasites in vitro and in vivo. In general, it is reported that T equi infection is much more difficult to clear than B caballi, and that in some cases, B caballi infection may self-clear over time.

ID is considered to be the treatment of choice for alleviation of clinical signs and clearance of either parasite. The drug is administered intramuscularly, and although it is rapidly eliminated from the plasma, it remains at high concentrations in certain tissues of the body.[59] A dose in the range of 2.2 to 4.4 mg/kg intramuscularly, given once, is generally effective in elimination or reduction of clinical signs. Lower doses can be repeated if necessary every 24 to 72 hours for two to three treatments. To accomplish clearance of B caballi from an animal residing in a nonendemic area, a dose of 4.0 mg/kg intramuscularly every 72 hours for four doses is effective.[60] Data support that for T equi, the same dose achieves clearance in experimental and natural infections.[4,61] Of 25 naturally infected horses cleared with ID, one remained positive after initial treatment and required an additional round of treatment before attaining clearance.[4] If clearance is determined to be the best option for a T equi–infected horse in the United States, the owner and veterinarian must enroll the horse in the USDA treatment program to ensure that appropriate quarantine, preclearance and postclearance testing, and release occurs. Currently, clearance and subsequent release from quarantine are defined as serial negative PCR results and the inability to transmit the parasite to a naive splenectomized horse via blood transfusion, or negative results on required serologic testing. Studies are underway to more clearly define parasite elimination and determine the ideal testing regimen. The extent of ID efficacy for all isolates of T equi and B caballi is not known.

Horses undergoing treatment with ID should be monitored carefully for signs of drug reactions or toxicity.[62,63] ID has anticholinesterase activity resulting in adverse cholinergic effects including include agitation, sweating, colic, and diarrhea. Usually these transient signs occur immediately after administration of the drug and are rarely life-threatening. Atropine and glycopyrrolate have been used successfully to prevent these adverse signs, yet both of these relatively long-acting drugs can have detrimental anticholinergic side effects, such as ileus. Administration of the shorter-acting anticholinergic drug n-butylscopolamine (Buscopan; Boehringer Ingelheim, Animal Health GmbH, Ingelheim, Germany) at a dose of 0.3 mg/kg intravenously immediately before ID administration can lessen and often prevent the onset of ID-associated adverse cholinergic signs without causing prolonged ileus.[4] Local injection site swelling and muscle inflammation are common following ID administration. Injection sites should be rotated with each dose and the areas should be monitored carefully. ID undergoes hepatic and renal clearance so toxicity can result in damage to these body systems. Hepatic enzymes and the urinary γ-glutamyl transferase/creatinine ratio may become transiently elevated during the dosing regimen, but these levels usually return to normal after therapy is discontinued.[62,63] It is reported that donkeys and mules are more sensitive to ID toxicity, indicating its use in these species may be unpredictable and potentially fatal.[64] Information regarding the use of this drug in pregnant mares and neonatal foals is lacking.

Acutely infected horses often require supportive care including, but not limited to, intravenous fluids, nonsteroidal anti-inflammatory drugs, pain management, and blood transfusions. Adequate hydration is essential on initiation of and during treatment with imidocarb.

CONTROL STRATEGIES

Prevention and control strategies differ tremendously between endemic and nonendemic countries. Prevention is virtually impossible in endemic regions and naivety is not desired because infection provides a degree of protection. In nonendemic countries, the foundation of prevention is supervised import and testing of horses from endemic areas. The guidelines for movement of horses are variable depending on the country but for the United States and Canada, a negative result on specific serologic tests is required for entry. If infected horses are allowed in for sporting events, the horses are examined thoroughly and treated for ticks and then carefully monitored and quarantined appropriately. Federal and state regulatory officials are notified if a horse within the United States tests positive and appropriate measures are taken to ensure the protection of the US horse population.

Nonendemic nations that border endemic nations cannot completely prevent introduction of ticks so diligent measures must be taken to reduce horses' contact with ticks. Several studies have investigated the use of vaccines to induce protective immunity yet none have been found to be completely effective in preventing infection.[65]

SUMMARY

Equine piroplasmosis has a major effect on the horse industry around the world. This insidious disease can cause significant economic losses to endemic countries making it very advantageous for nonendemic countries to remain free. Enhanced control through surveillance of equine and vector populations is of paramount importance. As more data about these parasites emerge, the way in which infected horses are tested, treated, and regulated will continue to change in North America and globally.

REFERENCES

1. Ueti MW, Palmer GH, Scoles GA, et al. Persistently infected horses are reservoirs for intrastadial tick-borne transmission of the apicomplexan parasite *Babesia equi*. Infect Immun 2008;76:3525–9.
2. de Waal DT. Equine piroplasmosis: a review. Br Vet J 1992;148:6–14.
3. Friedhoff KT, Soule C. An account on equine babesioses. Rev Sci Tech 1996;15:1191–201.
4. Ueti MW, Mealey RH, Kappmeyer LS, et al. Re-emergence of the Apicomplexan *Theileria equi* in the United States: elimination of persistent infection and transmission risk. PLoS One 2012;7:e44713.
5. Kappmeyer LS, Thiagarajan M, Herndon DR, et al. Comparative genomic analysis and phylogenetic position of *Theileria equi*. BMC Genomics 2012;13:603.
6. Mehlhorn H, Schein E. Redescription of *Babesia equi* Laveran, 1901 as *Theileria equi* Mehlhorn, Schein 1998. Parasitol Res 1998;84:467–75.
7. Hall CM, Busch JD, Scoles GA, et al. Genetic characterization of *Theileria equi* infecting horses in North America: evidence for a limited source of U.S. introductions. Parasit Vectors 2013;6:35.
8. Viljoen A, Saulez MN, Donnellan CM, et al. After-hours equine emergency admissions at a University Referral Hospital (1998-2007): causes and interventions. J S Afr Vet Assoc 2009;80:169–73.
9. Basset J, Auger L. Piroplasmose vraie du cheval (*P. caballi*) dans le Sud-Est. Comp Rend Soc Biol 1931;107:629.
10. Wise LN, Kappmeyer LS, Mealey RH, et al. Review of equine piroplasmosis. J Vet Intern Med 2013;27:1334–46.
11. Stiller D, Coan ME. Recent developments in elucidating tick vector relationships for anaplasmosis and equine piroplasmosis. Vet Parasitol 1995;57:97–108.
12. Scoles GA, Hutcheson HJ, Schlater JL, et al. Equine piroplasmosis associated with *Amblyomma cajennense* ticks, Texas, USA. Emerg Infect Dis 2011;17:1903–5.
13. Roby TO, Anthony DW. Transmission of equine piroplasmosis by *Dermacentor nitens* Neumann. J Am Vet Med Assoc 1963;142:768–9.
14. Schwint ON, Knowles DP, Ueti MW, et al. Transmission of *Babesia caballi* by *Dermacentor nitens* (Acari: Ixodidae) is restricted to one generation in the absence of alimentary reinfection on a susceptible equine host. J Med Entomol 2008;45:1152–5.
15. De Waal DT. The transovarial transmission of *Babesia caballi* by *Hyalomma truncatum*. Onderstepoort J Vet Res 1990;57:99–100.
16. Short MA, Clark CK, Harvey JW, et al. Outbreak of equine piroplasmosis in Florida. J Am Vet Med Assoc 2012;240:588–95.
17. Allsopp MT, Lewis BD, Penzhorn BL. Molecular evidence for transplacental transmission of *Theileria equi* from carrier mares to their apparently healthy foals. Vet Parasitol 2007;148:130–6.
18. Georges KC, Ezeokoli CD, Sparagano O, et al. A case of transplacental transmission of *Theileria equi* in a foal in Trinidad. Vet Parasitol 2011;175:363–6.
19. Phipps LP, Otter A. Transplacental transmission of *Theileria equi* in two foals born and reared in the United Kingdom. Vet Rec 2004;154:406–8.
20. Erbsloh JK. Babesiosis in the newborn foal. J Reprod Fertil Suppl 1975;(23):725–6.
21. Al-Saad K. Acute babesiosis in foals. J Anim Vet Adv 2009;8:5.
22. Thompson PH. Ticks as vectors of equine piroplasmosis. J Am Vet Med Assoc 1969;155:454–7.

23. World Organization of Animal Health. Equine prioplasmosis terrestrial manual. 2013. Available at: www.OIE.int. Accessed February 15, 2013.
24. Cantu-Martinez MA, Segura-Correa JC, Silva-Paez ML, et al. Prevalence of antibodies to *Theileria equi* and *Babesia caballi* in horses from northeastern Mexico. J Parasitol 2012;98:869–70.
25. Moltmann UG, Mehlhorn H, Schein E, et al. Fine structure of *Babesia equi* Laveran, 1901 within lymphocytes and erythrocytes of horses: an in vivo and in vitro study. J Parasitol 1983;69:111–20.
26. Schein E. Equine babesiosis. In: Ristic M, editor. Babesiosis of domestic animals and man. Boca Raton (FL): CRC; 1988. p. 197–208.
27. Ramsay JD, Ueti MW, Johnson WC, et al. Lymphocytes and macrophages are infected by *Theileria equi*, but T cells and B cells are not required to establish infection in vivo. PLoS One 2013;8:e76996.
28. Guimaraes AM, Lima JD, Ribeiro MF, et al. Ultrastructure of sporogony in *Babesia equi* in salivary glands of adult female *Boophilus microplus* ticks. Parasitol Res 1998;84:69–74.
29. Zapf F, Schein E. The development of *Babesia (Theileria) equi* (Laveran, 1901) in the gut and the haemolymph of the vector ticks, Hyalomma species. Parasitol Res 1994;80:297–302.
30. de Waal DT, van Heerden J, Potgieter FT. An investigation into the clinical pathological changes and serological response in horses experimentally infected with *Babesia equi* and *Babesia caballi*. Onderstepoort J Vet Res 1987;54:561–8.
31. Allen PC, Frerichs WM, Holbrook AA. Experimental acute *Babesia caballi* infections. II. Response of platelets and fibrinogen. Exp Parasitol 1975;37:373–9.
32. Donnellan CM, Marais HJ. Equine piroplasmosis. In: Mair TS, Hutchinson RE, editors. Infectious diseases of the horse. Fordham, Ely (United Kingdom): EVJ Ltd; 2009. p. 333–40.
33. Holbrook AA. Biology of equine piroplasmosis. J Am Vet Med Assoc 1969;155: 453–4.
34. Maurer FD. Equine piroplasmosis—another emerging disease. J Am Vet Med Assoc 1962;141:699–702.
35. Pitel PH, Pronost S, Scrive T, et al. Molecular detection of *Theileria equi* and *Babesia caballi* in the bone marrow of asymptomatic horses. Vet Parasitol 2010;170:182–4.
36. Kuttler KL, Gipson CA, Goff WL, et al. Experimental *Babesia equi* infection in mature horses. Am J Vet Res 1986;47:1668–70.
37. Guimarães AM, Lima JD, Tafuri WL, et al. Clinical and histopathological aspects of splenectomized foals infected by *Babesia equi*. J Equine Vet Sci 1997;17: 211–6.
38. Ambawat HK, Malhotra DV, Kumar S, et al. Erythrocyte associated haematobiochemical changes in *Babesia equi* infection experimentally produced in donkeys. Vet Parasitol 1999;85:319–24.
39. McGuire TC, Banks KL, Poppie MJ. Combined immunodeficiency in horses: characterization of the lymphocyte defect. Clin Immunol Immunopathol 1975; 3:555–66.
40. Knowles DP Jr, Kappmeyer LS, Perryman LE. Specific immune responses are required to control parasitemia in *Babesia equi* infection. Infect Immun 1994; 62:1909–13.
41. Cunha CW, McGuire TC, Kappmeyer LS, et al. Development of specific immunoglobulin Ga (IgGa) and IgGb antibodies correlates with control of parasitemia in *Babesia equi* infection. Clin Vaccine Immunol 2006;13:297–300.

42. Kappmeyer LS, Perryman LE, Hines SA, et al. Detection of equine antibodies to *Babesia caballi* by recombinant *B. caballi* rhoptry-associated protein 1 in a competitive-inhibition enzyme-linked immunosorbent assay. J Clin Microbiol 1999;37:2285–90.

43. Zobba R, Ardu M, Niccolini S, et al. Clinical and laboratory findings in equine piroplasmosis. J Equine Vet Sci 2008;28:301–8.

44. Taylor WM, Bryant JE, Anderson JB, et al. Equine piroplasmosis in the United States: a review. J Am Vet Med Assoc 1969;155:915–9.

45. Allen PC, Frerichs WM, Holbrook AA. Experimental acute *Babesia caballi* infections. I. Red blood cell dynamics. Exp Parasitol 1975;37:67–77.

46. Oladosu LA, Olufemi BE. Haematology of experimental babesiosis and ehrlichiosis in steroid immunosuppressed horses. Zentralbl Veterinarmed B 1992;39:345–52.

47. Hailat NQ, Lafi SQ, al-Darraji AM, et al. Equine babesiosis associated with strenuous exercise: clinical and pathological studies in Jordan. Vet Parasitol 1997;69:1–8.

48. De Waal DT, Van Heerden J, Van den Berg SS, et al. Isolation of pure *Babesia equi* and *Babesia caballi* organisms in splenectomized horses from endemic areas in South Africa. Onderstepoort J Vet Res 1988;55:33–5.

49. Rudolph W, Correa J, Zurita L, et al. Equine piroplasmosis: leukocytic response to *Babesia equi* (Laveran, 1901) infection in Chile. Br Vet J 1975;131:601–9.

50. Brüning A. Equine piroplasmosis an update on diagnosis, treatment and prevention. Br Vet J 1996;152:139–51.

51. Knowles DP Jr, Kappmeyer LS, Stiller D, et al. Antibody to a recombinant merozoite protein epitope identifies horses infected with *Babesia equi*. J Clin Microbiol 1992;30:3122–6.

52. Lewis MJ, Wagner B, Woof JM. The different effector function capabilities of the seven equine IgG subclasses have implications for vaccine strategies. Mol Immunol 2008;45:818–27.

53. Donnelly J, Phipps LP, Watkins KL. Evidence of maternal antibodies to *Babesia equi* and *B caballi* in foals of seropositive mares. Equine Vet J 1982;14:126–8.

54. Weiland G. Species-specific serodiagnosis of equine piroplasma infections by means of complement fixation test (CFT), immunofluorescence (IIF), and enzyme-linked immunosorbent assay (ELISA). Vet Parasitol 1986;20:43–8.

55. Bhoora R, Quan M, Zweygarth E, et al. Sequence heterogeneity in the gene encoding the rhoptry-associated protein-1 (RAP-1) of *Babesia caballi* isolates from South Africa. Vet Parasitol 2010;169:279–88.

56. Nicolaiewsky TB, Richter MF, Lunge VR, et al. Detection of *Babesia equi* (Laveran, 1901) by nested polymerase chain reaction. Vet Parasitol 2001;101:9–21.

57. Bhoora R, Franssen L, Oosthuizen MC, et al. Sequence heterogeneity in the 18S rRNA gene within *Theileria equi* and *Babesia caballi* from horses in South Africa. Vet Parasitol 2009;159:112–20.

58. Bernasconi NL, Traggiai E, Lanzavecchia A. Maintenance of serological memory by polyclonal activation of human memory B cells. Science 2002;298:2199–202.

59. Belloli C, Crescenzo G, Lai O, et al. Pharmacokinetics of imidocarb dipropionate in horses after intramuscular administration. Equine Vet J 2002;34:625–9.

60. Schwint ON, Ueti MW, Palmer GH, et al. Imidocarb dipropionate clears persistent *Babesia caballii* infection with elimination of transmission potential. Antimicrob Agents Chemother 2009;53:4327–32.

61. Grause JF, Ueti MW, Nelson JT, et al. Efficacy of imidocarb dipropionate in eliminating *Theileria equi* from experimentally infected horses. Vet J 2013;196:541–6.

62. Meyer C, Guthrie AJ, Stevens KB. Clinical and clinicopathological changes in 6 healthy ponies following intramuscular administration of multiple doses of imidocarb dipropionate. J S Afr Vet Assoc 2005;76:26–32.
63. Adams LG. Clinicopathological aspects of imidocarb dipropionate toxicity in horses. Res Vet Sci 1981;31:54–61.
64. Frerichs WM, Allen PC, Holbrook AA. Equine piroplasmosis (*Babesia equi*): therapeutic trials of imidocarb dihydrochloride in horses and donkeys. Vet Rec 1973;93:73–5.
65. Kumar S, Malhotra DV, Dhar S, et al. Vaccination of donkeys against *Babesia equi* using killed merozoite immunogen. Vet Parasitol 2002;106:19–33.

Infectious Diseases of Working Equids

Andrew P. Stringer, BVSc, PhD, MRCVS

KEYWORDS

- Working • Equid • Infectious disease • Morbidity • Mortality

KEY POINTS

- Most of the world's 112 million equids are working equids, residing in low-income countries where they have an essential role in the livelihoods of their owners.
- Key infectious diseases affecting the health of working equids include African horse sickness (AHS), epizootic lymphangitis (EZL), equine infectious anemia (EIA), gastrointestinal nematodes, glanders, piroplasmosis, tetanus, and trypanosomosis.
- There are considerable technical, social-behavioral, and institutional impediments globally to reducing the burden of infectious diseases on working equids.

INTRODUCTION

Working equids (working horses, mules, and donkeys) have an essential role in the livelihoods of millions of people worldwide.[1,2] These equids perform numerous activities on a daily basis, including the transportation of goods, people, and construction materials, as well as being used in agricultural and tourism activities.[3,4] It is estimated that the total world equid population is approximately 112 million (approximately 58.5 million horses, 43.0 million donkeys, and 10.5 million mules), although this is very likely to be a gross underestimate.[5] These equids are found across the globe: 46 million in the Americas, 7 million in Europe, 33 million in Asia, and 25 million in Africa. Most of the world's equids are working equids, many residing in low-income, net food-importing countries (more than one-third of all equids, and >50% of all donkeys).

Working equids have a role in reducing poverty, providing food security, enhancing rural development, and promoting gender equity across the globe. These animals are especially important to vulnerable groups, landless communities, and to women, where they can provide an effective entry point to income-generating activities.[6,7] Working equids currently have a limited place within many animal health systems, and are largely absent from agricultural policy, research, and education programs.[3] They are frequently not included in disease eradication and vaccination campaigns,

Society for the Protection of Animals Abroad (SPANA), 14 John Street, London WC1N 2EB, UK
E-mail address: astringer@spana.org

Vet Clin Equine 30 (2014) 695–718
http://dx.doi.org/10.1016/j.cveq.2014.09.001
0749-0739/14/$ – see front matter © 2014 Elsevier Inc. All rights reserved.

vetequine.theclinics.com

and despite many equine diseases featured on the World Organisation for Animal Health's (OIE) notifiable disease list, these diseases are not often included in government disease surveillance systems.

Working equids suffer from low productivity as a result of prevalent infectious diseases, and diseases associated with poor management practices. The health and welfare of working equids is often compromised in many low-income countries as a result of the impoverished situations their owners live in, the challenging environmental and climatic conditions,[8] the unavailability of appropriate medications and vaccines, and the widespread use of ineffective or harmful traditional therapies.

INFECTIOUS DISEASES OF WORKING EQUIDS

Infectious diseases are an important constraint to the health and productivity of working equids.[9–18] However, there are often limited or no data quantifying the occurrence, prevalence, and distribution of many infectious diseases in working equids in low-income countries. Many countries known to have large populations of working equids do not have an OIE official status for certain diseases, and many countries have no reporting history regarding many infectious diseases. Numerous viral, bacterial, fungal, and parasitic diseases affect working equids. These diseases are widely distributed and cause considerable morbidity and mortality. Key infectious diseases of working equids are proposed in **Box 1**.

Although the reader is referred to other articles in this issue for additional comprehensive discussions of 2 of these diseases (see the articles equine infectious anemia by Issel et al and piroplasmosis by Wise et al else where in this issue), information with particular relevance to working equids is provided in the following sections.

AFRICAN HORSE SICKNESS

African horse sickness (AHS) is a noncontagious, infectious, insect-borne disease of equids caused by African horse sickness virus (AHSV). The course of the disease is usually peracute to acute and is associated with high morbidity and mortality in working equid populations in affected countries, causing significant economic losses for owners.

Etiology

AHSV is a member of the genus Orbivirus in the family Reoviridae. Nine antigenically distinct serotypes have been described, with some cross-relatedness between the

---

Box 1
Key infectious diseases of working equids (in alphabetical order)

- African horse sickness (AHS)
- Epizootic lymphangitis (EZL)
- Equine infectious anemia (EIA)
- Gastrointestinal nematodes
- Glanders
- Piroplasmosis
- Tetanus
- Trypanosomosis

serotypes.[19,20] The distribution of these serotypes is different in each region of the African continent. All 9 serotypes have been documented in eastern and southern Africa, with serotype 9 more widespread in the northern areas of sub-Saharan Africa.[21]

Epidemiology

AHSV is biologically transmitted by the *Culicoides* spp. *Culicoides imicola* and *Culicoides bolitinos* have been shown to play an important role in Africa.[22,23] The disease has a seasonal occurrence and its prevalence is influenced by climatic and other conditions that favor the breeding of *Culicoides* spp. A continuous transmission cycle of AHSV between *Culicoides* midges and zebras has been shown to exist, and therefore a sufficiently large enough zebra population can act as a reservoir for the virus.[24] Donkeys may play a similar role in parts of Africa where there are large donkey populations.[25]

AHS is endemic in many countries in central and eastern Africa and spreads regularly to southern Africa.[9,26–30] In endemic areas, different serotypes may be active simultaneously, but one serotype is usually dominant during a particular season. The disease is occasionally reported in countries in North Africa, from where it has also entered the Middle East and Spain.[21] Two countries on the African continent with large working horse populations are Ethiopia and Senegal. Outbreaks of AHS have been documented in Ethiopia, including reports of serotype 6[31] and serotypes 2, 4, and 8.[9,26] Previous to these reports, serotype 9 was the predominate serotype found. In one study in Ethiopia, the cardiac form accounted for 52.8% of cases, followed by the African horse sickness fever form (31.9%), pulmonary form (8.4%), and mixed form (6.9%).[26] A retrospective study of the 2007 AHS epidemic in Senegal identified AHSV-2 as the serotype responsible for the outbreak and mortality in horses.[27]

Clinical Signs and Pathologic Findings

Clinically, AHS is characterized by pyrexia; edema of the lungs, pleura, and subcutaneous tissues; and hemorrhages on the serosal surfaces of internal organs. There are 4 clinical presentations of the disease: the pulmonary form, the cardiac form, the mixed form, and the horse sickness form (**Boxes 2–5**).

Box 2
Clinical signs of the pulmonary form of AHS

- Peracute form of AHS and occurs when AHSV infects fully susceptible horses.

- Short incubation period followed by a rapid rise in temperature.

- Characterized by marked and rapid respiratory failure. Elevated respiratory rate and forced expiration.

- Animal stands with forelimbs apart, head extended, and nostrils dilated.

- Profuse sweating is common.

- Paroxysmal coughing may be observed terminally, accompanied by frothy, serofibrinous fluid from the nostrils.

- The onset of dyspnea is occurs suddenly and death follows quickly.

- Mortality for the pulmonary form of AHS is greater than 90%.

Data from Long MT, Guthrie AJ. African horse sickness. In: Sellon DC, Long MT, editors. Equine infectious diseases. St Louis (MO): Saunders; 2014. p. 181–8.

Box 3
Clinical signs of the cardiac form of AHS

- Longer incubation period than the pulmonary form followed by pyrexia.
- Filling of the supraorbital fossa above the level of the zygomatic arch.
- Edema can extend to conjunctiva, lips, cheeks, tongue, intermandibular space, laryngeal region, and potentially down the neck.
- Dyspnea and cyanosis may follow edema.
- Unfavorable prognostic signs include petechial hemorrhages on conjunctivae and ventral tongue.
- The cardiac form is more protracted and milder than the pulmonary form, with a mortality of greater than 50%.

Data from Long MT, Guthrie AJ. African horse sickness. In: Sellon DC, Long MT, editors. Equine infectious diseases. St Louis (MO): Saunders; 2014. p. 181–8.

Box 4
Clinical signs of the mixed form of AHS

- The most common form of AHS, although rarely diagnosed clinically.
- Often diagnosed at post mortem in fatal AHS cases.
- Initial mild pulmonary signs followed by edematous swelling, effusions, and cardiac failure.
- Commonly, the subclinical cardiac form is followed suddenly by marked dyspnea and clinical signs consistent with the pulmonary form.

Data from Long MT, Guthrie AJ. African horse sickness. In: Sellon DC, Long MT, editors. Equine infectious diseases. St Louis (MO): Saunders; 2014. p. 181–8.

Box 5
Clinical signs of the horse sickness form of AHS

- Horse sickness fever is the mildest form of AHS and rarely diagnosed clinically.
- Following the incubation period, the temperature rises before returning to normal.
- Other clinical signs are rare, apart from the febrile reaction.
- Horse sickness fever is usually observed in donkeys and zebras, or in immune horses infected with a heterologous serotype of AHSV.

Data from Long MT, Guthrie AJ. African horse sickness. In: Sellon DC, Long MT, editors. Equine infectious diseases. St Louis (MO): Saunders; 2014. p. 181–8.

The pathologic findings associated with AHS infection in horses have been extensively described in other texts.[21] In the pulmonary form of AHS, the most striking pathologic finding is the diffuse, severe, subpleural, and interlobular edema of the lungs. Severe hydrothorax is common, with the pleural cavity containing large quantities of transparent, pale-yellow, gelatinous fluid. The trachea and bronchi usually contain large volumes of froth and yellow serous fluid, which is often seen at the nostrils (**Fig. 1**). One of the most characteristic findings in the cardiac form of AHS is the presence of yellow edema of the subcutaneous and intramuscular connective tissues, and generalized edema of the head region (**Fig. 2**). Severe hydropericardium is almost always present (**Fig. 3**).

Diagnosis

A presumptive diagnosis of AHS is often possible once the characteristic clinical signs have developed. The typical macroscopic lesions of AHS on postmortem are often sufficiently specific to allow a provisional diagnosis of the disease.[21] Virus isolation is currently the gold standard diagnostic test for AHS, although other serologic and molecular tests are now accepted by the OIE. Serotyping of AHSV isolates is performed using virus neutralization tests.

Therapeutic Strategies

There is no specific therapy for AHS. Supportive therapy, nursing, and rest are essential, as any exertion has the potential to cause death.

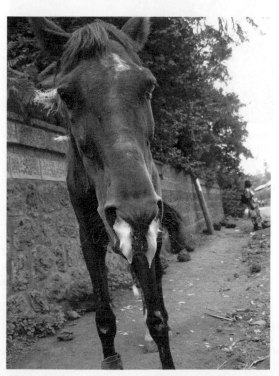

Fig. 1. Pulmonary form of AHS, with nasal discharge caused by severe alveolar edema. (*Courtesy of* Dr Nigatu Aklilu, SPANA, Debre Zeit, Ethiopia.)

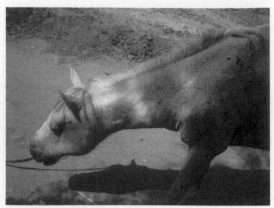

Fig. 2. Cardiac form of AHS, with generalized edema of the head region. (*Courtesy of* Dr Nigatu Aklilu, SPANA, Debre Zeit, Ethiopia.)

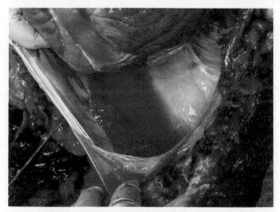

Fig. 3. Extensive effusion within the pericardium due to AHS. (*Courtesy of* Dr Nigatu Aklilu, SPANA, Debre Zeit, Ethiopia.)

Control Strategies

In endemic areas, vaccination of horses at the appropriate time of the year is a practical means of control. Some countries (South Africa and Ethiopia) currently have polyvalent vaccines containing attenuated strains that offer protection against the circulating serotypes. The risk of infection in susceptible horses can be reduced by stabling before dusk until after sunrise, as *Culicoides* spp. are nocturnal. The application of insect repellents and the use of insecticides on animals also reduces the risk of infection.

EPIZOOTIC LYMPHANGITIS

Epizootic lymphangitis (EZL) is caused by the fungal agent *Histoplasma capsulatum* var. *farciminosum* and affects horses, mules, and donkeys. EZL has been eradicated from large areas of the world but is still a major cause of morbidity and mortality in working equids in many countries, particularly in Africa.

Etiology

The fungus has 2 distinct phases: the mycelial form is present in the environment and the yeast is the pathogenic phase found in lesions.[32] The mycelial phase favors humid, moist environments and is thought to persist in the environment where the disease is endemic. Dissemination of the organism from discharging lesions of affected animals is likely to contribute to environmental contamination. The soil phase is considered to be an important part of the organism's pathogenesis.

Epidemiology

Currently the disease remains endemic in parts of North, East, and West Africa; the Middle East; and Far East.[32] However, up-to-date surveillance information is scarce. Studies in the carthorse populations within Ethiopia show both the mycelial and yeast forms are present.[11,33–35] Cross-sectional studies have reported the overall prevalence of EZL in Ethiopia to be between 18.8% and 30.1%.[11,35] EZL has severe economic consequences for the carthorse population in Ethiopia, particularly those based in towns between 1500 and 2300 m above sea level.[11,35,36] Although EZL has been reported in all equid species, traditionally it has been thought that donkeys are less susceptible to infection than horses and mules.[32] There have been a number of risk factors reported to be associated with particular forms of the disease; however, no large-scale epidemiologic cohort studies have been carried out to provide further evidence for these.[32]

Pathogenesis and Clinical Signs

Following invasion, *H capsulatum* var. *farciminosum* disseminates through the lymphatic system to regional lymph nodes, and in severe cases to organs.[37] Nodular lesions develop in the skin along the lymphatics and in the lymph nodes. These nodules ulcerate, and produce a thick, purulent discharge containing yeast cells. Four different clinical presentations of EZL have been described[32]: the cutaneous form (**Box 6**), ocular form (**Box 7**), respiratory form (**Box 8**), and asymptomatic carriers. These are not necessarily considered distinct clinical entities and combinations may occur with one form of the disease leading to development of another.

Diagnosis

EZL can be identified in the purulent discharge from nodules (or the mucopurulent ocular discharge) using Gram or Giemsa staining. The yeast form is characterized as a Gram-positive pleomorphic ovoid to globose structure with a "halo" appearance due to a nonstaining capsule.[32] Samples for diagnosis should be taken if possible from an unruptured nodule after clipping and disinfecting the skin to reduce contamination. It is also possible to visualize the organism in stained histologic sections of matured or developing lesions. Culture of the organism is necessary to confirm the presence of *Histoplasma* species.[32]

The "Histofarcin" test was evaluated in the field and the sensitivity of the test found to be 90.3%; however, specificity in endemic areas was only 69%.[33] This test is similar to the "mallein" skin test for glanders, where a delayed, intradermal, type IV hypersensitivity reaction indicates previous exposure to the organism. There is need to improve the sensitivity and specificity of the current diagnostic tests available for the diagnosis of EZL to allow for improved early detection of infection and for differentiating EZL from other diseases.

> **Box 6**
> **Clinical signs of the cutaneous form of EZL**
>
> - Most widely reported form of the disease.
> - Insidious onset with variable incubation period.
> - Disease characterized by chronic suppurative, ulcerating pyogranulomatous dermatitis and lymphangitis.
> - Nodules may be present on any part of the body, but most commonly originate around the lower limbs, chest, neck, and head.
> - The lesions spread from the primary lesion along the lymphatics, creating a characteristic cording pattern on the affected limbs (**Fig. 4**).
> - The fungus migrates to the local lymph nodes; from here the organism can potentially disseminate to other regions of the body.
> - There is a repeated cycle of nodule development, discharge, and ulceration.
> - In early cases, the animal's working ability and appetite are largely unaffected. As the disease progresses, the animal gradually becomes debilitated, and lameness, anorexia, and loss of body condition are common.
>
> *Data from* Scantlebury C, Reed K. Epizootic lymphangitis. In: Mair TS, Hutchinson RE, editors. Infectious diseases of the horse. EVJ Ltd; 2009.

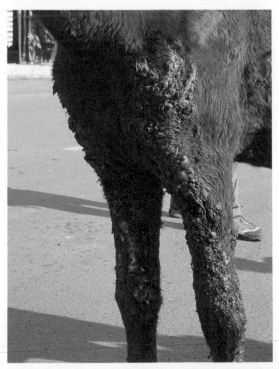

Fig. 4. Cutaneous form of EZL in a carthorse. (*Courtesy of* Dr Nigatu Aklilu, SPANA, Ethiopia.)

Box 7
Clinical signs of the ocular form of EZL

- Characterized by a kerato-conjunctivitis with a serous to mucopurulent discharge.

- Intradermal swellings present within the palpebrae. There may be characteristic button ulcers on the outer margins of the conjunctivae.

- The infection may extend to the periorbital tissues where a granulomatous reaction may develop, and to the lacrimal ducts where the infection can communicate with the external skin of the face **(Fig. 5)**.

- The secondary effects of the condition include corneal ulceration, lacrimal duct occlusion, panophthalmitis, myiasis, and bacterial infection.

Data from Scantlebury C, Reed K. Epizootic lymphangitis. In: Mair TS, Hutchinson RE, editors. Infectious diseases of the horse. EVJ Ltd; 2009.

Therapeutic Strategies

Numerous therapeutic strategies have been used in an attempt to treat horses with EZL. Amphotericin B is the listed drug of choice for the treatment of clinical cases of EZL by the OIE, and has been used successfully; however, the use of antifungal preparations in many low-income countries is not economically viable. The standard treatment protocol used by one nongovernmental organization (Society for the Protection of Animals Abroad [SPANA]) in the field is outlined as follows. This treatment protocol is labor intensive, expensive because of the cost of the drugs (not sourceable in large quantities within many countries), and efficacious only in the early stages of the disease.

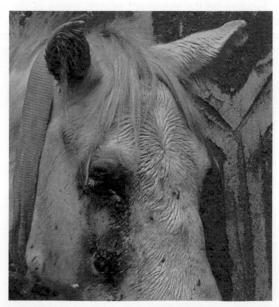

Fig. 5. Ocular form of EZL in a carthorse. (*Courtesy of* Dr Claire Scantlebury, University of Liverpool, Ethiopia.)

> **Box 8**
> **Clinical signs of the respiratory form of EZL**
>
> - Respiratory form thought to occur through inhalation of the organism either as spores from the environment or through extension of infection from the external mucous membranes of the nares or from the naso-lacrimal duct.
> - Nodules can present around the mucocutaneous junction of the nose and at *postmortem* are commonly seen to extend from the nasal passages, through the trachea and into the lung parenchyma.
> - There is often an accompanying viscid mucopurulent nasal discharge (**Fig. 6**), and in advanced stages, affected animals will show increased respiratory effort and have a stertuous noise during respiration.
> - This form causes severe debility, cough, and progressive weakness.
>
> *Data from* Scantlebury C, Reed K. Epizootic lymphangitis. In: Mair TS, Hutchinson RE, editors. Infectious diseases of the horse. EVJ Ltd; 2009.

- On initial presentation, the animal is sedated and all nodules are incised and flushed with topical 4% tincture of iodine.
- Potassium iodide (KI, 30 g) in solution is administered by nasogastric tube (for a horse of 200–250 kg).
- Oral KI is given at the same dose daily, for 5 days, and then every other day for a further 3 to 4 weeks, or as long as there is compliance from the owner.

Control Strategies

Because of the important role working equids play in the livelihoods of their owners, the euthanasia of all infected animals is often impracticable, and therefore the control of EZL in Ethiopia focuses on the treatment of mild cases of the disease and the euthanasia of the more moderate and severely infected animals (**Fig. 7**). Control also should focus on addressing some of the assumed risk factors of EZL, and, therefore, basic hygiene, fly control, wound prevention, and management should be promoted.

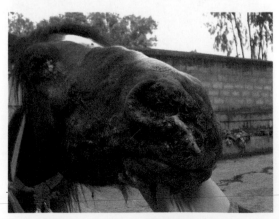

Fig. 6. Respiratory form of EZL in a carthorse. (*Courtesy of* Dr Claire Scantlebury, University of Liverpool, Debre Zeit, Ethiopia.)

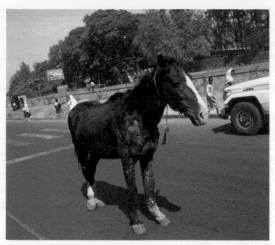

Fig. 7. Abandoned carthorse affected by severe EZL. (*Courtesy of* Dr Nigatu Aklilu, SPANA, Ethiopia.)

EQUINE INFECTIOUS ANEMIA

Equine infectious anemia (EIA) is an infectious disease of equids characterized by recurrent episodes of fever, lethargy, inappetence, thrombocytopenia, and anemia.

Etiology

Equine infectious anemia virus (EIAV) is a lentivirus of the family Retroviridae. In contrast to other lentiviruses, EIAV infection results in an acute phase of the disease, followed by recurrent clinical disease episodes that subside in most horses. These horses become persistently infected lifelong carriers.

Epidemiology

Equine infectious anemia is a disease affecting all species of working equids and is found worldwide.[38] The prevalence of this disease is higher in regions with warm climates because of its transmission by insect vectors.[39] Transfer of blood from infected horses to susceptible horses via blood-feeding insects is the predominate means of natural transmission. The important insect vectors for natural transmission are members of the family of Tabanidae, specifically horseflies and deer-flies.[40–42] Stable flies (*Stomoxys calcitrans*) also have been shown to transmit the virus.[42]

Pathogenesis and Clinical Signs

Thrombocytopenia is one of the earliest and most consistent abnormalities in EIAV-infected horses and closely correlates with pyrexia and viremia.[43] Anemia is a consistent clinical abnormality and its severity directly correlates with the frequency and duration of febrile episodes.[44] The clinical course of EIA is variable and depends on the dose and the virulence of the virus strain, and the susceptibility of the horse.[45] Clinical disease may be less severe in donkeys and mules than in horses.[46] Infections can result in a variety of clinical and pathologic abnormalities, with 3 characteristic clinical stages of EIA.

- Acute EIA occurs following initial infection with a virulent strain of EIAV. After exposure, pronounced viremia can develop, resulting in pyrexia, thrombocytopenia, lethargy, and inappetence.
- Following the initial disease episode, most infected horses experience recurrent episodes of acute clinical disease.
- If clinical disease episodes become frequent and severe, the horse develops the classical signs of chronic EIA (a "swamper"), characterized by anemia, thrombocytopenia, weight loss, and dependent edema.

Diagnosis

Definitive diagnosis is made through serologic testing, as EIAV is a persistent virus that is not cleared by the host. The agar gel immune-diffusion (AGID) test, also known as the Coggins test, is the test prescribed by the OIE and the most widely accepted procedure for the diagnosis of EIA. See the article by Waller, elsewhere in this issue, for additional information on diagnostic testing.

Therapeutic and Control Strategies

There is no specific therapy for EIAV infection. If elected, supportive therapy and isolation from other horses is recommended. Equine infectious anemia is an OIE-listed reportable disease. Control programs often focus on maintaining a low prevalence by detecting EIAV-infected horses and removing them from exposure to naïve populations, therefore decreasing the likelihood of transmission.

GASTROINTESTINAL NEMATODES

The etiology, epidemiology, pathogenesis, clinical signs, diagnosis, and therapeutic and control strategies relating to gastrointestinal nematodes in equids have been extensively documented.[47] Helminthiasis has been documented as a significant issue in working equids, many having a polyparasitism problem.[15,48–57] One study[55] revealed the following findings from a 2-year survey into gastrointestinal parasites in working donkeys in Ethiopia: "Coprological examination revealed 99% strongyle, 80% Fasciola, 51% Parascaris, 30% Gastrodiscus, 11% Strongyloides westeri, 8% cestodes and 2% Oxyuris equi infection prevalence. Over 55% of donkeys had more than 1000 eggs per gram of feces (epg). Forty-two different species of parasites consisting of 33 nematodes, 3 trematodes, 3 cestodes and 3 arthropod larvae were identified from postmortem examined donkeys." Interestingly, a study in Mexico found no correlation between fecal worm egg count (EPG) and body condition score in 140 randomly selected working equids.[56] The study concluded that despite the high prevalence and parasite burdens, these equids did not appear seriously affected, and that more emphasis should be placed on other interventions to improve health (eg, nutrition), with anthelmintic treatments reserved only for those equids with the highest EPG or showing clinical signs.

GLANDERS
Etiology

The causative agent of glanders is Burkholderia mallei, a short, rod-shaped, gram-negative, aerobic, facultative, intracellular, nonmotile non–spore-forming bacteria, which can survive outside the host for varying lengths of time.

Epidemiology and Pathogenesis

The principal hosts for B mallei are horses, mules, and donkeys. Both acute and chronic forms of the disease are found; horses are typically chronically infected, whereas donkeys and mules are more likely to develop the acute form. Chronically infected equids are the known reservoir for *B mallei*. Human infections can occur by aerosol transmission from infected animals and are frequently fatal if untreated. Glanders is considered endemic in many countries with large populations of working equids.[58,59] The increasing number of outbreaks in recent years led to the classification of glanders as a reemerging disease.

Clinical Signs

Glanders has been described as either acute or chronic, although clinically it may be difficult to distinguish between the 2 forms. Donkeys are most likely to die from the acute disease within 7 to 10 days, whereas horses may either die rapidly, or live for several years with chronic abscessation.[60]

Acute glanders is characterized by bronchopneumonia and septicemia with a moderate to high fever, depression, and rapid weight loss. Frequently, highly infectious mucopurulent to hemorrhagic nasal discharge forms crusts on the external nares.[60] Chronic glanders is typically described in 1 of 3 forms, cutaneous (farcy), nasal, or pulmonary, although there is much overlap among the 3 forms.[60] The clinical signs of these 3 forms are described in detail in other texts,[60] but include ulcerations, swollen cutaneous lymphatic nodules, and nasal discharge.

Diagnosis

The test for glanders as listed by the OIE is the complement fixation test (CFT). Historically, the mallein test has been used to eradicate glanders. The intradermal-palpebral test is acknowledged as the most sensitive, reliable, and specific of the mallein tests for glanders. The CFT is currently the test used for international trade. Numerous other serologic and molecular diagnostic tests also are available for glanders diagnosis.

Therapeutic Strategies

Euthanasia and slaughter of equids with glanders is strongly recommended. *B mallei* appears to be resistant to many antimicrobial drugs,[61] and the difficulty in treating horses is in determining whether the infection has been eliminated.

Control Strategies

Glanders has been successfully eliminated from many countries through the slaughter of animals with a positive mallein test. A wide variety of national and international regulations exist, and glanders is a reportable disease of the OIE. Glanders is a rare but serious zoonotic disease.

PIROPLASMOSIS

Equine piroplasmosis (EP) is an infectious, noncontagious, tick-borne disease caused by the hemoprotozoan parasites, *Theileria equi* and *Babesia caballi*.[62] This disease affects all equid species, including horses, mules, donkeys, and zebras.[62] Equine piroplasmosis is found globally where the tick vectors are present and is endemic in many regions.[63–65]

Etiology

The genera *Babesia* and *Theileria* belong to the family Piroplasmidae within the phylum Apicomplexa. Piroplasmosis occurs in many countries, and with more than 850 tick species worldwide, the potential for transmission is high.[63] For *T equi*, the reservoir of infection is the persistently infected equid; however, for *B caballi*, both the infected horse and the primary tick vector serve as reservoirs for transmission.[63] Multiple ixodid tick species have been identified as vectors of equine piroplasmosis.[63] Parasitemia typically does not exceed 1% in *B caballi* infections and may be as low as 0.1% in clinical cases.[62] Reported parasitemia in natural *T equi* infections usually range from 1% to 7%.[65]

Epidemiology

The OIE Web site is continually updated to provide the most up-to-date information regarding available infectious disease epidemiologic information.[38] However, for many countries (many of which have large working equid populations), reliable and accurate information is not available. One study in Brazil of 88 donkeys found that 31.8% and 20.5% were positive for *T equi* and *B caballi*, respectively, as determined by nested polymerase chain reaction (PCR) assays,[66] whereas another study in Ethiopia of 395 working donkeys found a seroprevalence of *T equi* and *B caballi* of 55.7% and 13.2%, respectively.[67] Both *B caballi* and *T equi* are usually present in the same geographic regions (tropical and subtropical climates), and can share vectors and co-infect horses.[62] Most horses in endemic areas are infected within their first year of life, although outbreaks of overt clinical disease are uncommon in these areas, with acute clinical disease most often observed in naïve horses moved into endemic areas.[62]

Pathogenesis and Clinical Signs

The life cycle of both *B caballi* and *T equi* involve distinct stages that occur in both the host and the tick. In both parasites, regardless of tick species variation, infectious sporozoites are transmitted through the tick saliva to the equid host, causing erythrocyte lysis resulting in variable degrees of hemolytic anemia.[63] Immune responses to infection remain poorly defined. It is widely accepted in endemic areas that protective immunity is present after an initial infection, yet no studies have been performed proving this phenomenon.[63] There are 3 presentations of equine piroplasmosis: acute (**Box 9**), chronic, and the inapparent carrier.

Chronically infected horses usually exhibit signs of nonspecific chronic inflammatory conditions, including weight loss, poor body condition, partial anorexia, malaise, and decreased performance.[68] The vast majority of *B caballi* and *T equi* seropositive horses are inapparent carriers. These horses have low levels of parasitemia, no obvious clinical signs, and are reservoirs for the parasite.

Diagnosis

Various diagnostic modalities can be used alone or in combination to diagnose infection. Diagnosis of acute equine piroplasmosis can be made on the basis of clinical

---

Box 9
Clinical signs of acute equine piroplasmosis

- Initially characterized by nonspecific signs of infection, including pyrexia, lethargy, decreased appetite, and peripheral edema.

- Petechiations on mucous membranes due to profound thrombocytopenia may be observed.

- Signs of hemolytic anemia follow, with pale/icteric mucous membranes, tachycardia, tachypnea, weakness and pigmenturia.

- In severe cases, systemic involvement results in disseminated intravascular coagulopathy, renal failure, liver disease, and multiple organ dysfunction.

Data from Wise LN, Knowles DP, Rothschild CM. Piroplasmosis. In: Sellon DC, Long MT, editors. Equine infectious diseases. St Louis (MO): Saunders; 2014. p. 467–74.

signs and the careful examination of blood smears.[62] Serologic tests are necessary to diagnose chronically infected horses. Diagnosis by microscopic examination of blood smears is possible only in the acute phase of equine piroplasmosis. During this acute phase, *B caballi* and *T equi* can be easily distinguished from one another within infected erythrocytes by using microscopy. Several serologic tests exist to increase diagnostic sensitivity especially for horses demonstrating no clinical signs. See the article by Waller elsewhere in this issue for additional information on diagnostic testing.

Therapeutic Strategies

Therapeutic strategies for equids infected in endemic areas should focus on alleviating the clinical signs and decreasing recovery time. Clearance of the organism serves little purpose in endemic areas, as lifelong immunity is assumed to be conferred with chronic infection.[63] Imidocarb dipropionate is considered the drug of choice to alleviate clinical signs, and for this purpose, a dose in the range of 2.2 to 4.4 mg/kg, intramuscularly, given once, is generally effective. Lower doses can be repeated if necessary every 24 to 72 hours for 2 to 3 treatments. See the article by Waller, elsewhere in this issue, for additional information on treatment. Other drugs, including diminazene aceturate and diminazene diaceturate, also have been used to alleviate clinical signs.

Control Strategies

No vaccine is currently available for the prevention of infection or disease caused by *B caballi* or *T equi*. Currently, prevention of the disease in endemic areas is virtually impossible, so it is essential for young animals in these populations to be infected early in life, as it is assumed that early infection confers immunity for subsequent infections.

TETANUS

Tetanus is caused by exotoxins produced by *Clostridium tetani*. *C tetani* is a motile, anaerobic gram-positive bacillus found ubiquitously in soil.

Etiology

The most common route of infection is inoculation of wounds with *C tetani* spores. Puncture wounds contaminated by soil or rusty metal are especially likely to cause tetanus. Injuries around the pastern associated with hobbling were prevalent sites of *C tetani* infections in working horses, mules, and donkeys in Morocco.[69]

Epidemiology

Tetanus occurs in all regions of the world. Tetanus cases are seen frequently in Morocco and Ethiopia,[12,69] both countries with large working equid populations. A retrospective analysis of tetanus case records of one nongovernmental organization in Ethiopia reported 22% fatality.[70] Another retrospective study of 45 tetanus cases treated in Ethiopia between 2008 and 2009 revealed a survival rate of 66.3%.[12]

Pathogenesis and Clinical Signs

The clinical signs of tetanus are caused by exotoxins. The pathogenesis of tetanus in equids has been extensively described in other texts.[71] The most commonly recognized form of tetanus in horses is generalized tetanus. In horses, the clinical signs associated with tetanus have been classified as a result of the clinical severity of the disease.[71] The proposed classification is shown in **Box 10.**

> **Box 10**
> **Classification of clinical severity**
>
> **Mild**
>
> Anxious expression
>
> Prolapsed nictitans
>
> Trismus
>
> Extended head
>
> **Moderate (as for mild, plus)**
>
> Dysphagia
>
> Hyperresponsiveness
>
> Muscle spasms
>
> Tail-head extension
>
> "Saw-horse" stance (**Fig. 8**)
>
> Stiff gait
>
> **Severe (as for moderate, plus)**
>
> Lateral recumbency
>
> Frequent severe spasms
>
> Respiratory difficulties
>
> Cardiovascular instability
>
> *Data from* Mackay R. Tetanus. In: Sellon DC, Long MT, editors. Equine infectious diseases. St Louis (MO): Saunders; 2014. p. 368–72.

Diagnosis

A diagnosis of tetanus is presumptive and based on clinical signs in the context of a history of poor, absent, or unknown vaccination against tetanus. An early and sensitive test in the horse is transient prolapse of the nictitans membrane provoked by stimulation of the head.[71]

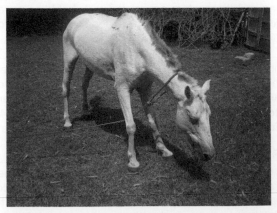

Fig. 8. Carthorse in Ethiopia with generalized tetanus showing classic "saw-horse" stance. (*Courtesy of* Dr Nigatu Aklilu, SPANA, Debre Zeit, Ethiopia.)

Therapeutic Strategies

Therapeutic strategies for tetanus cases have been widely described.[71] Therapy for tetanus should have the following objectives: provision of safe, quiet environment; elimination of *C tetani* and unbound toxin; sedation; muscle relaxation and relief of pain; and general support.

Box 11
Dourine

Etiology

Dourine is a chronic trypanosomal disease of horses that is transmitted predominately by coitus and characterized by genital edema, neurologic dysfunction, and death.

Epidemiology and Pathogenesis

Currently dourine is considered a reportable disease by the OIE and is present in most of Asia, southeastern Europe, South America, and Africa. Equids are considered the only natural host for *T equiperdum*. Clinical signs are less obvious in donkeys than in horses, and these animals may be a reservoir for infection. Transmission is considered most likely during the early stages of the disease.

Clinical Signs

The initial sign of dourine in mares are vaginal discharge, with edema of the vulva, perineum, mammary gland, and ventral abdomen. Abortion may occur if the mares are infected with a virulent strain. In stallions, the initial signs include edema of the external genitalia and perineum and potentially paraphimosis. Cutaneous plaques (silver plaques) are considered pathognomonic for dourine; however, these plaques do not occur with all strains of the parasite. Chronically infected horses develop signs of neurologic dysfunction with progressive weakness and ataxia, leading ultimately to recumbency and death. Clinical signs may wax and wane for many months or years before death, depending on the strain of infecting parasite.

Diagnosis

In endemic areas, the diagnosis of dourine is usually made on the basis of characteristic clinical signs. The OIE-prescribed test for diagnosis is the complement fixation test (CFT), although this test does not distinguish between infection with *T equiperdum* and infection with the closely related *T evansi*, *T gambiense*, or *T brucei*. A range of alternative serologic tests also exist.

Therapeutic Strategies

In many cases, the treatment of horses with dourine is not recommended because it may result in an inapparent carrier state. A number of treatments have been used, including neoarsphenamine and suramin in large-scale eradication programs.

Control Strategies

Dourine has been successfully eradicated from a number of areas and countries around the world based on CFT testing.

Data from Walden HS, Ness SA, Mittel LD, et al. Miscellaneous parasitic diseases. In: Sellon DC, Long MT, editors. Equine infectious diseases. St Louis (MO): Saunders; 2014. p. 505–7.

Control Strategies

Tetanus can be prevented by vaccination. Currently, tetanus vaccines are not available in many of the countries where there are large populations of working equids.

TRYPANOSOMOSIS

Trypanosomes are spindle-shaped protozoal parasites. Infection of horses with *Trypanosoma equiperdum*, *Trypanosoma evansi*, and *Trypanosoma brucei brucei* has traditionally been associated with the diseases dourine (**Box 11**), surra (**Box 12**), and

---

Box 12
Surra

Etiology

Surra is caused by infection with the hemoparasite *T evansi*. Surra is characterized by anemia, weight loss, recurrent fever, and death.

Epidemiology and Pathogenesis

Surra can affect numerous species, but is most severe in horse and camels. The etiologic agent is transmitted mechanically by hematophagous biting flies of the *Tabanus* and *Stomoxys* species. The mortality rate in horses can be high in areas where the disease has been newly introduced. There is no known age, breed, or sex predilection.

Clinical Signs

Horses with surra present with pyrexia, progressive anemia, weight loss, and neurologic abnormalities. The disease is usually acute, although some horses will experience chronic manifestations. Intermittent fever correlates with intermittent episodes of parasitemia. Urticarial lesions and edematous plaques may appear on the ventral abdomen, and distal limb edema and petechial hemorrhages are common. Neurologic signs when they occur lead to progressive weakness and ataxia, most evident in the hind limbs.

Diagnosis

A diagnosis of surra is suspected on the basis of compatible clinical signs in a horse residing in an endemic area. In the early stages of the disease, a diagnosis is confirmed by observation of typical trypanosomes in blood or tissue fluids. This is more difficult in the equids with chronic disease. A number of serologic tests are available, although information on their specificity and sensitivity for the field diagnosis of surra is largely lacking.

Therapeutic Strategies

Suramin is the drug that has been most frequently used to treat surra in horses. A number of other drugs, including quinapyramine sulfate, isometamidium chloride, melarsen oxide, and diminazene, also have been suggested.

Control Strategies

There are currently no vaccines available for the prevention of surra in horses. Prevention relies on the identification and treatment of infected horses, appropriate vector control, and good hygiene. Repeated treatment with an antitrypanosomal medication has been suggested.

Data from Walden HS, Ness SA, Mittel LD, et al. Miscellaneous parasitic diseases. In: Sellon DC, Long MT, editors. Equine infectious diseases. St Louis (MO): Saunders; 2014. p. 505–7.

African animal trypanosomiasis (AAT, **Box 13**). The other trypanosomes that infect horses, *Trypanosoma congolense* and *Trypanosoma vivax*, along with *T brucei brucei*, are etiologic agents of AAT. Because of the considerable overlap in clinical disease between infections with these specific parasites, the following section discusses clinical syndromes (dourine, surra, and AAT) instead of individual agents.

Box 13
African animal trypanosomosis (AAT)

Etiology

AAT is a disease complex caused by the single or combined infection with *T congolense*, *T vivax*, or *T brucei brucei*.

Epidemiology and Pathogenesis

Infections in horses and other animals with AAT results in disease that ranges from subclinical to mild to chronic to fatal. Ruminants are considered reservoirs for infection. Within Africa, the most important vectors for transmission of AAT are the 3 species of tsetse flies (*Glossina morsitans*, *Glossina palpalis*, and *Glossina fusca*). The natural range of AAT infection is largely defined by the range of the tsetse fly (the principal vector). Cycles of parasitemia, antibody production, parasite death, immune complex formation, and glycoprotein coat antigenic changes occur.

Clinical Signs

Clinical signs of AAT, regardless of the specific trypanosome involved, include anemia, intermittent fever, edema, and weight loss. Increased stress due to malnutrition or concurrent disease increase the likelihood and severity of the disease. Infection with *T congolense* causes severe disease in the horse, and in donkeys may cause chronic infection with longer persistence in the blood. *T vivax* causes relatively mild disease in horses, whereas *T brucei brucei* causes severe, frequently fatal infections in horses.

Diagnosis

AAT should be suspected in horses residing in endemic areas with anemia and poor body condition. The diagnosis is usually confirmed by demonstration of the organism in the blood or lymph node smears. Both serologic and molecular diagnostic tests have been used to detect the disease.

Therapeutic Strategies

A number of antitrypanosomal medications have been used for the treatment and prevention of AAT; however, increasing drug resistance has complicated this approach to disease control. Drugs used include quinapyramine derivatives, isometamidium chloride, homidium bromide, diminazene aceturate, and melarsen oxide.

Control Strategies

The most effective way to control AAT is to control vector populations. Numerous approaches for vector control have been used. The trypanosomes associated with AAT are considered nonpathogenic for humans.

Data from Walden HS, Ness SA, Mittel LD, et al. Miscellaneous parasitic diseases. In: Sellon DC, Long MT, editors. Equine infectious diseases. St Louis (MO): Saunders; 2014. p. 505–7.

The presence of *T equiperdum* has been studied in Ethiopia, using enzyme-linked immunosorbent assays (ELISAs) for the detection of both the trypanosomal antigen and antibody.[10] The study revealed that the seroprevalence increased with the severity of the observed clinical signs and that there was a positive correlation between the presence of circulating trypanosomal antigen and clinical evidence of infection. Serologic screening of 646 horses in the highlands of Ethiopia showed a *T evansi* seroprevalence of 28%, 25%, and 19% using the card agglutination test, LATEX (latex agglutination) test, and ELISA, respectively.[72] The presence of drug-resistant *T congolense* in naturally infected donkeys also has been documented in Ethiopia.[73] In 241 equids from the Central River Division in The Gambia (183 horses and 58 donkeys), the overall trypanosome prevalence was 91%, with an infection rate of 31% for *T congolense*, 87% for *T vivax*, and 18% for *T brucei*.[74]

SUMMARY

Most of the world's equids are working equids, residing in low-income countries where they have an essential role in reducing poverty, providing food security, enhancing rural development, and promoting gender equity for millions of people worldwide. Numerous infectious diseases negatively impact the health and productivity of these working animals. There are, however, considerable technical (eg, lack of epidemiologic data), social-behavioral (eg, limited equine-specific owner knowledge and education), and institutional (eg, the low recognition of the role of working equids) impediments globally to reducing the burden of infectious diseases on working equids. One the greatest remaining challenges is the lack of funding for research, resulting from the relatively low priority assigned to working equids by funding bodies. Changing the attitudes of decision makers will require data-driven advocacy, and global networks of collaborators have a vital role in building this more robust evidence base.

ACKNOWLEDGMENTS

The author acknowledges Dr Nigatu Aklilu and Dr Claire Scantlebury for the use of their images, and Dr Adele Williams for her comments and feedback on the article while in preparation.

REFERENCES

1. Perry B, Randolph T, McDermott JJ, et al. Investing in animal research to alleviate poverty. Nairobi (Kenya): International Livestock Research Institute (ILRI); 2002.
2. Thornton P, Kruska RL, Henninger L, et al. Mapping poverty and livestock in developing countries. Nairobi (Kenya): International Livestock Research Institute (ILRI); 2002.
3. Pritchard JC. Animal traction and transport in the 21st century: getting the priorities right. Vet J 2010;186:271–4.
4. Garuma S, Lemecha F, Sisay A, et al. Study on gender distribution of ownership of animal-drawn carts and its effect on women's life in Adami Tulu and Dugda Bora districts. Edinburgh (Scotland): Draught Animal News. Centre for Tropical Veterinary Medicine (CVTM); 2007.
5. FAO. Available at: http://faostat.fao.org/site/573/DesktopDefault.aspx?PageID=573#ancor. Accessed October 31, 2013.

6. Curran MM, Feseha G, Smith DG. The impact of access to animal health services on donkey health and livelihoods in Ethiopia. Trop Anim Health Prod 2005;37:47–65.
7. Marshall K, Ali Z. Gender issues in donkey use in rural Ethiopia. In: Starkey P, Fielding D, editors. Donkeys, people and development. A resource book of the Animal Traction Network for Eastern and Southern Africa (ATNESA). ACP-EU Technical Centre for Agricultural and Rural Cooperation (CTA), Wageningen, The Netherlands. 1997. p. 62–8.
8. Pritchard JC, Lindberg AC, Main DC, et al. Assessment of the welfare of working horses, mules and donkeys, using health and behaviour parameters. Prev Vet Med 2005;69:265–83.
9. Aklilu N, Batten C, Gelaye E, et al. African horse sickness outbreaks caused by multiple virus types in Ethiopia. Transbound Emerg Dis 2014;61:185–92.
10. Alemu T, Luckins AG, Phipps LP, et al. The use of enzyme linked immunosorbent assays to investigate the prevalence of *Trypanosoma equiperdum* in Ethiopian horses. Vet Parasitol 1997;71:239–50.
11. Ameni G. Epidemiology of equine histoplasmosis (epizootic lymphangitis) in carthorses in Ethiopia. Vet J 2006;172:160–5.
12. Ayele G, Bojia E, Getachew M, et al. Important factors in decision making in tetanus cases in donkeys: experience of donkey health and welfare project, Ethiopia. In: The 6th International Colloquium on Working Equids: Learning from Others. New Delhi (India): The Brooke; 2010. p. 195–9.
13. Biruhtesfa A, Yilikal A, Bojia E, et al. Aerobic bacterial isolates in equids and their antimicrobial susceptibility pattern. Int J Appl Res Vet Med 2007;5:107–12.
14. Duguma B. Seroprevalence and risk factors for equine herpes virus 1 (EHV-1) and 4 (EHV-4) in working equids, central Ethiopia [MSc Thesis]. London (UK): University of London; 2007.
15. Fikru R, Reta D, Teshale S, et al. Prevalence of equine gastrointestinal parasites in western highlands of Oromia, Ethiopia. Bull Anim Heal Prod Africa 2005;53:161–6.
16. Okell CN, Pinchbeck GP, Stringer AP, et al. A community-based participatory study investigating the epidemiology and effects of rabies to livestock owners in rural Ethiopia. Prev Vet Med 2012;108(1):1–9.
17. Pearson R, Alemayehu M, Tesfaye A, et al. Use and management of donkeys in peri-urban areas of Ethiopia. Edinburgh (Scotland): CVTM; 2001.
18. Yilma J, Gebreab F, Svendsen E, et al. Health problems of working donkeys in Debre Zeit and Menagesha regions of Ethiopia. In: Fielding D, Pearson R, editors. Donkeys, mules and horses in tropical agricultural development. Edinburgh(Texas): Centre for Tropical Veterinary Medicine (CVTM), University of Edinburgh; 1990.
19. Howell PG. The isolation and identification of further antigenic types of African horsesickness virus. Onderstepoort J Vet Res 1962;29:139–49.
20. McIntosh BM. Immunological types of horsesickness virus and their significance in immunization. Onderstepoort J Vet Res 1958;27:465–539.
21. Long MT, Guthrie AJ. African horse sickness. In: Sellon DC, Long MT, editors. Equine infectious diseases. St Louis (MO): Saunders; 2014. p. 181–8.
22. Meiswinkel R, Baylis M, Labuschagne K. Stabling and the protection of horses from *Culicoides bolitinos* (Diptera: Ceratopogonidae), a recently identified vector of African horse sickness. Bull Entomol Res 2000;90(6):509–15.
23. Venter GJ, Graham SD, Hamblin C. African horse sickness epidemiology: vector competence of South African *Culicoides* species for virus serotypes 3, 5 and 8. Med Vet Entomol 2000;14:245–50.

24. Lord CC, Woolhouse ME, Barnard BJ. Transmission and distribution of African horse sickness virus serotypes in South African zebra. Arch Virol Suppl 1998; 14:21–8.
25. Hamblin C, Salt JS, Mellor PS, et al. Donkeys as reservoirs of African horse sickness virus. Arch Virol 1998;14:37–47.
26. Ayelet G, Derso S, Jenberie S, et al. Outbreak investigation and molecular characterization of African horse sickness virus circulating in selected areas of Ethiopia. Acta Trop 2013;127:91–6.
27. Diouf ND, Etter E, Lo MM, et al. Outbreaks of African horse sickness in Senegal, and methods of control of the 2007 epidemic. Vet Rec 2013;172(6):152.
28. Bitew M, Andargie A, Bekele M, et al. Serological survey of African horse sickness in selected districts of Jimma zone, Southwestern Ethiopia. Trop Anim Health Prod 2011;43:1543–7.
29. Scacchia M, Lelli R, Peccio A, et al. African horse sickness: description of outbreaks of the disease in Namibia. Vet Ital 2009;45:255–64.
30. Kazeem MM, Rufai N, Ogunsan EA, et al. Clinicopathological features associated with the outbreak of African horse sickness in Lagos, Nigeria. J Equine Vet Sci 2008;28:594–7.
31. Zeleke A, Sori T, Powell K, et al. Isolation and identification of circulating serotype of African horse sickness virus in Ethiopia. J Appl Res Vet Med 2005; 3(1):40–3.
32. Scantlebury C, Reed K. Epizootic lymphangitis. In: Mair TS, Hutchinson RE, editors. Infectious diseases of the horse. Fordham (UK): EVJ Ltd; 2009. p. 397–406.
33. Ameni G, Terefe W, Hailu A. Histofarcin test for the diagnosis of epizootic lymphangitis in Ethiopia: development, optimisation and validation in the field. Vet J 2006;171:358–62.
34. Ameni G, Terefe W. A cross-sectional study of epizootic lymphangitis in cartmules in Western Ethiopia. Prev Vet Med 2004;66:93–9.
35. Ameni G, Siyoum F. Study on histoplasmosis (epizootic lymphangitis) in carthorses in Ethiopia. J Vet Sci 2002;3:135–40.
36. Jones K. Epizootic lymphangitis: the impact on subsistence economies and animal welfare. Vet J 2006;172:402–4.
37. Al-Ani FK. Epizootic lymphangitis in horses: a review of the literature. Rev Sci Tech 1999;18(3):691.
38. OIE. Disease information 2012. Available at: http://www.oie.int/wahis_2/public/wahid.php/Wahidhome/Home. Accessed June 14, 2014.
39. Mealey RH. Equine infectious anaemia. In: Sellon DC, Long MT, editors. Equine infectious diseases. St Louis (MO): Saunders; 2014. p. 232–8.
40. Issel CJ, Foil LD. Studies on equine infectious anemia virus transmission by insects. J Am Vet Med Assoc 1984;184(3):293–7.
41. Foil LD, Meek CL, Adams WV, et al. Mechanical transmission of equine infectious anemia virus by deer flies (Chrysops flavidus) and stable flies (Stomoxys calcitrans). Am J Vet Res 1983;44(1):155–6.
42. Hawkins JA, Adams WV, Cook L, et al. Role of horse fly (Tabanus fuscicostatus Hine) and stable fly (Stomoxys calcitrans L.) in transmission of equine infectious anemia to ponies in Louisiana. Am J Vet Res 1973;34(12):1583–6.
43. Sellon DC, Fuller FJ, McGuire TC. The immunopathogenesis of equine infectious anemia virus. Virus Res 1994;32(2):111–38.
44. McGuire TC, O'Rourke KI, Perryman LE. Immunopathogenesis of equine infectious anemia lentivirus disease. Dev Biol Stand 1990;72:31–7.

45. Kemeny LJ, Mott LO, Pearson JE. Titration of equine infectious anemia virus. Effect of dosage on incubation time and clinical signs. Cornell Vet 1971;61(4): 687–95.

46. Cook SJ, Cook RF, Montelaro RC, et al. Differential responses of *Equus caballus* and *Equus asinus* to infection with two pathogenic strains of equine infectious anemia virus. Vet Microbiol 2001;79(2):93–109.

47. Nielsen MK, Reinemeyer CR, Sellon DC. Nematodes. In: Sellon DC, Long MT, editors. Equine infectious diseases. St Louis (MO): Saunders; 2014. p. 475–89.

48. Crane MA, Khallaayoune K, Scantlebury C, et al. A randomised triple blind trial to assess the effect of an anthelmintic programme for working equids in Morocco. BMC Vet Res 2011;7:1.

49. Upjohn MM, Shipton K, Lerotholi T, et al. Coprological prevalence and intensity of helminth infection in working horses in Lesotho. Trop Anim Health Prod 2010; 42:1655–61.

50. Getachew M, Gebreab F, Trawford A, et al. A survey of seasonal patterns in strongyle faecal worm egg counts of working equids of the central midlands and lowlands, Ethiopia. Trop Anim Health Prod 2008;40:637–42.

51. Getachew AM, Innocent GT, Trawford AF, et al. Equine parascarosis under the tropical weather conditions of Ethiopia: a coprological and postmortem study. Vet Rec 2008;162:177–80.

52. Getachew M. Endoparasites of working donkeys in Ethiopia: epidemiological study and mathematical modelling [PhD Thesis]. Glasgow: University of Glasgow; 2006.

53. Yoseph S, Smith DG, Mengistu A, et al. Seasonal variation in the parasite burden and body condition of working donkeys in East Shewa and West Shewa regions of Ethiopia. Trop Anim Health Prod 2005;37:35–45.

54. Getachew M. Epidemiological studies on the health and welfare of the Ethiopia donkey, with particular reference to parasitic disease [MVM Thesis]. Glasgow: University of Glasgow; 1999.

55. Getachew M, Trawford A, Feseha G, et al. Gastrointestinal parasites of working donkeys of Ethiopia. Trop Anim Health Prod 2010;42:27–33.

56. Valdez-Cruz MP, Hernandez-Gill M, Galindo-Rodriguez L, et al. Gastrointestinal nematode burden in working equids from humid tropical areas of central Veracruz, Mexico, and its relationship with body condition and haematological values. Trop Anim Health Prod 2013;45:603–7.

57. Burden F, du Toit N, Hernandez-Gill M, et al. Selected health and management issues facing working donkeys presented for veterinary treatment in rural Mexico: some possible risk factors and potential intervention strategies. Trop Anim Health Prod 2010;42:597–605.

58. Hornstra H, Pearson T, Georgia S, et al. Molecular epidemiology of glanders, Pakistan. Emerg Infect Dis 2009;15(12):2036–9.

59. Krishna L, Gupta VK, Masand MR. Pathomorphological study of possible glanders in soliped in Himachal Pradesh. Indian Vet J 1992;69:211–4.

60. Kettle AN, Nicoletti PL. Glanders. In: Sellon DC, Long MT, editors. Equine infectious diseases. St Louis (MO): Saunders; 2014. p. 333–6.

61. Thibault FM, Hernandez E, Vidal DR, et al. Antibiotic susceptibility of 65 isolates of *Burkholderia pseudomallei* and *Burkholderia mallei* to 35 antimicrobial agents. J Antimicrob Chemother 2004;54:1134–8.

62. de Waal DT. Equine piroplasmosis: a review. Br Vet J 1992;148:6–14.

63. Wise LN, Knowles DP, Rothschild CM. Piroplasmosis. In: Sellon DC, Long MT, editors. Equine infectious diseases. St Louis (MO): Saunders; 2014. p. 467–74.

64. Knowles D. Equine babesiosis (piroplasmosis): a problem in the international movement of horses. Br Vet J 1996;152:123–6.
65. Friedhoff KT, Tenter AM, Muller I. Haemoparasites of equines: impact on international trade of horses. Rev Sci Tech 1990;9:1187–94.
66. Machado RZ, Toledo CZP, Teixeira MR, et al. Molecular and serological detection of *Theileria equi* and *Babesia caballi* in donkeys (*Equus asinus*) in Brazil. Vet Parasitol 2012;186:461–5.
67. Gizachew A, Schuster RK, Joseph S, et al. Piroplasmosis in donkeys – a hematological and serological study in central Ethiopia. J Equine Vet Sci 2013;33: 18–21.
68. Donnellan CM, Marais HJ. Equine piroplasmosis. In: Mair TS, Hutchinson RE, editors. Infectious diseases of the horse. Fordham (UK): EVJ Ltd; 2009. p. 333–40.
69. Kay G, Knottenbelt DC. Tetanus in equids: a report of 56 cases. Equine Vet Educ 2007;9:107–12.
70. Boija E, Gebreab F, Alemayehu F, et al. A comprehensive approach to minimise the fatal effects of tetanus and colic in donkeys in Ethiopia. In: Pearson R, Muir C, Farrow M, editors. Fifth International Colloquium on Working Equines. Addis Ababa (Ethiopia); 30 October - 2 November, 2006.
71. Mackay R. Tetanus. In: Sellon DC, Long MT, editors. Equine infectious diseases. St Louis (MO): Saunders; 2014. p. 368–72.
72. Hagos A, Abebe G, Buscher P, et al. Serological and parasitological survey of dourine in the Arsi-Bale highlands of Ethiopia. Trop Anim Health Prod 2009; 42:769–76.
73. Assefa E, Abebe G. Drug-resistant *Trypanosoma congolense* in naturally infected donkeys in north Omo Zone, southern Ethiopia. Vet Parasitol 2001;99: 261–71.
74. Pinchbeck GL, Morrison LJ, Tait A, et al. Trypanosomosis in the Gambia: prevalence in working horses and donkeys detected by whole genome amplification and PCR, and evidence for interactions between trypanosome species. BMC Vet Res 2008;4:7.

Index

Note: Page numbers of article titles are in **boldface** type.

A

AAT. *See* African animal trypanosomosis (AAT)
Abortion
    EHV-1–related, 495
African animal trypanosomosis (AAT), 713
African horse sickness (AHS), 696–700
    causes of, 697
    clinical signs of, 697–699
    control strategies for, 699–700
    described, 696
    diagnosis of, 697, 699
    epidemiology of, 697
    pathologic findings in, 697
    therapeutic strategies for, 699
AHS. *See* African horse sickness (AHS)
Anemia
    equine infectious, **561–577,** 704–706. *See also* Equine infectious anemia (EIA)
Anti-inflammatory drugs
    in EPM management, 668
Arteritis
    equine viral, **543–560**. *See also* Equine viral arteritis (EVA)

B

Biologic response modifiers
    in EPM management, 668

C

Chorioretinopathy
    EHV-1, 497

D

Dourine, 711

E

Eastern equine encephalitis (EEE), **523–529**
    causes of, 523–524
    clinical signs of, 524
    control strategies for, 529
    diagnosis of, 525–527

http://dx.doi.org/10.1016/S0749-0739(14)00083-2
0749-0739/14/$ – see front matter © 2014 Elsevier Inc. All rights reserved.

Moving?

Make sure your subscription moves with you!

To notify us of your new address, find your **Clinics Account Number** (located on your mailing label above your name), and contact customer service at:

Email: journalscustomerservice-usa@elsevier.com

800-654-2452 (subscribers in the U.S. & Canada)
314-447-8871 (subscribers outside of the U.S. & Canada)

Fax number: 314-447-8029

Elsevier Health Sciences Division
Subscription Customer Service
3251 Riverport Lane
Maryland Heights, MO 63043

*To ensure uninterrupted delivery of your subscription, please notify us at least 4 weeks in advance of move.

Printed and bound by CPI Group (UK) Ltd, Croydon, CR0 4YY